Conceiving Histories

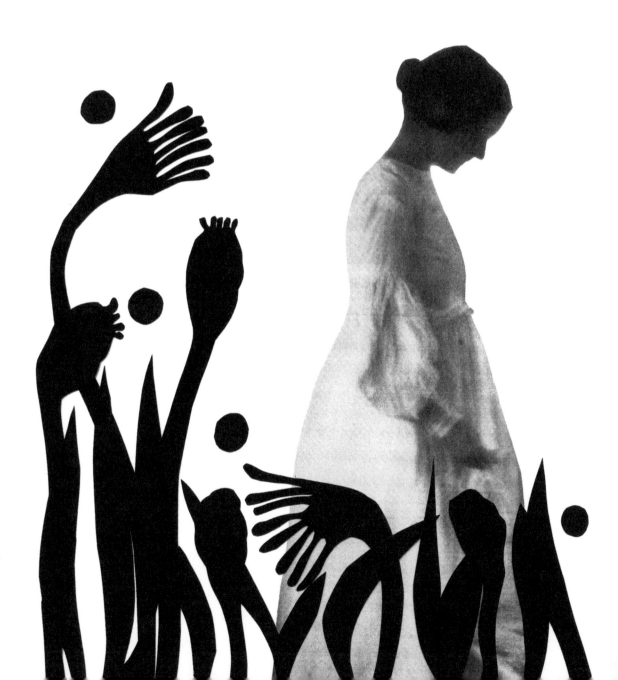

Conceiving Histories

Trying for Pregnancy, Past and Present

Isabel Davis

illustrated by Anna Burel

The MIT Press
Cambridge, Massachusetts
London, England

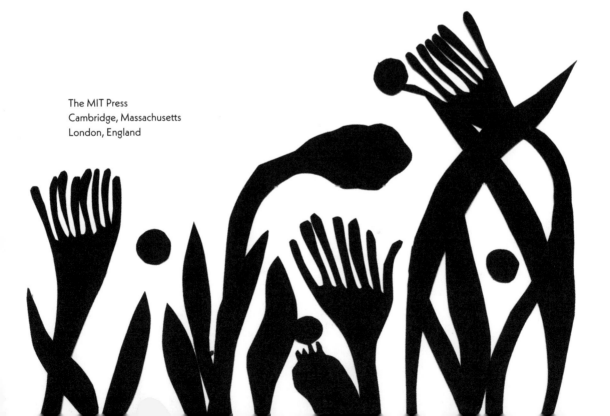

The MIT Press would like to thank the anonymous peer reviewers who provided comments on drafts of this book. The generous work of academic experts is essential for establishing the authority and quality of our publications. We acknowledge with gratitude the contributions of these otherwise uncredited readers.

This book was set in Plantin and Neue Kabel by the MIT Press. Printed and bound in the United States of America.

Library of Congress Cataloging-in-Publication Data

Names: Davis, Isabel, author. | Burel, Anna, illustrator.
Title: Conceiving histories : trying for pregnancy, past and present / Isabel Davis ; illustrated by Anna Burel.
Description: Cambridge, Massachusetts : The MIT Press, [2025] | Includes bibliographical references and index.
Identifiers: LCCN 2024017231 (print) | LCCN 2024017232 (ebook) | ISBN 9780262049481 (hardcover) | ISBN 9780262381604 (pdf) | ISBN 9780262381611 (epub)
Subjects: LCSH: Conception—Social aspects—History—Popular works. | Human reproduction—Social aspects—History—Popular works. | Fertility, Human—Social aspects—History—Popular works.
Classification: LCC RG133 .D383 2025 (print) | LCC RG133 (ebook) | DDC 618.2—dc23/eng/20241120
LC record available at https://lccn.loc.gov/2024017231
LC ebook record available at https://lccn.loc.gov/2024017232

10 9 8 7 6 5 4 3 2 1

For Mark (I.D.)

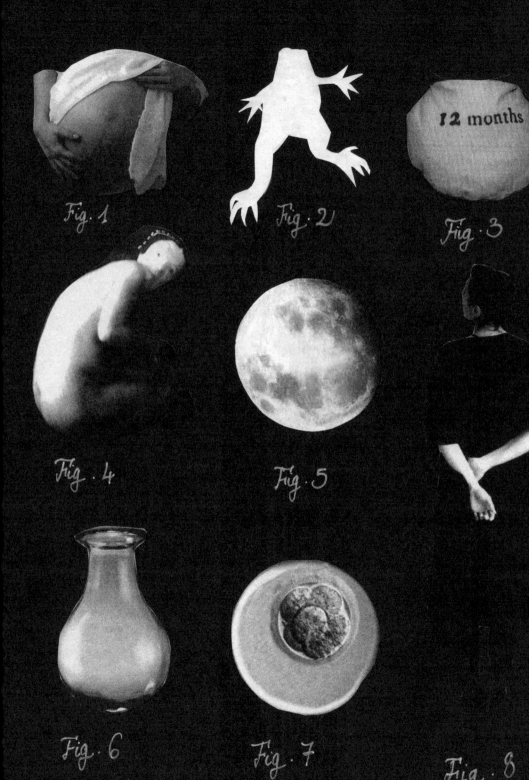

Table I

Fig. 1   Fig. 2   Fig. 3

12 months

Fig. 4   Fig. 5

Fig. 6   Fig. 7   Fig. 8

Contents

Introduction: Annunciations

Jane is no more pregnant than I; I suspect less so.
—Angela Carter, unpublished journal (1961)[1]

Just Buy a Fish and Put It In

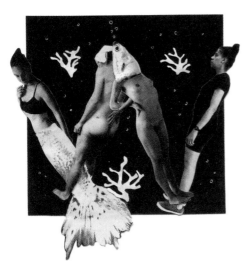

HEN I STOPPED TRY-
ing for a baby, I bought a
tropical aquarium. Before I
stocked it with fish, I tried to
establish a nitrogen cycle by
growing the bacterial colony
which would turn the fish
waste into fertiliser for the
plants I wedged under rocks.
I went about it scientifically.
I dripped in some ammonia
and waited for life, invisible
microscopic life, to drop into
the tank. Daily I was testing
the ammonia, nitrite, and
nitrate levels, watching for change, counting out drops of chemical
reagents, holding coloured test tubes and dipsticks up against the
rainbow wheels on different packets. Time on the x axis, milligrams
of ammonia per litre of water on the y axis. An aquarist keeps water,
not fish. Wait two weeks, those in the know said, and it would be ready.
But a month later, life had still not arrived as expected. Where does it
come from? How would it come? By what transport?

A friend with an established tank brought over some gravel and
bits of dirty filter sponge in an old stocking. This would spawn
life, for sure, but still there was nothing. My tank was inhospitable. Another month passed. I squinted at chalky motes drifting in
the filtering water. Could they be a bacterial bloom? The stones
all looked beautiful, and the plants were thriving, but I needed
another element, an invisible force to make the tank habitable for
fish. The wait stretched to three months. The constant hum of the
filter was soothing, but I hadn't planned on having a water feature.
The orange, emerald, and blue test-tubes of water would have been
beautiful, like liquid stained-glass, if they had been the right colours
and signalled success.

I

I spent a small fortune on the internet, buying bacterial spores and different filter media. They came: clear fluids, old rocks, snake oil. Perhaps this one didn't work because it had been dispatched and delivered in the snow, freezing the bacteria on route, and another, because I had got the quantities wrong. Drawing up and accurately measuring a few drops in a tiny syringe isn't easy. That's the mountebank's defence: "Don't tell me that you made the mistake of administering the dose at full moon?"

"We didn't have all these tests and bottles of stuff in my day," my Mum said. "Just buy a fish and put it in."

The two little fish that were selected to tough out this hostile environment were beautiful male guppies with bright floating tails, one red and one yellow. Most days, I spent an hour siphoning off and replacing a third of the water to keep them safe, even though they seemed to resent it, and my life was busy. "You're cleaning it out too much," my parents suggested. My care had become sterility. The internet too was alive with advice, belief, science, and pseudo-science. Then, to add a new layer of confusion, my friend, the one with a working tank, told me she was trying to conceive and not having any luck, as if we'd swapped lanes and batons in a relay.

I seemed to have chosen a pet whose care very much resembled the magical-religious adventure of trying to get pregnant. What was it about me, I wondered: why was I so jinxed? The fishes' foetal forms began to swim through my dreams. In one dream, I had an aquarium so large that it accommodated the local war memorial, and the fish swam through the names cut out of sheet metal; in another, the thermostat broke, and the fish boiled. Months passed, and the ammonia continued to squat uncycled in the water. The test-tubes of tank water treated with drips of reagent still glowed kryptonite-green, and my friend had an unsuccessful round of intrauterine insemination.

Months later, my partner, M., and I were about to go on a holiday, and because I wasn't sure that the fish could survive in their water whilst we were away, they had their own holiday in my friend's tank. When we returned, my tank was green with algae; little translucent snails beetled through it. Now the test-tube turned only a washed-out lemon yellow rather than radioactive green; the water had finally come right. There was a little nitrate, but no more than the water from the tap and no trace of ammonia or nitrite.

"It just didn't like being watched," M. said. "You had to go away and leave it." When I went to pick up my two little fish from their holiday, my friend told me she was finally pregnant, with twins.

■

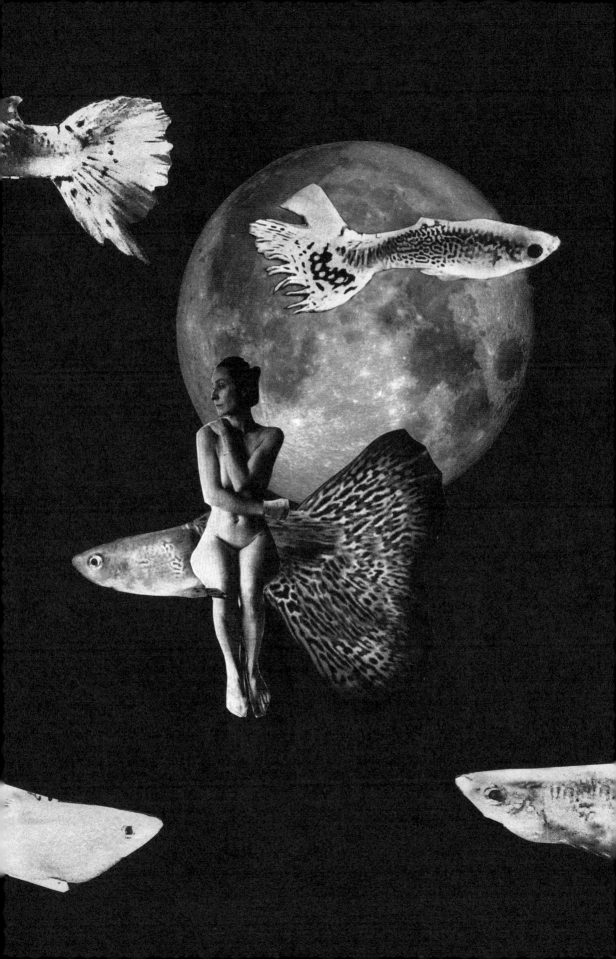

Actually, I did have a baby, but the point of this book is not to chart my fertility journey, which is not an especially unusual one. I could have written the same book, whatever the outcome for me personally, because it is about the periods of time before endings are known, about wanting, trying, and struggling to get and stay pregnant.

The longer it took me to conceive, the more I noticed time in both its largest and smallest revolutions: small portions of time swelled as I waited, yet my childbearing years were rushing by. I had to hurry up . . . but only to wait. The present expanded and became ill defined, yet the prospect of an inflexible nine months persistently loomed. The rhythms of the passing months and seasons of the natural world took on new significance. My interest in the future was intensified and with it, paradoxically, my curiosity about the past. If this is modernity, I wondered, what on earth was trying for a baby like in history? In the past, when even less was known and when there were fewer things that could be done, what suffering there must have been. That was my starting assumption. What I found in the historical archives, though, challenges the accustomed thinking about history as progress which informed my initial assumption. Like many other historians of the body and medicine, I will be charting historical differences and changes but not necessarily improvements.

Alongside the deep-rooted belief about history as progressive, there is another entrenched narrative which this book also challenges: that trying wasn't such an issue for people in the past. This narrative is an effect of the high profile of family planning in our cultural indices, which has cast other fertility concerns into comparative obscurity. Childbirth was so frightening and birth rates so high, our presiding take on history goes, that the main struggle for historical women was to avoid unwanted pregnancies and, if they couldn't do that, to terminate them. Women didn't have to *try* because they married and came to motherhood younger. For the few it afflicted, infertility was often a blessing. Modern thought-worlds do not always stretch to imagine that women might willingly volunteer for an enclosed religious life, so we bundle this into our assumptions about the fear that women felt about a secular, reproductive lifecycle. The choice of a contemplative life, this narrative suggests, was largely taken up—where it was available—by those who wanted a get-out from the expectations of marriage and motherhood.

This book stands in oblique relation to these two strong, interconnected, but opposed narratives: that we have reached an apex of power where much more is known and people's fortunes are more controllable and, at the same time, that in places like the UK, where I am writing, we are now uniquely culturally infertile. I am not suggesting that all or any of this is completely wrong. Historically, childbirth *was* frightening; women typically wrote their wills before they went into labour. Just like lots of women today, many in the past didn't want to have children or to experience childbirth, and some of the women in convents may have answered that description. Contraception and abortifacients, often described as "menstrual regulators," were in demand and use by women who applied available knowledge actively to shape their lives.[2] All that is true. But there are also other stories we can tell.[3] Some women and men wanted to become parents despite the risks. Lots of couples *did* have to try; women didn't always just fall pregnant. Although shrouded in cultural silence, there are records and ways to tell the history of pregnancy and baby loss.[4] If we, just temporarily, quieten the important topics of contraception and childbirth, we can pick out other themes and dignify them with a history. And whilst in some historical writing trying to conceive has been seen as a life-stage to be covered in a narrative sweep towards the more evidently dramatic story of childbirth, this book stops at the trying stage and looks around.

I wrote *Conceiving Histories* because of what we still don't know about the history of trying to conceive. At the same time, though, we don't fully know about trying in the present. I am just a few years older than the first baby conceived through in virto fertilization (IVF), Louise Brown. She and I are now approaching fifty and the menopause—a good time, then, to take stock. My generation grew up and came to parenthood (or not) with a trust in scientific solutions for fertility problems; the promise was that assisted reproductive technologies would be improved and made universal. Excited media reports about discoveries and breakthroughs give us the impression that that promise is being kept. Yet, whilst the triumphs of modern technology and knowledge are eagerly reported, more humdrum experiences—waiting around, not being sure, hoping, being disappointed—inevitably get less press. Assisted reproductive therapies *are* awe inspiring, especially at their high-profile end, and have helped people to be parents who wouldn't have been in the past. Yet still most IVF embryo transfers are unsuccessful, and infertility medicine has not been democratised.[5] And what about knowledge outside of the clinic? If you Google "am I . . . ," then "am I pregnant?" will be a top suggested search, despite its being a question that Google cannot definitively answer. We use Google like women of early seventeenth-century England used astrologer-physicians like Simon Forman and Richard Napier. "Am I pregnant?" is the most-asked question in their surviving case notes.[6] People still live with

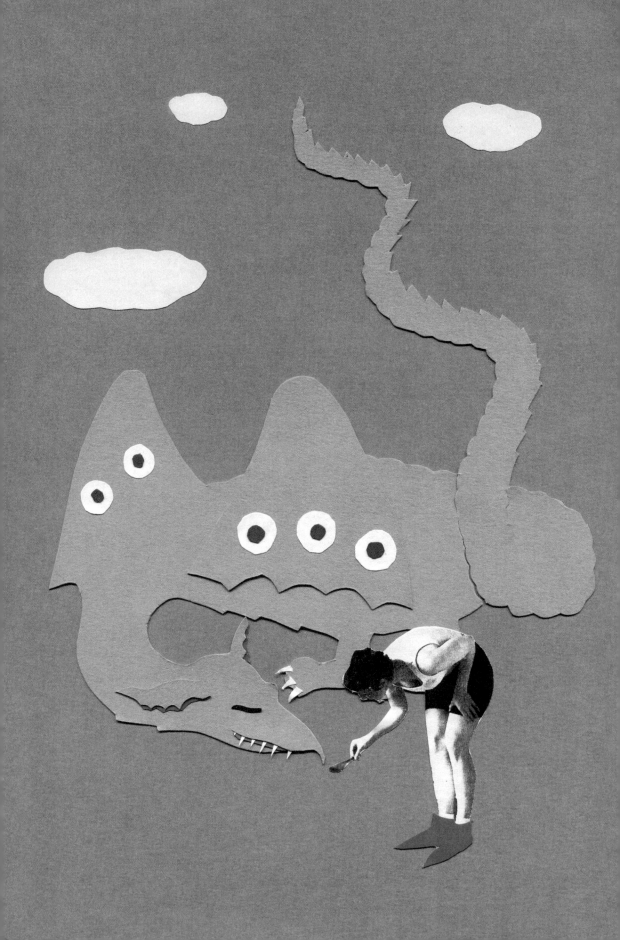

the unknown. Modernity must lay claim to disappointment, delay, and uncertainty and not pretend these are things of the past.

Trying to conceive is a considerable topic in contemporary women's memoirs. Often a work will spare a passing thought for the past or comment on a sense of anachronism. For example, in her memoir, *Adrift: Fieldnotes from Almost-Motherhood*, Miranda Ward describes the experience of fertility treatment "as a kind of mapping," and yet, she writes, "there still seems to be an awful lot of *here be dragons* about it."[7] In her metaphor, fertility medicine cannot effectively survey the wilder regions of the body, beyond the limits of scientific cartographic practice. Ariel Levy, reminiscing about her sex education, also turns to the image of the dragon to talk about fertility.[8] She was taught, she says, to chain up the dragon and leave it to slumber, reassured that it could be awakened by the wizardry of modern science. Fertility "treatments on the very edge of modern technology," she writes, seemed oddly "medieval," because they promised access to an ancient power—dragon whispering, perhaps. Dragons have not stayed in the premodern past, then, even stalking hygienic and high-tech clinics which seem so inhospitable to their ancient scaly forms. Facing the reproductive unknown triggers a retrospective reflex for modern memoirists like these; it places us back into history.

I think of this tug of the past in the encounter with the unknown as the Frankenstein reflex, evoking that most famous of novels about human ingenuity and reproduction: Mary Shelley's *Frankenstein; or, the Modern Prometheus* (1818/1831). Victor Frankenstein's education is an amalgam of both very modern and very ancient science. His discovery of the "cause of generation and life" and his ability to bestow "animation upon lifeless matter" rely on his university curriculum but also his youthful reading adventures in medieval science: Albertus Magnus (1200–1280), Heinrich Cornelius Agrippa (1486–1535), and Paracelsus (1493–1541).[9] Without this early research in medieval studies, Frankenstein reflects, he would "never have received the fatal impulse that led to my ruin."[10] The alchemical tradition is an animating impulse that galvanises the body Frankenstein builds using his practical research physics and anatomy. Just as we do, when historical people faced mysteries unsolved by modern science, they responded with a backwards glance. It is as if the questions "What was it like in the past?" and "Are we as modern as we think?" inevitably occur when plumbing the considerable depths of the reproductive unknown. Historical commentators similarly expressed surprise that anachronistic unmapped dragon-infested wildernesses persisted. Those before us also felt modern and were similarly impatient that the body was still sometimes resistant, hard to read and know, despite awe-inspiring innovations and new scientific information. The Frankenstein reflex exposes as myth the idea that a greater historical familiarity with uncertainty and loss hardened people to it.

Just like us, historical people lived with the unknown, but they were also more explicitly able to acknowledge it.[11] We have paid a price for modern scientific gains. Whilst high-tech and pharmaceutical tools have multiplied, social tools have been lost. In the nineteenth century, for example, when it wasn't known whether a woman was pregnant or not, she was said to be in an "interesting condition."[12] This uses the literal sense of *interesting*, from the Latin *inter* + *esse*, "to be between or within." We have lost that sense of the word *interesting*, of living in an in-between, and with it a concept that it would be useful to have kept.

We congratulate ourselves on how far we have come from the past. But turn on the internet to look down the other end of the telescope. In trying-to-conceive internet forums, women respond with the same blend of science, pseudo-science, magical thinking, and religious belief as people always did. As I will discuss, you don't have to delve far, for example, to find threads in those forums in which women swap notes on which internet astrologers are best to consult on fertility. In true modern form, the exchanges across trying-to-conceive chat forums are machine hyperlinked, but to unregulated markets of the kind that historians tell us mushroomed in the past, bustling with private medical services and suppliers, with ample virtual space for predatory quacks and charlatans. *Conceiving Histories* uses the internet as it would a cache of historical documents containing rare snippets of female life writing like those found in court depositions or letters. The present is also part of history, and the unfiltered chatter of the online world is archival evidence of our times.

Driving along one day with our baby asleep in his car seat in the back, M. said, his eyes on the road, "So I did become a parent after all." Then, after a pause, he added, "And you did be one too." I still can't work out the tense of this or even whether it's correct grammatically. The tenses are all tangled up, imagining us now as revelations of the futures we once didn't know. The histories in this book are also tangled up in time. I don't tell a chronological or comprehensive story in the order in which things happened, moving from discovery to discovery, invention to invention, and the careers of era-defining scientists. Just as my life isn't a progression towards my son's birth, this book is not about the incremental advancement that has been made in the knowledge of reproduction across time.

Struggling to conceive, losing pregnancies, and then researching the history of those experiences have taught me a great deal as a professional historian about the movements and habits of time, or at least this process has backed up with experience what I appreciated before only in theory. But it has also taught me more about the present. It is easy to see the reproductive past as far off in the distance. Twentieth-century innovations—the pregnancy test, the Pill, sonography, IVF—represent a reproductive revolution, an apparently clean break with the world that existed before. Change is undeniable, but there is also continuity. Whilst some historians will tell you that historically women were often able to intuit and to know their bodies, my work has turned up different but co-existing stories: of women and men, too, who were just as clueless and as curious about the workings of the body as I am. Because people in the past weren't idiots, I find both their bewilderment and their eager reaching for knowledge heartening. The question—"What on earth was it like in the past?"—has taken me out of myself into a new world where everything is shifted but also curiously familiar. In this looking-glass world, we can see afresh problems we face but struggle to articulate, to the extent that we are literally losing the language we once had for them.

(Not So) Instant Pregnancy

How convenient, in a time before the pregnancy test, for an angel to arrive from the sky and deliver a definitive, authoritative diagnosis. The Annunciation, when the angel Gabriel announces Mary's conception of Jesus, is such a familiar scene in Western art because it offers a point, an event around which Christian history pivots. Gabriel's intervention isn't only a message, an after-the-fact diagnosis. In the medieval world which elaborately embroidered the Gospel stories, Mary conceives at nearly the same moment of the Annunciation. After she hears Gabriel's words—"Hail, thou that art highly favoured, the Lord is with thee; blessed art thou among women" (Luke 1:28)—she has a blink of time to consent, and then a ray of light shines through the glass of a window, carrying Christ as a little homunculus or the Holy Spirit as a dove into her womb.

As light through glass, the spirit passes into Mary, leaving her virginity intact. She conceives and instantly knows that she has, in the way that light and sound are perceived: immediately, without the clumsy and delayed intervention of diffuse inner sensation. The messiah doesn't emerge from the kind of body that you or I might have, one that is reluctant to conceive, that has to "try" or is hard to diagnose. His descent into flesh is so astonishing and revolutionary that he is perfectly formed at once and immediately

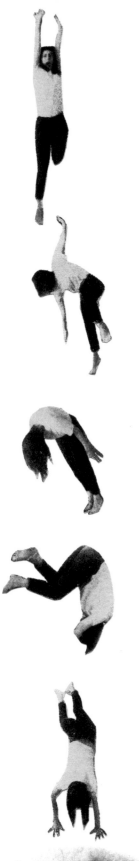

known. Whilst medieval science writers understood that natural embryos developed over time, Christ was an exception who arrived ready-made.[13] The Annunciation as a fantasy of objective pregnancy diagnosis has been able to hide in open view, painted on walls and in books, displayed in windows, carved on pillars and benches, embedded in sermons and prayers. Yet how often do we think about the wish: to see inside, as if through glass, and evade waiting and unknowing? Gabriel also announces the pregnancy of Mary's cousin Elizabeth. Medieval sculptors frequently showed the pair together with see-through bumps. Their wombs have windows, and everyone can look in.

For some, pregnancy and knowledge of a pregnancy *can* come like an annunciation, a bolt from the blue, suddenly and with certainty. Now and in the past, lots of people just do and did fall pregnant and have little or no doubt about it, having children without complication. Mundane annunciations happen all the time. But we also amplify that experience into a norm, part of what historian Lara Freidenfelds calls "the myth of the perfect pregnancy."[14] We surround ourselves with the impression of the immediacy and simplicity of pregnancy. Our common phrase "fall pregnant," a vestige of older theological habits of mind, describes conception as a slip, a mere nothing, a misplaced footing on your way to the shops. Sex education is careful to stress, because it is true, that even one half-cocked sexual encounter could result in a pregnancy. And because that education impresses on us the life-changing revolutionary nature of this "fall," it's easier to think of it as a single event, determined in a moment. In films set in a time before the test, two characters have sex in one scene, and in the next she's suffering with morning sickness. It will be clear that it's the morning (though morning sickness can be an all-day or anytime affliction): she'll tumble straight out of the bed you just saw her have sex in to the bathroom. In films set after the test, the cinematic shorthand is the blue line on a white stick. The test produces the impression of conception as a binary with a switch point: pregnant or not pregnant, true or false, pass or fail. Some tests are literally digital. Drama needs events and so favours the annunciation-style pregnancy revelation. Only existential French cinema has managed to make waiting and nothing much happening cinematic.

The wait that is most often isolated and remarked on in the whole endeavour of trying to conceive is the so-called two-week wait, which has even crystalised into an abbreviation in internet discussion forums: the 2WW. The term started off as an IVF phrase, referring to the two weeks between embryo transfer and the time when a pregnancy test result will be reliable. It is now used more widely to

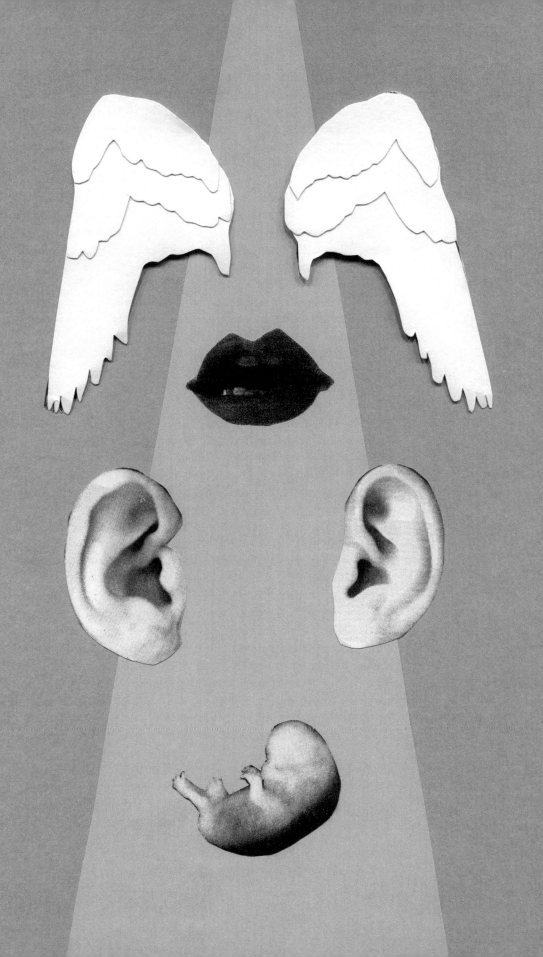

mark out the approximate time between ovulation and pregnancy testing. In the online forums, the 2WW is the part of trying that has a particular reputation for being hard, seeming interminable, feeling longer than it should. Yet two weeks drastically underestimates its duration. Two weeks doesn't reckon with the extra time it takes to diagnose a negative or the time lost to irrational trust, doubt, or the raw disbelief of it. Two weeks doesn't allow for the time after a positive result, when the test stick is beyond use and the hospital's early pregnancy unit is on speed dial. If you multiply these various strung-out waits by the number of months or years spent trying, you come to quite a different time estimate that differs from person to person. Eventually, chronic failure to conceive may be diagnosed as infertility, a historically and culturally variable condition often defined by time spent trying and "by what it is not."[15] Many sufferers are given the diagnosis of unexplained infertility, which is really no diagnosis at all.

Waiting and not knowing are reiterative and refuse to stay in neat two-week pockets, spilling out and becoming the condition of life, part of the larger unknown that is the future, joining with the wider wait to meet a life partner, find suitable accommodation, secure an income, or whatever other nest building seems necessary. For me as for many others, once trying began in earnest, for sizeable periods I existed in an in-between, where I could have been, could soon have been, or thought I was pregnant but wasn't sure. I began to think about the most intense phase of the trying-to-conceive experience, when this curiosity was at its peak, as "the am-I-aren't-I time." Yet all my trying to conceive years were an in-between. "Am I pregnant?" blurred into "Am I *ever* going to be pregnant?" The two-week wait, then, is one small part, a core, of the larger object that concerns this book. Whilst the phrase emerges from the normalisation of the pregnancy-test stick, it fails to appreciate the expansive blind spots that gape around that object. The test stick may cap the intense heart of the am-I-aren't-I time, but it doesn't remove conception uncertainty as completely as we sometimes imagine it does. In the great swathes of time when home pregnancy tests and other technologies are of no use, women are in a position similar to those in the past who lived before their invention.

In Miriam Stoppard's *Conception, Pregnancy and Birth: The Childbirth Bible for Today's Parents*, a diagram of the female reproductive organs depicts all the moving parts of conception on one double-page spread where they are all happening simultaneously.[16] We laugh that you can't be a little bit pregnant, but perhaps you can, given that conception relies on sex, ejaculation, ovulation, fertilization, implantation, the development and then the viability of an egg, a sperm, a blastocyst, an embryo, a foetus. Stoppard's diagram even shows a baby, smiling, holding up its head: the end point of a logical progression. Given that babies generally can't hold up their heads and smile about it until they are at least four months old, this page charts a process which takes, at absolute best, thirteen months. For those, like me, who spend any time trying to get from one side of the page to the other (or to a later section of the book, "You and Your Developing Baby"), this image's narrative of pregnancy—its collage of all the processes of conception happening perfectly all at once, from start to successful finish—looks alien and uncomfortably funny. A process with so many parts has multiple ways of going wrong and is difficult to monitor, and it is particularly challenging to get a clear picture of its not being underway, of the process not beginning or not being sustained.

The home test kit is useful but only as a snapshot, a postcard from a process. In the past, before that handy blue line, people found other ways to isolate still frames within a moving picture. We still use the first day of the last period to roughly date a pregnancy in advance of a scan; that's a habit we inherited from the past. Historically, though, that marker was trusted more for dating than diagnosis, for which it was thought notoriously misleading given that some women could bleed throughout a pregnancy and others didn't bleed at all, whether pregnant or not. The historical idea of "quickening," the term for the fluttering sensations that are felt when a pregnant woman first notices foetal movement, was often preferred and was much more significant in the past than the present. The term *quicken* means "to come to life," and it described the moment when the child was physically perfected and "ensouled." This is the account of that event in the encyclopaedia of all knowledge written by Bartholomaeus Anglicus (1203–1272) in the thirteenth century:

> And whan þe body is þus maad and ischape with membres and lymes, and disposed to fonge þe soule, þan it fongiþ soule and lif, and bigynnyþ to meue itself and sprawle, and puttiþ wiþ feet and hondes.[17]

> [When the body is made and shaped with members and limbs, and disposed to receive the soul, then it receives soul and life and begins to move itself and to jerk [sprawle] and knock [puttiþ] with feet and hands.]

This expressive sentence is perfectly poised on the fulcrum of the word "then": beforehand the foetus is passive (it is "made" and "disposed"), and afterwards it takes on agency (it "begins to move

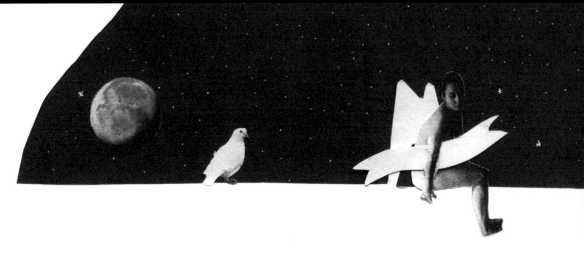

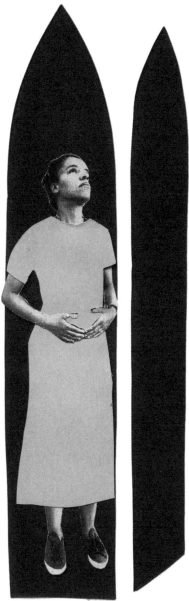

itself"). Although foetal movements are first sensed diffusely and become defined only in time, quickening was nonetheless forced into the mould of a sudden event—*then*—one moment this and another moment that, off and then on. Nothing . . . and then the foetus is "sprawling" and "putting"—jerking and hitting—alive with independent life. Over time, quickening came to be redescribed as foetal movement rather than the investiture of the soul, yet it still represented a discernible moment, a switch point. The emphasis on quickening, occurring well within the second trimester, reminds us that pregnancy ambiguity could be prolonged in the past. Nonetheless a moment, an annunciation, was looked for and consequently carved out of a conception process with duration.

Despite this search for a single moment, I will consider later how ready historical midwifery writing was to admit to the difficulty of detecting very early pregnancy. Our books notice that there is an uncertain time before a diagnosis. They see that Google-search am-I-aren't-I 2WW time, but they have odd things to say about it. The fact of uncertainty seems hard to admit. Appropriately enough, the first word in the best-seller *What to Expect When You're Expecting* is "Maybe," and the first page describes a diverse community of readers all with the same question: "Am I pregnant?" However, the first dilemma that the book presents is curious: "My doctor said the exam and pregnancy test showed I wasn't pregnant, but I really feel I am." In answer it offers this:

As remarkable as modern medical science is, when it comes to pregnancy diagnosis, it still sometimes takes a backseat to a woman's intuition. The accuracy of the different pregnancy tests varies, and many do not indicate pregnancy as early as some women begin to "feel" that they are pregnant.[18]

Stoppard's *Childbirth Bible* suggests something similar: "Many women 'know' when they've conceived," she writes. "This intuitive feeling is probably due to the early outpouring of female hormones."[19] A woman's intuition, intuitive feelings: what are those things? Both these statements implicitly recognise that intuition is in tension with science. In *What to Expect When You're Expecting*, "women's intuition" is directly opposed to and even trumps modern medical science. For Stoppard, "intuitive feelings" need a physiological explanation: they are a part or product of the endocrine system. Intuition has become a secular word, but it started in theology. It isn't a word which can be found in medical materials until the nineteenth century, when we usually tend to think of science and belief becoming increasingly separated. Intuition began in English as the mechanism by which angels and saints appreciate God: immediately, with no gap between sight and knowledge, like an annunciation.[20] Angels and saints are not beset by the clumsy struggles of the ordinary pedestrian human mind. Clearly, I am no saint, as my intuition is very out of true.

Anyway, intuition is true only in retrospect. Only those women who come to discover that they are pregnant can say, "I just knew straightaway." And the idea of women's special knowledge of their bodies can go both ways. What if women know but are not letting on? Robert Lyall, a nineteenth-century medic who comes up later in the book, tried to imagine what conception would feel like: "the sting of a wasp, or like the bite of some other insects," he speculated, swapping angelic intervention for a more up-to-date entomological idea of conception.[21] His work on pregnancy diagnosis stems from a deep distrust of women, whom he accuses of systematic mendacity. Lyall doesn't doubt that pregnancy *is* immediately obvious, that annunciation-style recognition is the norm: women know but are naturally untruthful. Feminists and antifeminists alike want to believe in women's special insight. Comforting or not, the idea that a woman's intuitive and secret knowledge can transcend or outfox medical science is remarkably persistent, suggesting women have special access to some sort of ancient magic which exceeds rational thought.

We habitually turn to magico-religious terms to articulate our awe at reproduction. Phrases like "the miracle of birth" and "the miracle of life" are so commonplace we miss their devotional cast. Children are "miracle babies," particularly when their pregnancy or birth has been precarious or they are premature and need neonatal care. I will be thinking in this book about how we create parenthood as a hallowed space overseen by spiritual powers and, in the terms of the metaphor, about how entry to that space depends on grace. What about those left out in the very unmiraculous cold despite their best efforts? What if you snap your fingers to activate the magic and watch eagerly . . . as absolutely nothing happens?

In my trying-to-conceive years, I periodically had the refrain of Thom Gunn's poem "Lazarus Not Raised" on a loop in my head: "the scheduled miracle did not take place."[22] There are Lazarus's friends and family, waiting expectantly around the grave at which Jesus has indicated they may witness a miracle, a resurrection. For what? Nothing happens. Lazarus demonstrably does not rise from his grave. The word *schedule* gained currency in the nineteenth century with the coming of the railways. It marks the standardisation of time made necessary by timetables. But it looks awkward in a miracle story; mythic or supernatural narratives are in a different temporal plane. The question is: into which temporal frame, the mythic or the mundane, does conception fit?

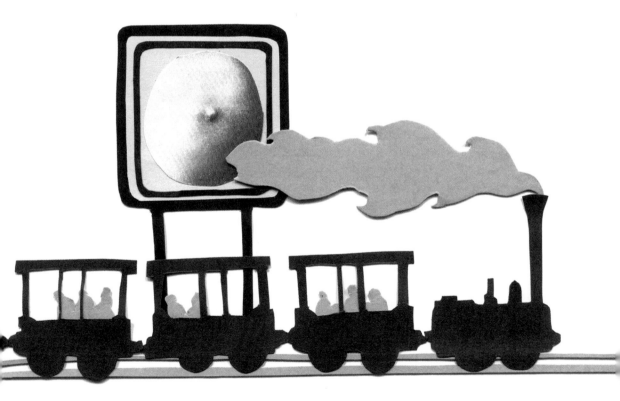

Introduction

In Saint Émilion's Cell

I once went on holiday to the Bordeaux region of France and visited a place called Saint-Émilion. As well as eating and drinking, tourists can book a guided tour of its extraordinary medieval subterranean buildings: a church carved out of the hill around which the village sits, atmospheric as an Indiana Jones set, and the hermitage of St. Émilion himself, a little-known eighth-century monk. Within his tiny sandy cell, lit by a small glassless window, is, according to the guide who led my tour, a fertility seat. Women who wanted to be pregnant, she said, should sit on the seat, and they would conceive within a year. The shrine received letters and cards, she said cheerfully, from women who had successfully tried it out. There were about fifteen in my party, and as they filed out of the cave, I and a handful of others hung back to take a turn sitting on the seat. As I waited, I wasn't sure whether to fill in the instructions that our tour guide had left out: you can't just sit on the seat, you must also offer a prayer to St. Émilion. I know this from my training as a medievalist. That is how medieval shrines work: they are activated through prayer.

The others joked about our credulity. There we were, in the twenty-first century, relying on the miracle-working of an early medieval saint. As part of this jocular exchange, I could have offered my advice about the prayer, casually thrown it into the pool of their laughter. But I couldn't speak. I was so shocked by my urgent concern that these women should know how to use this rough stone seat. I had been thinking through the actual mechanics of an ancient technology and not only in my role as a professional historian. My research object, the culture of the Middle Ages, had always seemed distant, exotic, and otherworldly, and it fascinated me for being so. Just for a moment, I had entered a medieval symbolic world. I shuffled on and sat on the seat, cold and damp through my summer dress, and even offered a silent and unpractised prayer.

Perhaps you are wondering if it worked. Did I fall pregnant in the following year?

Why would you wonder *that* in this rational age? What would you say if I said that it did work? You might complain that there was no control me who didn't sit on the seat or that only tourists who do happily fall pregnant send cards, so the data is skewed. There are any number of ways you could dismiss the idea of a connection between sitting on the seat and outcomes. And yet there I was: an agnostic woman who hadn't previously signed up to saint cults, sitting on the seat in a line of others who did the same.

Why did I sit on the seat at all? The short and obvious response is, "Why not?" The long answer I give to you in the rest of this book.

As a matter of fact, I did get pregnant but then also miscarried. Curling up in the aftermath of that loss, I caught myself considering if it was me who had been ignorant of the proper workings of St. Émilion's seat, forgetting some important codicil or failing to read an appendixed small-print disclaimer.

I have never encountered anything that felt so intensely historical as trying to become a parent. My trying-to-conceive years were a drawn-out version of the convulsion I encountered in St. Émilion's cell: the shocking touch of the past in the present. This book has been generated by that extended encounter, and I offer it to sceptics and believers, to parents and unparents alike, as a reflection on the reproductive body in these supposedly modern times.

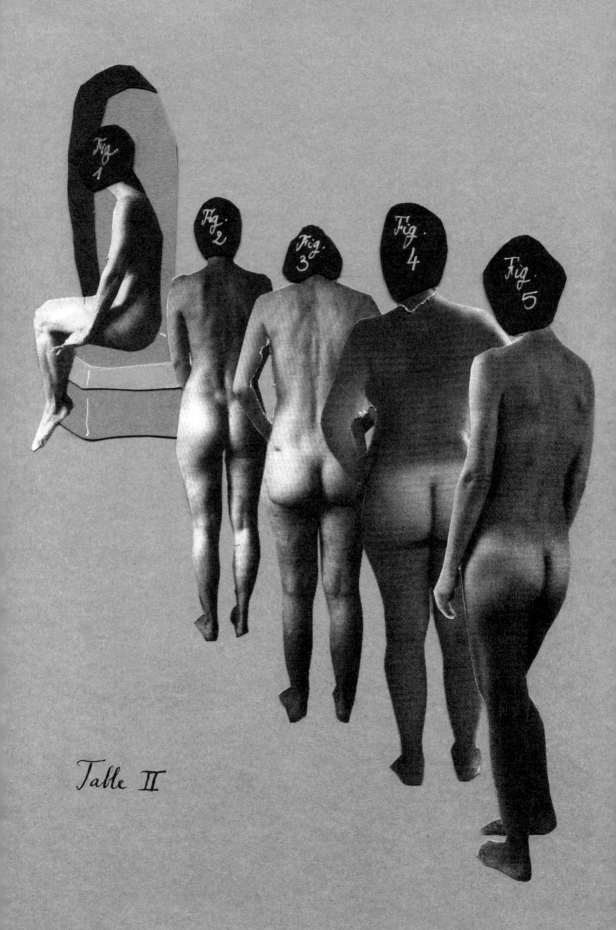

Table II

1 Frogs: What Your Sex Ed Never Taught You

Some againe doe write, that if a Woman take a Frogge and spit three times in her mouth, she shall not conceive with Childe that yeare.
—Edward Topsell, *The Historie of Serpents*, 1608[1]

Filth is listed [by the Nyakyuza people] as meaning excreta, mud, frogs.
—Mary Douglas, *Purity and Danger*, 1966[2]

An Amphibian ABC

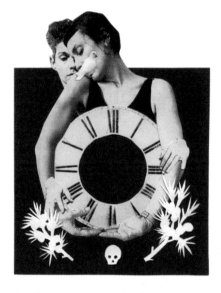

NCE UPON A TIME, my Granny gave me an illustrated collection of Grimms' fairytales. When I read the story "The Juniper Tree," I knew that she couldn't have read it herself. I was quite small, but even I could see that, with its detailed descriptions of child murder and cannibalism, it was not expressly for children. And so, of course, I loved it. It had got itself smuggled in; its illustrations were an invisibility cloak. Now I had a book which looked safe to the adults around me but really wasn't, a book that was in disguise, and only I knew what it said.

This is how "The Juniper Tree" starts:

> It is now long ago, quite two thousand years, since there was a rich man who had a beautiful and pious wife, and they loved each other dearly. They had, however, no children, though they wished for them very much, and the woman prayed for them day and night, but still they had none.[3]

The original German is more evocatively handwringing, more like "but they didn't get any, and they didn't get any," striking especially perhaps for the adult reader.[4] Fairytales look as if they're for children, but they emerged from the capacious historical genre of romance, which was never solely or even mainly for young readers. In the nineteenth century, long-form romance was repackaged as the adult novel, and short-form romance as fairytales. Mostly, the magical elements were absorbed by fairytales rather than novels. At the same time, illustration was increasingly being reserved for children's books and particularly for books of fairytales, when it hadn't been before. Illustrated fairytale books, then, offered the ultimate childish camouflage for adult themes.

Romance literally means "Roman-ish." These were stories low enough to be written in European vernaculars—the Romance languages, which were degraded forms of Latin. The subjects of romance were supposedly frivolous: magical beings and objects; animal and monstrous transformation; children lost and found; dangerous quests; exotic places and people; women, men, sex, and love. The word *romance* has attached itself to the human heart because love was an abiding romance topic, part of what made those tales lowbrow. The fairy story's power is in the mismatch between its structural simplicity and its psychological complexity. It looks like a story for children, whilst at the same time it enfolds our worst fears, dirtiest fantasies, and deepest revulsions. Story forms like these historically shaped the languages we speak, long before being pressed into service as literacy primers for young children. Language development, both historically and in infancy, was and is mixed up with the mythic packaging of sex education.

The fairytale, then, offers a starting point for this chapter on sex education and knowledge. This is what we teach to children—how we begin talking to them about sex and fertility, about the shape of their lives—without using any of the actual words or apparently talking about those things at all. What kind of knowledge do we foster when we approach only symbolically? In this chapter, I discuss knowledge and how it is shaped, how it is or isn't shared, and to whom it belongs. My theme is frogs and the slime that our thought-worlds often associate with them, considering the frog's curious enmeshment in the history of human reproductive knowing.

Frogs are frequent visitors in fairytales. A particularly slimy one is in the Grimms' "Frog King," which, like "The Juniper Tree," is also set in a time long ago "when wishing still helped."[5] The frog exploits a princess's wish (for the return of her golden ball, which has dropped down a well) to slime his way into the innermost parts of the castle, eating off her golden plate and sleeping in her bed. You've got to kiss a lot of frogs, we say, minimizing the repugnance that the Grimm brothers' story evokes: the princess "began to cry, for she was afraid of the cold frog which she did not like to touch, and which was now to sleep in her pretty, clean little bed."[6] The way the Grimms' version has it, the princess must do more than kiss the frog. Held to her rash promise by her father, the princess is forced into intimacy with the creepiest of the fairytale men-beasts. Surely a wolf would be better? You can see here how the fairytale encapsulates sexual themes in its metamorphic plotline, the boggy icky bits.

A frog is also mixed up in the infertile opening of "Briar Rose," better known as "Sleeping Beauty," an opening a bit like the one that begins "The Juniper Tree." There the frog takes on a role like angel Gabriel's in an inverted Annunciation:

> A long time ago there was a King and Queen who said every day: "Ah, if only we had a child!" but they never had one. But it happened that once when the Queen was bathing, a frog crept out of the water on to the land, and said to her: "Your wish shall be fulfilled; before a year has gone by, you shall have a daughter."
>
> What the frog had said came true, and the Queen had a little girl who was so pretty that the King could not contain himself for joy, and ordered a great feast.[7]

Who is this frog? How can it talk? How does it know what it knows? How does the conception happen? Why does the frog talk only to the queen and not the king? None of these questions is answered, of course. The frog just exists; it just can speak; it just has insight. The encounter is as miraculous and unmotivated as the Annunciation: Mary, holy and already halfway to heaven, meets an angel that has winged down out of the air. The childless queen in "Sleeping Beauty" gets into the pool as a frog emerges: fellow amphibians meeting between worlds. And somehow in those exchanges, in unspoken (perhaps unspeakable) ways, conception occurs.

"We don't have a baby in this family, do we?" my son said about this opening when we read it together.

"We have you," I pointed out.

"But we don't have a *real* baby, mummy."

"Shall we go on with the story?"

Let's let the frog stand in for those things we don't want to use plain language for—the inundating, wetter, and most alien ones. The frog archive is a slimy one, but if we can bear to, we can open it up and read its many secrets.

The Secret Secretion Syllabus

I start with the slime. The memoirist Mary Karr, writing about her girlhood in Texas in 1970, describes her teenage idea of what it took to be "one of those chipper, well dressed girls whose namebox on student ballots is automatically checked."[8] One of those girls, she reckoned, should not "give any evidence of knowledge concerning bodily functions or fluids." Some knowledge should be disowned. About two hundred years earlier, in 1792, feminist Mary

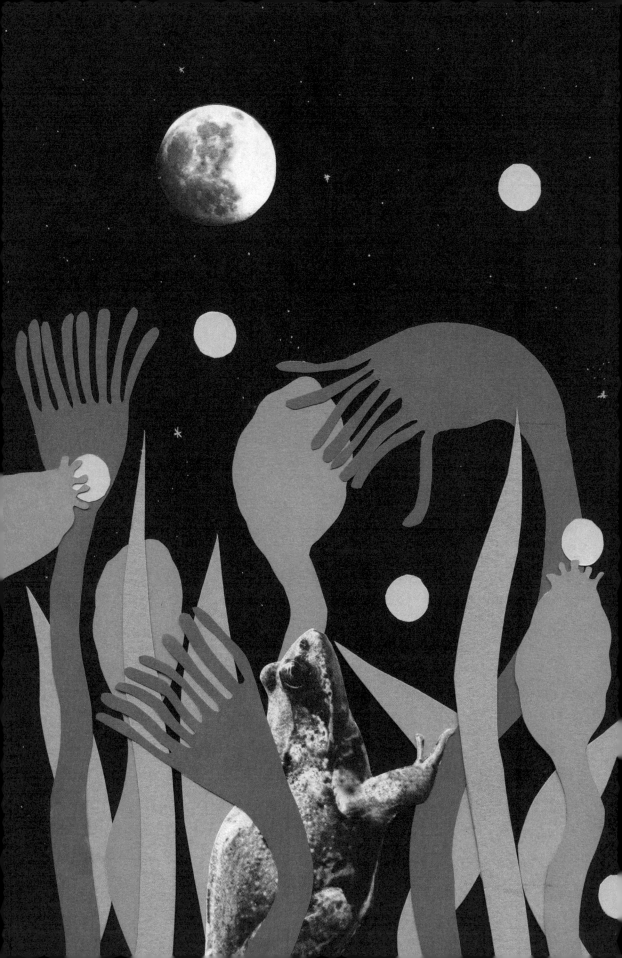

Wollstonecraft (1759–1797), wrote about similar forms of knowledge. Girls' boarding schools, she complains, are places where

> Secrets are told—where silence ought to reign; and that regard to cleanliness, which some religious sects have, perhaps, carried too far, especially the Essenes, amongst the Jews, by making that an insult to God which is only an insult to humanity, is violated in a brutal manner. How can DELICATE Women obtrude on notice that part of the animal economy, which is so very disgusting?[9]

Wollstonecraft is usually a crystal-clear writer but here is oblique and euphemistic. She won't use straight language for her topic: menstruation but also other ill-defined "secrets." As Wollstonecraft was an advocate for women's education, who notably railed against how it was inhibited by inappropriate modesty, her disgust here surprises me. Silence on bodily functions is clean, she suggests, whereas talking about them contaminating. Like Mary Karr's younger self, Wollstonecraft feels that nice women, "DELICATE Women," shouldn't let on about what they know about the wetter aspects of the female body. And she keeps these "secrets" herself by not expressly naming menstruation, although she makes it clear that that is what she means in her reference to Jewish ritual purity. Wollstonecraft founded and briefly co-ran a boarding school for girls a decade before; now she recoils from the disgusting whispered secrets that she imagines are coercively shared in girls' dormitories.[10]

These two astute female witnesses from very different points in time comment on biological reproduction and knowledge—schoolgirl knowledge—and pick out bodily fluids as the missing topic from official syllabuses. So let's stop there with them. There still isn't a vocabulary for talking easily about bodily fluids; perhaps there won't ever be. All the words we have for them are disgusting: mucus, discharge, excretion. *Secretion* is only marginally nicer. A secretion can be disgusting, or it can be exotic—a rare extraction, an essence or elixir, a delicacy; or both: the hallucinogenic secretions of the Colorado River toad licked straight from its warty back, perhaps. Secretion comes from the same root as the word *secret*, from the Latin secenere, "to separate or divide off." Secretions are those things which have left a secreting host and become separate; whereas secrets are things which are so profoundly separate as to have moved beyond ordinary knowledge. But bodily secretions are often also secret and kept so by disgust.

Wollstonecraft's use of the word *secrets* in the passage evokes a very old tradition of writing about the secrets of women and generation.[11]

This was a body of knowledge that included information about intimate facts like menstruation, sex, and generation, which had been repackaged for each new generation since the year dot. In the eighteenth century, when Wollstonecraft was writing, secrets writing had received a particular boost by the cheapening of print. Historians of reproduction have written a great deal about one particular secrets text, the best-seller *Aristotle's Masterpiece*, a compendium of medical, sexological, and pornographic writing from the late seventeenth century which went into multiple editions and was widely circulating well into the nineteenth century.[12] It built on, borrowed and anthologised older medieval and classical gynaecological materials, explicitly referred to as the secrets of women. Even if secrets texts gathered a female readership, they were written by men and emerged from a thoroughly masculine tradition of speculating about women's bodies and the mysteries of generation.[13] Wollstonecraft is complaining about women sharing rude, stickier forms of knowledge, but she is also recoiling from intrusive male curiosity about the female reproductive body of the kind on show in *Aristotle's Masterpiece*. She implicitly rails at how a pall of secrecy set up women's bodies as salacious problems for male science to investigate and so master.

Knowledge about women's bodily fluids, whilst not on the official syllabus for girls in 1970s Texas or 1790s London, circulated illicitly, compromising those discovered to have access. The copies of *Cosmopolitan* magazine passed around between girls at my school in the early 1990s, dog-eared from their multiple readers, were pored over for secrets of sex and bodies. We had a similar impression that we were gathering unauthorised insights of which our teachers and parents might not approve; magazines were our secrets texts. Now, the internet has taken up that role, generating knots of knowledge—official and unofficial, authorized and dissident, questionable and trustworthy—that need sophisticated critical untangling to be useful. The online knowledge revolution has put pressure on women's magazines to carry more "secrets" than they previously dared. Yet despite all these changes in the information landscape, there still seems to be a disinclination to be open about female fertility awareness and bodily fluids. There is nothing equivalent to the Bristol stool scale for blood and other discharges.[14] The sharp end of this ignorance is that we have no language to talk about bodily fluids, which has implications for whether or how we treat women in healthcare contexts. But, more generally, we still encounter a vestigial unwillingness to know and to teach the sticky slimy bits of female biology. What is all this stuff? What meaning can we make from it?

In my day, magazines restricted themselves to articles about periods, so it wasn't until I came to conceive myself that I discovered

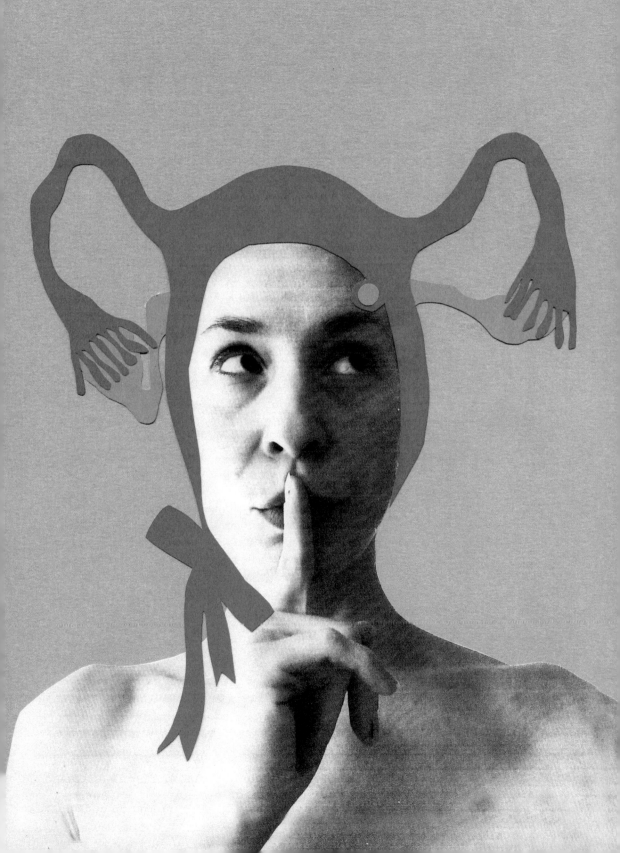

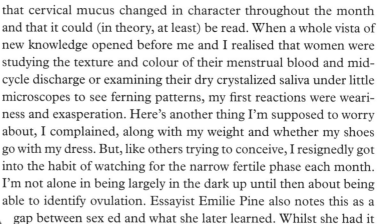

that cervical mucus changed in character throughout the month and that it could (in theory, at least) be read. When a whole vista of new knowledge opened before me and I realised that women were studying the texture and colour of their menstrual blood and mid-cycle discharge or examining their dry crystalized saliva under little microscopes to see ferning patterns, my first reactions were weariness and exasperation. Here's another thing I'm supposed to worry about, I complained, along with my weight and whether my shoes go with my dress. But, like others trying to conceive, I resignedly got into the habit of watching for the narrow fertile phase each month. I'm not alone in being largely in the dark up until then about being able to identify ovulation. Essayist Emilie Pine also notes this as a gap between sex ed and what she later learned. Whilst she had it impressed on her as a schoolgirl in the Republic of Ireland in the 1990s that sex at any point of the month might result in a pregnancy, "now that I want to get pregnant it's magically revealed to me that the baby-window is fucking tiny."[15] The facts never seem to be in our favour.

Knowledge in secrets writing (from medieval gynaecological writing to *Aristotle's Masterpiece*, *Cosmopolitan*, and the internet) has changed utterly. Their authors and readers are also unrecognisably different. Yet the idea of the secrets of women persists. There are still things that don't get onto the official syllabus, things we find out only in the process of trying to conceive. What comes first—embarrassment or ignorance? Do we label the things we cannot understand disgusting, or do intrinsically disgusting things inhibit our coming to knowledge of them? A great deal has been written by feminists about disgust and bodily fluids to understand the persistence of secrecy and mystery in relation to female sexuality and the reproductive body. Feminist philosopher Elizabeth Grosz, for example, understands female bodies to be culturally coded as "a leaking, uncontrollable, seeping liquid; as formless flow; as viscosity, entrapping, secreting; as lacking not . . . the phallus but self-containment."[16] For Grosz, the supposed mystery of female bodies is closely related both to this disorderly flow and its association with potential motherhood. Sperm, she suggests is understood differently, and the male body more associated with sexual pleasure than fatherhood.

The information gathering about how to find the fertility window has been particularly credited to male scientists like, for example, Kyusaku Ogino (1882–1975) and Hermann Knaus (1892–1970), who independently of each other put together very similar time-lines identifying when ovulation occurs in relation to menstruation. We should also, though, give credit to the nameless women whose bodies they used in their research. Knaus did his work by inserting a balloon with a recording device through the cervix of women with regular menstrual cycles to chart uterine contractions at different points across the month.[17] In Japan, women undergoing hysterectomies in the early 1920s gave occasion for Ogino's follicular, ovarian, and endometrial inspections. Ogino opened up the abdominal wall and physically looked inside women at different points in the month to establish what was happening when, what coincided with what, and when his patients should time sex to improve their chances of conception.

It turns out, then, that there is order in the ooze, that disgust screens an appreciation of intricate patterns revealed only in relation to time and/or under the microscope. That knowledge has become important for the so-called fertility awareness method of family planning, which can be used to try to both conceive and prevent conception. Fertility awareness should be distinguished from the rhythm method, which can also be used to optimise or avoid conception.[18] Both are "natural" family planning regimens; however, the rhythm method uses the calendar and relies on timing intercourse in relation to monthly bleeding, but the fertility awareness method also takes in other changes across the month, such as body temperature, relative position of the cervix, or the character of midcycle discharge. Women who choose the fertility awareness family planning method have been contributing test subjects to the project of developing this body of knowledge. The research done on saliva ferning has been assisted by those already charting their menstrual cycles and detecting ovulation and cross-checked using intrusive vaginal examinations.[19] Women entering their personal at-home observations about their bodily fluids into fertility apps are also feeding a scientific data collection process from which new technologies will be formed and marketed. There is a wealth of evidence too of women—and sometimes men—keeping close account of the menstrual cycle in the past. Women used nick sticks, wooden sticks that you notched, which were also used for other kinds of accountancy.[20]

Knowledge, though, can be hard to apply. Information about changes across the menstrual month has two potential applications: for optimising conception and for avoiding it. The use of fertility monitoring techniques as contraception is controversial because, whilst it works for some women, it has a bad reputation as unreliable. For any accuracy, it relies on several variables not being variable and, worst of all, on partial sexual abstinence. Before the smartphone fertility apps which chart women's cycles today, you could get cardboard volvelles, those spinning wheels that offer handy guides to all things—when to plant your allotment, what time it is in different world capitals, or when you should avoid or have sex, depending on your family plans. Ogino opposed the use of his method as a contraceptive because of its fallibility. But Catholic practice meant that "natural" family planning methods were the only ones available in some places in the world. In Italy, a whole generation is now known as the "Ogino-Knaus generazione," and in France, they refer to "les bébés Ogino." Concern about natural planning methods is still high: when fertility app makers broaden their market to attract those looking for contraception, they often come under fire for overselling. Conception knowledge and contraception knowledge don't fit easily together. Because "natural" methods of contraception, particularly the rhythm method, have a negative reputation, there is a hesitation about passing on knowledge of fertility awareness. This is knowledge from a hazard-strewn path. What knowledge can women, especially young women, be trusted with? What is it good for them to know? These hesitations mean that fertility awareness does not appear on the sex ed syllabus. What fertility is, how to look after it, and how to monitor it are currently gaps in young people's knowledge.

The internet, which is a knowledge soup, is often where people turn to fill knowledge gaps. In the Middle Ages, repositories of all knowledge, encyclopaedias, were described as mirrors, because they reflected the world. And if the book mirrored the world, the reader could become universally knowledgeable by mirroring the book, gathering all that was known into themselves and so becoming a mini world. The internet is our mirror and resembles the unsorted chaos out of which we make ourselves. All the intricacies of trying to conceive—inspecting one's secret secretions, for example—are being researched by everyone for themselves, using search engines and chat forums. Nutrition and other lifestyle issues, the timing and nature of sex, home technologies, staying sane, and ways to find support and treatment are largely self-taught. Within the online morass, there is a huge amount that is useful (who would want to live without it now?). We must sieve it out, though, from what is useless and harmful. Our mirrors are crazed mosaics, in which wannabe-parents must squint to make out their reflections as best they can.

What Nero Knew

After he murdered her, the emperor Nero had his mother, Agrippina, cut up so that he could see where he had gestated. Looking on his mother's dead corpse, he could not cry. Instead, he coolly evaluated her beauty: a 10 for legs but a 2 for her nose. As the butcher-surgeon removed her viscera, he hesitatingly pushed his fingers into the space below to find his own beginning, but his fingers closed around nothing. He stormed away into his private chambers, his hands dripping with his mother's blood. He had form. The blood of the Christian martyrs and his old trusty tutor, Seneca, was also on his hands.

Rather than withering, his desire grew and grew, until one day he heard a woman giving birth as he walked through the city, and he was struck with an idea. He called his physicians into his chamber and ordered them, on pain of death, to make him pregnant so he could experience giving birth.

A huddle of trembling robes, the physicians came up with a plan to save their own skins. One of them headed to the pond on the common land, where he knelt on the soggy edge amongst the rushes, leant over until he almost toppled in, and collected a mass of bright-eyed frogspawn in a pot. The physicians mixed the eggs into a potion, matured it for a whole moon, and brought it wriggling with black life to the emperor, who swallowed it down.

"Eating the right diet is important in pregnancy," the physicians said. "Your baby relies on you to provide the right balance of nutrients to help him grow and develop properly."

First, they gave him plants and small flies, then bigger and bigger flies, and finally they introduced some worms. The emperor swallowed them down.

After some time, when he put a wondering hand on his abdomen, he could feel the baby coming to life inside him, short hops here to there, and back.

Forty weeks were nowhere near up when Nero called his doctors again. They found him writhing in pain. "The baby's coming," he told them.

"But you aren't due yet."

"But the pain is too great," he said.

The physicians exchanged confederate glances and set to advising the emperor on birthing positions. One slipped back to his consulting rooms and prepared a new potion with shaking hands: egg white, mustard, salt, more salt. At first, he was selective, but soon he was grabbing at anything; if it looked disgusting, it went in. He stirred it with a long spoon, said a prayer

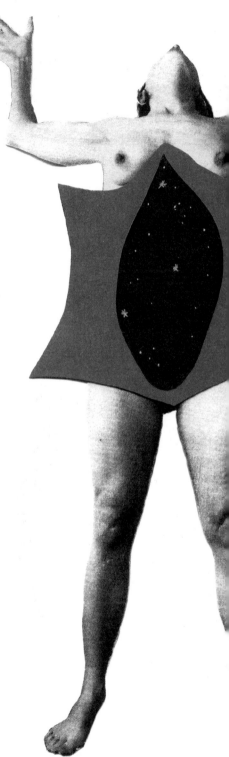

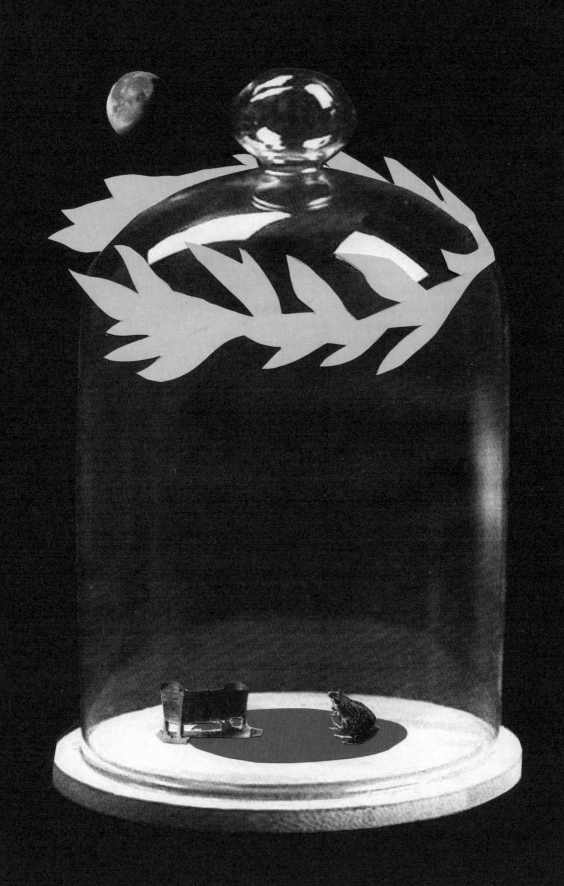

to Aesculapius, and returned to the palace. Snatching it from him in relief, the emperor swallowed it down.

Almost as soon as the potion hit his stomach, Nero was retching, choking out a large hopping frog, green and brownish and glistening. The physicians hopped about after it. It slipped from their hands several times before it could be captured and boxed. Nero got up from his knees, his chemise stained from his labours. He peered into the box but shrank revolted away. What a monster!

"Sire," they said, "the child is undershaped only because you were not willing to wait the full term."

"Was I ever as hideous as that?" he asked, and his thoughts moved back to Agrippina's bloody insides.

They reassured him: "Yes," carefully stressing "once upon a time."

Nero ordered that the frog be kept in a domed chamber, a bespoke incubator where it could be fed and looked after like any other premature baby. Every tyrant must have a beautiful enclosure with a rare creature inside. And the frog lived in its vivarium reliquary and watched its parent's depraved life play out: acting and singing, sleeping with men, sleeping with women. It has my eyes, Nero thought when the animal caught his occasional attention.

After Nero lit the taper and burnt Rome to the ground, the emperor was chased to the city's suburbs where he committed suicide, and his corpse was devoured by wolves.

The Romans returned to the city, dusting off their hands, and found the frog-child still squatting in its gilded nest, and they chased that out of the city, too, and set it on fire.

Nero's soul, departing from him, was swallowed down into the place where the demons work refitting old souls to new bodies. They have a particular job to do with evil souls, like Nero's, which require wrenching amputations and vigorous filing down with sharp tools, sometimes into little more than powder, to make them go into the hideous forms set aside for them.

The demons first attempted to get Nero into the body of a viper, one which would be reborn by eating its way out of its mother's womb; but because Nero had once oiled the right palm, a gentler form was finally chosen: the snug skin of a frog. Nero had always been pondlife, so it wasn't such a difficult shift. He liked to sing, too, just as frogs do; but in his case, audiences were forced to applaud, because he was the emperor.

Nero had once lived in a grand palace and afforded every luxury (it is said that he fished with golden nets). But he was reborn into a single eye winking in a clump of gelatinous frogspawn, in a pond on the common land on the edge of Rome. Not far away, busy workmen were whistling, getting on with the city's reconstruction after the fire that Nero had set.

∎

Frogs

I didn't make this story up. I gathered it together, as a medieval author would, from classical texts and medieval sources about Nero and frogs and retold it in my own way.[21] The medieval versions were the fullest renditions, and the fullest of those is in the ubiquitously popular anthology of saints' lives, Jacobus de Voragine's *Golden Legend*, where Nero is used to think about how things can be known.[22] Generation—where life came from and how—was the paradigmatic question, a question about God and how his creation was continuously managed and replenished. In that way, reproductive knowledge operated as an emblem for thinking about knowledge much more broadly: epistemology.

In these tales, Nero is shown trying or discarding research methods. He has little time for his first educators, his mother and tutor, putting them to death for their pains. So he is forced to experiential educational forms. Can he learn by seeing and touching, by human dissection, by hearing (listening to the woman whose labour cries can be heard from the street), or through painful firsthand experience? The dissection of Nero's mother and his looking inside her foreground the primary dilemma about pregnancy and conception knowledge: it happens out of sight inside a living body. A mother cannot be simultaneously cut up to reveal her maternal secrets and continue to exist as a functioning mother. Dissection, even vivisection, ends the living processes it hopes to discover.

The emperor's second research project—his frog pregnancy—is a travesty, a trick. Yet for all that, he does seem to identify the frog as his child and produce some fatherly feeling for it. Part of the joke is about how children look like their parents, about copies. He looks at the animal and recognises it, knows it. He finds out a truth: he is a creepy reptilian monster. There is consolation here: the truth will out in unexpected ways perhaps, but, one way or another, knowledge will come. We also see an interest in natural history in the Nero myth, in actual frogs and a recognition that, as oviparous animals whose embryological development was helpfully exteriorised, they provided rich clues to reproductive mysteries. As far as classical and medieval authorities were concerned, frogs were always motherless creatures, being spontaneously generated from rotting matter, like flies. This stood to reason because adult frogs have long hopped it by the time frogspawn can be observed turning into tadpoles, froglets, and frogs. The doctors use their true knowledge of the natural world to facilitate Nero's mad research. They also use it to cover themselves, reassuring the emperor that all preterm babies look like frogs.

Nero is the maddest scientist that the Middle Ages could imagine. He's not sure whether he wants to be a man, woman, lover, father, mother, son, or foetus; perhaps he wants to be all these at once. Some of the texts in which his story appears are interlaced with debates about sexuality; they display a revolted homophobic fascination in Nero's queer desires. He's obviously supposed to be a villain; often the Nero stories asked the question: why does evil prosper? He overreaches for knowledge, trying to know things illegitimately.

Although the Nero legends are a critique of prurient knowledge hunting, the main point of the story is not disapproval. Disapproval licences their fascination. The Nero legends become elaborate because of their curiosity about curiosity; they express anxieties about but also the draw of contemporary secrets writing, with its potentially unhealthy interest in female reproductive anatomy and function. The story was lavishly illustrated in some of the most beautiful manuscripts of the late Middle Ages. Agrippina's dissection was presented as a colourful juxtaposition of her naked and open abdomen with bloody viscera next to the high-fashion textiles of the clothed characters around her.[23] The tale draws a shocking contrast between well-heeled women and the perverse speculations which reduce them to their sexual and biological functions. At the same time, the stories celebrate the ingenuity of the emperor's doctors, their application of professional skills and wisdom. And there is an attraction both to natural historical knowledge and the idea of human investigations, inventions, and discoveries. *The Golden Legend* is very particular about the vivarium that Nero orders be constructed for the frog he "births." It has two "stones" in it for some sort of ovarian structure (ovaries and testicles were sometimes referred to as stones). So this enclosure is an artificial womb but also signals an interest in keeping animals for display, observation, and study. By pushing into disgusting territory beyond ethical limits, the Nero narratives playfully imagined professional human dissection emerging over the late-medieval horizon; the zoological research institution and the incubator, which were still some centuries off; and pharmaceutical insemination for men, which has not yet come to pass.

And frogs? Frogs and their important role in experimental research about conception and embryology, because of their exterior metamorphosis, are imagined here with striking precocity. All oviparous animals have been crucial for the study of conception, frogs included.[24] The Nero story tells us that even medieval science saw their potential for the study of unseen mammalian, especially human embryology. The Nero story shows that, from premodern times, the metamorphosis of the frog offered an analogue for human embryological development, a thought that I return to when I look back at Nero in the conclusion of this book.

Cape Town to London

In 1959, when she was just sixteen and still at school, writer and literary critic Lorna Sage (1943–2001) found herself unexpectedly pregnant. In her memoir, *Bad Blood*, she describes having a pregnancy test:

> We called out our new doctor, a pale, prim man in his thirties, Dr Clayton. After taking my temperature, asking about bowel movements and looking at my tongue, he looked out of the window at the copper beech tree, cleared his throat and asked could I be—um—pregnant? No, I said, feeling hot suddenly, No. He recommended a urine test anyway. . . . I spent days at home. On one of them Dr Clayton turned up again, embarrassed and puzzled. How old was I? Sixteen. He'd heard I was a clever girl, doing well at school, didn't we ever have biology lessons? I must have known what I was up to . . . From his first words and his tone, which had weariness and contempt in it, I knew it was true, just as absolutely as until that moment I knew I couldn't be.[25]

Caught up in this paragraph is a mire of confusion. What Sage knows. What she *should* know. What she *must* have known. Is it her school's biology syllabus or her capacity for learning it which is insufficient? The doctor expects that sex ed was on the syllabus, but somehow Sage hadn't taken it in. She is reputed to be clever, the doctor says, but she really doesn't seem to realise she has had sex, rowing with her boyfriend about his "lies" to a mutual friend about their "going all the way." At the end of this extract, we see the binary switch from "knowing" this to knowing that, a switch forced by a professional opinion confirmed by an objective test.

As well as the advantage it gave him over female patients like Sage, Dr. Clayton had a powerful epistemological tool that his professional predecessors did not have.[26] Whilst, as I consider in chapter 3, nineteenth-century obstetric writers are voluminous and anxious about the vexed topic of pregnancy diagnosis, Dr. Clayton is in a much more comfortable position. Dr. Clayton is weary, contemptuous, embarrassed, and puzzled but not anxious. Because the pregnancy test is a knowledge technology, I'm going to use it here as a way of thinking more about how knowledge is acquired, for what purpose it is obtained, and who is given access to it.

Let's begin by filling in the part which happens between the two encounters with Dr. Clayton.[27] He probably sent her urine sample by post in a glass vial. Although Sage's arrived safely, the Royal Mail complained to pregnancy testing centres about the number of urine bottles that broke in transit. Her sample probably went to one of the UK National Health Service test facilities. On arrival, Sage's urine will have been injected into a female *Xenopus laevis* toad, a species native to Southern Africa. That toad would then have been isolated from the others in its tank and put in a jar with a gridded platform, with room for just one toad. Within a few hours, because Sage was pregnant, the injection will have stimulated the toad to emit eggs, which drifted down through the grid into the bottom of the jar, where they were observed and recorded by the lab technicians. The lab then sent the result back to Dr. Clayton, who turned up in Sage's bedroom with the result.

Being able to test for pregnancy like this was a considerable step forward. Yet whilst we narrate the advent of reliable testing as progress, there are strange lags: a man walked on the moon before a home pregnancy test was available in the 1970s. And frogs filled in until the mid-1960s, which feels surprisingly recent. Frogs don't strike us as modern, hopping through our fairytales (as we have seen), myths, and dreams as swarming biblical plagues or chopped-up additions to witches' brews. Once I had heard about the frogs, I wanted to know more. What I couldn't get from the standard history was a picture of the logistics. It sounded so outlandish. Where, what, who, when? I went to the Family Planning Association (FPA) archive, which is now at the Wellcome Collection in London, to get some answers. Although the archive is huge, comprising thousands of files, pregnancy testing was a relatively small part of what the Association did, so the frog files are few.[28] These files contain correspondence to the FPA, copies of letters that went out, internal notes, press clippings, and associated journal articles. The documentation relating to "supplies of toads" give an amazing picture of the logistical challenge of acquiring and keeping tropical South African toads for pregnancy testing in London from 1948 to 1963. What I found in this cache of mid-twentieth-century loose typed papers is partly, but not only, a narrative of progress.

That the frog test was news to me when I started this research is perhaps not surprising: many people at that time also had no idea that this was how pregnancy testing was done. Sage probably didn't know; if she did, she doesn't let on. It may be that Dr. Clayton himself didn't know. My mother, who trained as a nurse in London and then a midwife in the 1960s, didn't know. But the distance between a lay body and a clinical test was and is wide and widening. Techniques and technology are applied to our samples unseen, unknown. How those technologies function exactly is beyond us. Everything we consume, including biotech, participates in a huge international economy from which we cannot extract ourselves or fully comprehend. We live in cultures so bewilderingly immense and globally interconnected that full knowledge of them is impossible. What follows is one historical example of how knowledge flows or doesn't, how it is shared or isn't, and how our thirst for it unwittingly contributes to hardening inequalities.

For much of the twentieth century, pregnancy tests were animal tests. Gynaecologist Selmar Aschheim (1878–1965) and endocrinologist Bernhard Zondek (1891–1966) are credited with first demonstrating that follicular maturation occurs when animals are injected with the urine of pregnant women.[29] Animals injected with the urine of pregnant women produce an ovarian response. Frogs had an advantage over mammals like mice, rats, and rabbits in that they lay eggs externally, so they didn't have to be dissected to retrieve results and could be used about two weeks later for the same purpose. *In vivo* testing produced accurate results, as good as today's tests, although the results were slower. The discovery that female frogs would ovulate when injected with the urine of a pregnant animal is credited to scientists who in the late 1920s and 1930s were working in a University of Cape Town lab led by British scientist Launcelot Hogben (1895–1975).[30] Exactly whose name should be on the discovery has been controversial and spans the divide between British and South African science.[31]

The natural habitat of the *Xenopus laevis* frog or toad is in Southern and Central Africa. They are an aquatic species and like to hang in stagnant pools. They are bloated and without the bone structure of other more lovely frogs. They don't eat neatly with one of those sticky zipping tongues. In fact, they have no tongues at all and shovel their food into their mouths with the three clawed toes of their front feet. Scavengers rather than hunters, *Xenopus* are hard to catch. Not only do they dart down to the depths when alarmed, but they also exude the kind of slippery slime which we imagine reptiles all produce, when really reptilian skins are often quite dry.

The toad trade was possible because of the way that the South African natural environment had operated as a "commodity frontier" of the British empire since the nineteenth century.[32] *Xenopus* frogs hopped about unsuspecting in their pools on the Cape flats, part of a rich but much-monetised ecosystem. South African tourism has

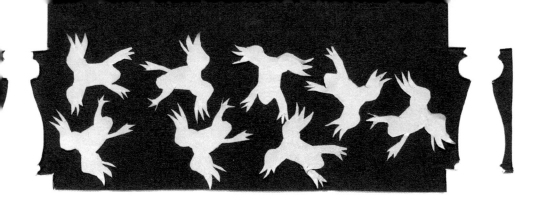

always foregrounded the natural world. Safaris are still the number one tourist attraction. In the nineteenth century, the hunting safari was especially pulling in British tourists, such as colonial administrators and military personnel stopping off on their way between India and Britain.[33] At the same time, British manufacturing was bulk buying South African ivory to make piano keys, billiard balls, and art objects.[34] Later in the century, those exports gave way to diamonds and gold, whose discovery triggered prospector rushes and formed the context for the Anglo-Boer wars (1880–1881 and 1899–1902).

A parallel extraction process saw knowledge flow back to the colonial centre in the form of zoological and botanical specimens headed for British universities and natural history collections like the one in the Natural History Museum in London, where I now work. The historian Nick Hopwood and scientist John B. Gurdon have described how the development of the frog pregnancy test fed *Xenopus* into international science practice, making it the standard laboratory frog.[35] Yet those shifts depended on *Xenopus* having become "known to nineteenth-century science through European anatomical and natural historical investigations of imperial fauna." They add, "laboratory animals are not just found, they are made" by cultures of knowledge.

The story of how *Xenopus* captive colonies were established for pregnancy testing in Britain is told by historian Jesse Olszynko-Gryn.[36] By the time that the Family Planning Association opened its pregnancy diagnosis lab in 1948, there was proof of concept both of the frogs' reliability as pregnancy test animals and also of their ability to be kept in captivity in labs in the chilly north, using the equipment developed by and for professional and amateur aquarists, for example, to optimise temperatures. One of the figures that Olszynko-Gryn credits with popularising the test is the doctor and herpetologist Edward Elkan. In an unpublished memoir, a copy of which is in the Wellcome Collection, Elkan describes how he kept a large aquarium containing a hundred or more *Xenopus* frogs on his balcony overlooking Regent's Park.[37] He managed to breed them himself, no small feat. At one point, he fed the tadpoles partly with his patients' blood, which they donated for a discount on their treatment. Elkan was a German Jewish émigré who came to England to escape Nazi violence in 1933. He was given help to get settled by Dr. Helena Rosa Wright, a family planning pioneer whom he'd met at a birth-control conference in Zurich in 1929. Elkan read about the frog pregnancy test in the science journal *Nature* and decided to try it, sending off for frogs by mail order. When war broke out in 1939, he was interned, first at Huyton near Liverpool and then on the Isle of Man. He was particularly sorry that his frogs were confiscated. He suggests that his international telegraphic order of one hundred *Xenopus* frogs had aroused the authorities' suspicions: "what kind of secret and probably dangerous war material was I ordering to the detriment of old England?"[38] The FPA facility opened after the war and principally served private medical practitioners. It ran alongside National Health Service pregnancy testing services and was the brainchild of Helena Wright's son, Henry Beric Wright, who had had laboratory experience with Elkan before the war. The scientific networks around the birth-control movement brought the FPA testing facility to life.

The Association's pregnancy testing was sited at 64 Sloane Street in London's Chelsea area in a several-story eighteenth-century townhouse whose basement was converted into a "froggery" and laboratory for pregnancy testing. The house is now grade II listed and houses a boutique investment bank. A 2015 application for planning permission refers to the basement at 64 Sloane Street as "nondescript and . . . not an area of high significance."[39] It is nondescript because it was stripped of any period features to make room for the FPA's froggery, although basements, being the servants' quarters, were perhaps more aesthetically basic than other parts of houses anyway. The upper floors at 64 Sloane Street are more characterful and more obviously historic than the basement. Jane Austen stayed on a couple of occasions to visit her brother, Henry. In the hierarchies of history writing, just as in the house itself, the basement froggery is low, whilst any room where Austen once breakfasted is high. The planning application is for the installation of air conditioning to manage the heat generated by modern computer servers. Ventilation was always an issue, although in the frogs' days, the smell was more unpleasant than the heat. One of the ongoing issues documented in the FPA "frog files" is about whether the finance committee can find the funds for a fan. Wright was ambivalent: "I feel hardly competent to give positive advice on this as I long since ceased to notice the smell."[40]

The frogs that ended up in the FPA's froggery came from the wild and after capture were taken to Cape Town's Peers Snake Park and Zoo. They were collected by children singly or by farmers who trapped them in larger numbers in dams.[41] Peers Snake Park was a tourist attraction on Adderley Street, Cape Town's main drag.[42] Tourists especially went to see its collection of venomous snakes, shown off by the famous snake handler, Christian. The proprietor of the Cape Town park was a Mrs. Peers, "whoever she may be," Wright wrote on an FPA office memorandum. I too can find out little about her, except that she took over running of the park in 1939 when her husband Bertie, the park's founder, died from a cobra bite. Bertie Peers, the founder of Peers Snake Park, was the son of botanist Victor Peers, who had initially come to South Africa as part of an Australian military contingent that fought with the British in the second Anglo-Boer war.[43] Victor was a botanist, and his encounter with African plants during his Cape convalescence after a war wound encouraged his later emigration, moving from one outpost of the British empire to another. The snake park was already a supplier of venom for antidote development to medical and military research institutions. Supplying animals to meet the new demand for pregnancy certainty was an obvious step but also shows the close relation of wildlife for tourism and wildlife for science with medical applications.

The frogs were difficult to breed in captivity, and, like many labs, the FPA preferred to order regular consignments to keep up stock levels and meet growing demand. A typical FPA consignment was for five hundred frogs. The order was placed by letter to Thomas Cook and Son, the FPA's live-animal transport agent, which cabled its Cape Town office to purchase the animals and arrange for their transport. The snake park was a stone's throw from the busy docks to which the animals were taken. At the docks, the frogs were loaded onto one of the Union Castle mail ships in large custom-built metal containers, a hundred or more frogs in each one. The FPA files also give us information about the flow of frogs during the war before the FPA facility was operating. Because of the dilemma about whether it was cheaper to buy new containers each time or send back the same ones empty, the FPA fruitlessly ask Thomas Cook if the frogs could be transported in four-gallon petrol cans, as was the practice in the war.[44]

The institutional infrastructure that enabled the flow of knowledge and the frogs themselves to Britain was also the legacy of empire. The telegraphic cables laid by British companies at the end of the nineteenth century conveyed the orders, and the mail ships carried those orders north. The Union Castle fleet offered a weekly service from Cape Town to Southampton. Regular mail ships went

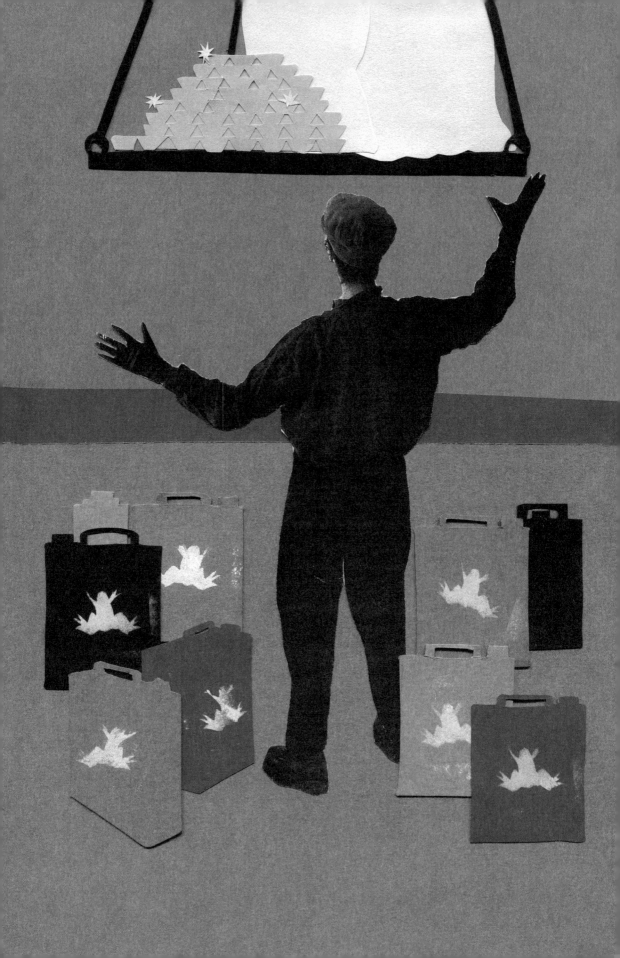

back and forth like this from at least the middle of the nineteenth century. An example letter from Thomas Cook in 1949, following up with the FPA on an order, gives the frogs' typical itinerary:

> With further reference to the three containers of live Frogs which arrived from Cape Town by the s.s. "STIRLING CASTLE," we confirm that these were duly placed on the 3.10 p.m. train from Southampton Central Station, consigned to your order at Waterloo Station, to be called for. We trust that they have arrived safely.[45]

Like the other Union Castle liners, the *Stirling Castle* had an iconic lavender keel and black and red funnel and was fitted with a wooden interior, like a "floating English country house."[46] There was room for around 175 first-class passengers, 500 tourist class, and 400 crew. Passengers had a hairdresser, a library, a swimming pool and gym, bars, and dining areas for their two-week voyage. They dressed for dinner and took part in organised entertainment: dances and games (including frog racing). Meanwhile, below the passenger decks, frogs destined for UK labs shared the ship's cargo hold with frozen meat, citrus fruit, other foodstuffs, and gold from the Transvaal goldmines on its way to British bank vaults.[47] This same fleet of ships served as troop carriers in the war; indeed, my paternal grandparents met on one and married on a stop in Durban. The Mediterranean was an extensively mined battle zone, and the route around the Cape of Good Hope was crucial for moving soldiers, medics, and support services to and from Britain and its Middle and Far Eastern commands. So the frogs bound for British labs were in these same holds in their petrol cans throughout the war.

The frog test emerges from an older imperial mindset which viewed the natural world as an unlimited resource. According to historians William Beinart and Lotte Hughes, in nineteenth-century South African colonial law, "Wildlife was free goods, not owned by anyone."[48] Indeed, Elkan writes about how easily *Xenopus* were to capture in large numbers: "So far supplies seem to be unlimited and export unrestricted."[49] Although at the end of the 1930s protective legislation did put an end to uncontrolled collection, hundreds of thousands of *Xenopus* were still collected from the wild and exported.[50] The FPA archive has evidence of times when the toads were in short supply. In 1954, for example, Thomas Cook wrote to the FPA that it was difficult to get toads. Demand was very high, and there were fewer frogs being captured because of heavy rainfall: "stocks are exhausted."[51] The FPA contacted an alternative supplier, but that plan fell through because the proprietor seemed to be off on a prolonged hunting trip. South African conservationist Douglas Hey put *Xenopus*'s population depletion in the 1940s and 1950s down to irresponsible overcollection.[52] Nowadays *Xenopus* is far from being endangered. Indeed, the frog's success threatens the survival of other species in South Africa and in countries which accepted *Xenopus* imports and where feral populations have become established, threatening biodiversity in another way. The *Xenopus* trade, as with other live animal transports, opened out a "significant invasion pathway, . . . increasingly implicated for movement of disease."[53]

The frog trade and transport for pregnancy testing predate the international protocols that have since been adopted to try to ensure that the benefits of knowledge generated from bioprospecting are fairly distributed.[54] But even if those protocols had been in place, the history of empire and apartheid made it impossible for South Africa's rich natural resources and the knowledge that has accrued from them to be equally shared. As well as enriching scientific knowledge within the British empire, South Africa's long colonial history also disenfranchised South Africa's majority Black populations, removing their rights to political self-determination.[55] In 1948, the same year that the first FPA consignment left Cape Town docks bound for the FPA's froggery, the general election was won by Daniel Malan's National Party, which came to power on an apartheid platform. Apartheid was an extension and systemisation of the racial discrimination that had always characterised South African colonial politics. In the decades after the FPA consignments stopped, apartheid policies eventually displaced millions of people into "townships" and "homelands," and their residents were then accepted in white areas only as cheap labour. A case in point is Cape Town's once-cosmopolitan District Six, which abutted the area surrounding Peers Snake Park and the docks and was cleared of inhabitants as part of the fantasy of an exclusively white city.

To focus on one aspect of how this political context manifested itself even before these mass displacements, we can look at the way that colour-bar politics did not stop at the gangway of the Union Castle ships but increasingly took hold of the passenger experience. In 1914, Solomon Plaatje—a founder member of the organisation which was to become the African National Congress—was able to describe his time aboard *Norseman* on route to Southampton as a momentary vision of a better world than existed onshore, in which people of different skin colours mixed and where he had "the full run of the ship."[56] But in his accounts of later voyages, he testifies to the encroachment of segregation policies on board. Interior design historian Harriet McKay has described the very English interiors and marketing materials of the Union Castle ships as a "constructed oblivion," an expression of British apartheid denial.[57]

In the same month that the FPA's first consignment of frogs was despatched, the British Transport Minister, Alfred Barnes, was being asked in the Westminster parliament to intervene to prevent race apartheid on board Union Castle liners; Barnes preferred to leave it to the discretion of the shipping company.[58] The problem was that the shipping company, although it was British-owned, was not independent of the South African government. The company needed the contract to deliver and collect the mail, which left it actively collaborating with the racist demands of white passengers and the South African government. The South African political economy was "unusually dependent" on shipping to connect it to international capital and to bring in tourists.[59] But, equally, international shipping was dependent on the nationalist government to maintain market leadership. The frogs played their part in this collusion over shipping. From 1948 to 1960, when *Xenopus* were sourced for pregnancy diagnosis, northbound cargo from South Africa was charged a lower freight rate than cargo going south. This means that South African exports were increasingly protected and facilitated, even in a climate of growing international political and diplomatic hostility.

South Africa's traumatic history casts a long dark shadow into the present. The frog pregnancy test came into use in South Africa earlier than in Britain—because the question about how to keep *Xenopus* in a northern climate delayed the test's adoption—but it also continued to be used later. A South African friend tells me that her last pregnancy in 1974 was diagnosed by frog, whilst by then pregnancies in the UK were diagnosed using a chemical reagent test, more like the ones we use today. The hassle and cost of the transport were strong drivers in developing an alternative in Britain, whereas in South Africa the frogs were easier to get and keep. My friend, though, is a white South African and had access to a private health-care system in which a reliable diagnosis of pregnancy was available on demand, albeit for a fee. Private health-care services like these were and still are disproportionately accessed by white people.[60] But even within the public health-care system, more was invested in white people's health care than that of Black people's, whose health was also worse because of the lack of investment in housing, sanitation, and other infrastructure in the overcrowded areas in which they lived.

These inequalities necessarily extended into sexual and reproductive health care for women and girls, although it was complicated by racist fears of being demographically "swamped," which meant that there were well-funded contraception programmes for Black populations, alongside explicit inducements for white people to have larger families.[61] Women were rightly suspicious of approaching a "care" system with discriminatory motivations, even though they may have wanted family planning support. In a survey of the state of South African public health care in 1984, Aziza Seedat recorded that compulsory sterilisation and abortion were being threatened "unless 'certain ethnic groups' accepted family planning measures."[62] Under apartheid, South African medicine presented itself as cutting edge (the world's first heart transplant was undertaken in a Cape Town hospital in 1968), but that image of modernity was a propaganda narrative for the statistically poor health outcomes for a majority of the population.

Despite South Africa's shift to multiracial governance in 1994, inequalities are still in evidence, even by some measures widening, in part because of the drag of history. Sticking with the question of reproductive health care: in South Africa, Black African women have the poorest access to antenatal health care in comparison to others, and maternal mortality is described by Amnesty International as unacceptably high.[63] Early pregnancy diagnosis and antenatal care are especially important in the context of the South African HIV crisis and for protecting the lives of pregnant women and girls living with the virus. Whilst in theory pregnancy testing is freely available for all, in practice coverage is not universal, especially in impoverished rural parts of the country.[64] Women's knowledge about pregnancy testing—what it is and when it can be useful—is not always good, returning us to the questions about the education of women and girls with which this chapter began.

Frogs were not directly responsible for the injustice of apartheid, of course, and the frogs could have been transported in a more just world. But as it happens, they moved through cultures of injustice. The frog transports are part of a picture of a world which is not progressive and in which knowledge has been acquired and commodified in ways which reinforce structural oppression. So knowledge and techniques advance but at what cost? Who benefits? Who owns knowledge? With whom is it shared?

Idle Curiosities

So far I have painted a picture of how the demand for pregnancy certainty intersected with the politics of early apartheid in South Africa. Keeping in mind the topic of knowledge and whom it benefits, I turn to women in Britain, who were less in the know than their white South African counterparts. An unpublished story from the early 1960s by the British novelist Angela Carter (1940–1992) begins with this imagined patient-doctor encounter:

> As soon as the doctor told her she was pregnant, she felt frail and nauseous, although she had not done so before.
> "But are you sure?" she asked, foolishly, she felt, picking up her skirt and stockings. The doctor was washing his hands.
> "Oh yes," he said. "No doubt. Better book you into a maternity hospital."
> She laid a hand wonderingly on her stomach.[65]

Because the story starts in the middle of the scene, it isn't clear how the narrator's test has been done. She has removed her skirt and stockings, which suggests an internal examination. Whilst it is possible to diagnose relatively early pregnancy by an internal examination, it wasn't a popular method. Most people didn't have a pregnancy test at all. Lorna Sage's pregnancy, which I discussed earlier in this chapter, qualified because it was a hard case; she was in denial. It was more common for practitioners to do an external exam of their patient and then suggest a two-week wait to confirm their hunch.

If Carter imagines a urine test, she doesn't realise that tests had to be sent away. But the story is a fiction, a fantasy about a dramatic life moment. In that, it shares something with the Annunciation scene; the Virgin Mary is also frequently depicted in that pose with her hand on her stomach. The doctor is like the all-knowing angel with "no doubt." Indeed, his diagnosis brings on symptoms which don't seem to have been previously felt. Like the illuminated pages of a medieval book of hours whose narrative jumps precipitously from the annunciation to the nativity, the doctor initiates a maternity hospital booking at once. Carter was a well-read and politically aware twenty-something woman. She was older than Lorna Sage was in the scene from *Bad Blood* I discussed earlier. Whilst Sage was a girl living with parents on the Welsh borders, Carter lived in a city, had been to university, and was married. Yet she isn't clear on how pregnancy testing was done. Knowledge about diagnosis might as well have come from the sky and been conveyed by angels.

The power dynamic between doctor and patient is all too clear in Carter's story, as in Sage's real-life scene. Carter's imaginary protagonist feels foolish, which perhaps you always do without clothes on your bottom half. Sage's scene is even more excruciating. The balance of power is tipped as much by access to knowledge as by gender and age. The emergence of a reliable pregnancy test built a wider gulf between women's lay knowledge and that of their medical consultants than there had ever been before. Whilst practitioners

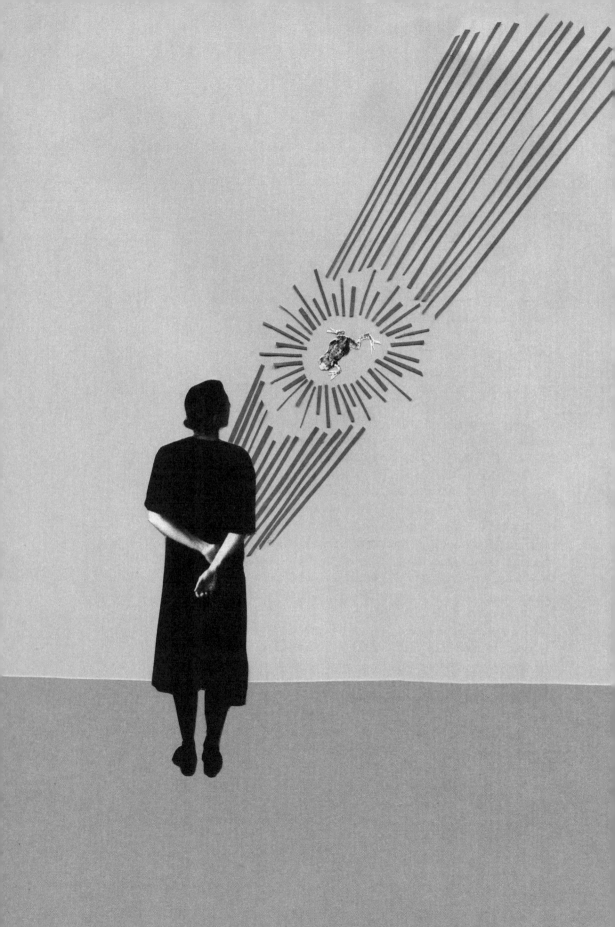

had historically struggled to know in hard cases, now they had access to something objective which liberated them from women's subjective reports about their own conditions. On the other hand, women became even more beholden to practitioners, who had a major new tool to supplement the professional judgement on which medics had previously had to rely.

The FPA didn't have a free rein in how it communicated with the women whose tests were being undertaken; it had to answer to powerful professional organisations. The Association was in correspondence with members of the central ethics committee at the British Medical Association, who were concerned about how women received their results and didn't want them to receive results directly.[66] General practitioners, like Sage's Dr. Clayton, were considered crucial to the care of women and their unborn children. A letter to the *Pharmaceutical Journal*, extracted and preserved in the FPA archive, gives the context of contemporary attitudes. The letter's author can think of only two reasons for a pregnancy test: "to satisfy ordinary curiosity" or "to establish grounds for illegal interference with pregnancy"; "I consider the performance of animal tests to gratify the curious or the person with illicit designs, to be somewhat uncivilised . . . and an abuse of the Home Office licence."[67] The "illicit designs" fear here is of an abortion epidemic, which pregnancy testing was supposed to herald, although it didn't. In a later issue of the same journal, Wright responded by letter that because no frogs were dissected, no Home Office licence was required and that he wanted every woman to be able to use the service and to bypass her doctor if she chose (a shocking thought). The FPA files confirm what we know about birth-control activists across the twentieth century: there were many who would have liked to put knowledge and, with it, a measure of self-determination straight into women's hands. Whatever the FPA might have wished for women, though, the compromise made with professional bodies placed a distance between women and knowledge of their own bodies.

Documents in the FPA files show that women did not always have sympathetic general practitioners who were prepared to request a test. One woman writes to the Association saying that she thinks she is pregnant and, because of a medical condition, fears it could be life threatening. Her doctor has refused her a test. The Association is forced to write back that it is unable to help. So she must live—or die—with not knowing. Such an extreme case wasn't typical, but it shows that the need to know was determined by practitioners. GPs routinely rejected "curiosity cases," dismissing women's ordinary concern to know what was happening in their own bodies as frivolous. At evil worst, they would plan to abort; at silly best, they would just be planning to knit booties. Many women preferred to seek out private medical services because of this NHS resistance.[68] The dismissal of women's curiosity meant that the FPA's advertising had to be publicly cautious. An article in the British tabloid paper *Reveille* in the summer of 1949, for example, carries the headline "Radar for the Stork" and includes a quotation from the FPA suggesting a proper use for the knowledge one of their tests could provide: "A serviceman about to leave for overseas can make proper arrangements for his wife's confinement."[69] Radar and a serviceman on active duty: pregnancy testing had to be keyed into the recent war effort to make it look decent. Women's curiosity about their futures and bodies did not carry respectable weight.

The frogs were decommissioned as pregnancy-test animals in the UK in the mid-1960s, when chemical reagent tests became readable and accurate enough to be useful. Once those were available as portable kits and pregnancy testing moved out of the test centres, the British Medical Association and other organisations had less control over access. Olszynko-Gryn has looked at how the women's liberation movement in the 1970s responded to the new technology by offering free or at-cost testing.[70] The volunteers who staffed those services expected to help a lot of women who dreaded pregnancy but were surprised that they also saw women who wanted to be pregnant and "just wanted to know." They hadn't anticipated that women would come out of curiosity or that the desire for knowledge would be so strong because those desires had previously been private. After all, there was no remedy for them. Rather than being dismissive, these activists saw curiosity and the desire for children as a happy break in otherwise emotionally difficult work. And that work played a significant part in forcing public health-care systems to expand their understanding of "need to know" and to satisfy women's legitimate curiosity. Just knowing, that's sometimes all one wants.

■

In adolescence, I wrote a lot of embarrassing poetry, probably because I listened incessantly to the music of Suzanne Vega, played and rewound until the brown loopy cassette tape stretched. "I didn't invite you, parasite," one poem began, "a shivered winter in my covert cave." Mercifully, I forget the rest now, but you get the gist. And that was how it seemed to me then. I could tell by my English teacher's cocked eyebrow that she found it disturbing, bad, or both. My juvenilia imagined pregnancy as a foreign occupation or an infestation by a creepy frog, perhaps, that chose me as its secret hibernacula.

In my defence, that was the message we were fed. Emilie Pine writes: "we were terrorised with the idea of getting pregnant." The word *terrorised* is a strong but fair interpretation of the message that we were given. Every time and any time, pregnancy might leap out and bite.

Struggling to conceive, on the other hand, was the stuff of fairy-tales, something that used to happen, before science, once upon a time. And ignorance about conception: that, too, was a thing of the past. And so I had no idea.

Dear teenage me,

At the moment, pregnancy fills you with horror, but imagining it also gives you a frisson, a shivery sense of secret inner knowledge. This book gives you a place to start thinking about those secrets, which you will need to learn about later.

Lots of love,
Your future self

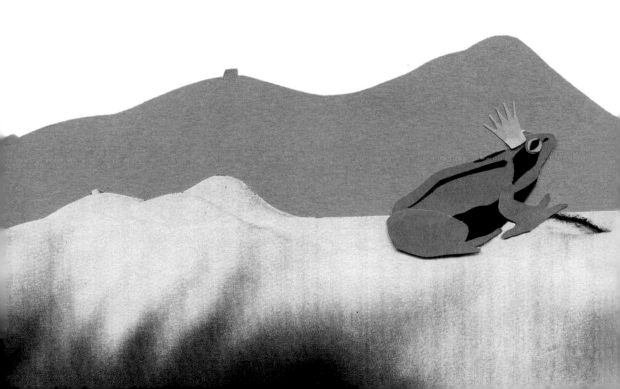

2 Pads: How to Join the Bump Club

Cynthia walked about . . . in a loose silk gown edged with dead wisps of marabou; the skirt strained and billowed outwards over her big belly on which she wore a bow, partly as decoration but rather more as a signpost to indicate what was already obvious. They used to refer to it, my uncle and she, as *the sprog*; and he would pat the bow as the ears of a good retriever.
—Isobel English, *Every Eye* (1956)[1]

Yet of course, the main dressing up always goes on in the mind.
—Naomi Mitchison, *You May Well Ask: A Memoir 1920–1940* (1979)[2]

Belts and Blessings

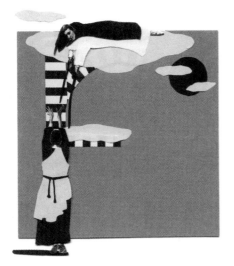

RONTED BY A WIDE piazza awaiting crowds of pilgrims, the cathedral in the Italian city of Prato is small and pretty, with black and white stripes. The square was nearly empty on the day I went but for a small group of North African migrants clustered in the shade on one side and the customers of the piazza café on the other. A raised pulpit faces out into the square from the south-west corner, wearing a conical roof as protection against the weather, purpose-built to show the cathedral's famed relic: the Virgin Mary's belt, a long thin green material strip embroidered with gold. Round the pulpit, pudgy stone-relief puti play, snatching toys, marching in time, dressing up.

In the story of the relic, Mary returned to earth after her assumption into heaven, literally on a flying visit to give her girdle to the apostle Thomas. This is the same Thomas, Doubting Thomas, who needed to touch Jesus's wounds for himself before he would believe in the Resurrection. Mary's girdle gives Thomas similar material proof for her assumption, which he also could not take on faith. In images of the scene, Mary emerges from parting clouds, and her belt trails down like a kite string or dog lead, linking her to Thomas, his feet planted firmly on the earth, hands outstretched. The belt that had encircled a womb pregnant with God, foetal and human, is strung out, spanning the gulf between heaven and earth.

The relic is not ordinarily visible and is displayed publicly only on special feast days, when it is raised in the pulpit above the crowds

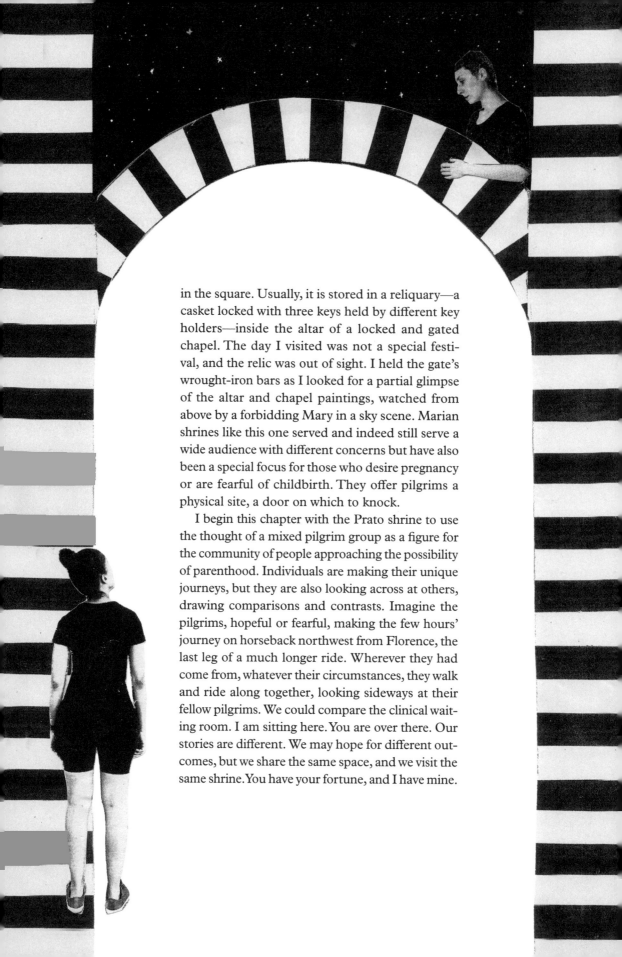

in the square. Usually, it is stored in a reliquary—a casket locked with three keys held by different key holders—inside the altar of a locked and gated chapel. The day I visited was not a special festival, and the relic was out of sight. I held the gate's wrought-iron bars as I looked for a partial glimpse of the altar and chapel paintings, watched from above by a forbidding Mary in a sky scene. Marian shrines like this one served and indeed still serve a wide audience with different concerns but have also been a special focus for those who desire pregnancy or are fearful of childbirth. They offer pilgrims a physical site, a door on which to knock.

I begin this chapter with the Prato shrine to use the thought of a mixed pilgrim group as a figure for the community of people approaching the possibility of parenthood. Individuals are making their unique journeys, but they are also looking across at others, drawing comparisons and contrasts. Imagine the pilgrims, hopeful or fearful, making the few hours' journey on horseback northwest from Florence, the last leg of a much longer ride. Wherever they had come from, whatever their circumstances, they walk and ride along together, looking sideways at their fellow pilgrims. We could compare the clinical waiting room. I am sitting here. You are over there. Our stories are different. We may hope for different outcomes, but we share the same space, and we visit the same shrine. You have your fortune, and I have mine.

Pilgrims seek access to a physical shrine but also to a less located, less defined condition of virtue. Although a lot of feminist work has gone into deconsecrating motherhood, it still carries cultural cachet and is hard fully to demystify.[3] So there still is a vestigial perception that pregnancy gives membership to an exclusive hallowed club, especially perhaps for those who can't get in and feel locked out, for those standing outside the shrine looking through the bars. I play my small part here in debunking the parenthood and pregnancy cults, bookending the chapter with two comedies of manners about the tussles at their thresholds. Those dramas pick up the themes of performance, fashion, and play which concern this chapter. Chapter 1 concerns knowledge and education—what we're brought up to know (or not)—and chapter 2 is about coming to the brink of putting that knowledge into practice in the glare of familial and community expectations and in cultures of competition. What if we could disrupt, once and for all, the competition and puncture the fake status categories it generates?

Women have always staged their rivalries through body shape, size, and fashion; that's as true in pregnancy as not. Pilgrims who travelled to Prato took their own belts, hoping that the relic's holy power to grant fertility or a pain-free labour would rub off onto them. Mary's maternal aura was wearable. Pilgrims returned not only with belts and bellies thus imbued but also with souvenirs: beautiful rings shaped like buckled belts, inscribed "O mater dei memento mei" (O, mother of God, remember me).[4] Belts were popular because they enunciate rather than conceal. The late medieval fashion for belting to emphasize a rounded stomach testifies to the influence that the Marian cult had on the female silhouette. Unusually in European historical fashions, medieval women were prepared to show off a pregnancy, just as we are today. In this chapter, I turn to a different era, the late eighteenth century, where the fashion for pregnancy took another step: not only was pregnancy *en vogue* for the pregnant, but the unpregnant could get the look, too. We live in a moment that has broken a lot of fashion taboos, but a fake baby bump is not yet a common accessory. In this chapter, we cross that last fashion barrier.

Let's dress up. Let's try pregnancy on for size and walk about in it.

THE MISCARRIAGE

A one-act farce

DRAMATIS PERSONÆ

MS. BLESSED
MS. CHILDLESS
MS. BELATEDLY
MR. SOMEONE
THE MOB
} played by members of the company

MS. MISCARRYING
played by me

SCENE: A WORK SOCIAL NETWORKING EVENT

[MS. MISCARRYING *and* MS. CHILDLESS *stand together, and* MR. SOME-
ONE *is pouring drinks. The rest of* THE MOB *are dotted round the room,
drinking and chatting.*]

MS. MISCARRYING
How are you, Ms. Childless? Well, I hope.

MS. CHILDLESS
I am still having infertility therapies and treatments.

MS. MISCARRYING
Of course, how is that going?

MS. CHILDLESS
Sadly, Mr. Childless and I have no luck. It's been very disappointing.

MS. MISCARRYING
I'm sorry to hear that, Ms. Childless.

[*Aside to the audience.*] She and I both. I know—from a scan and, now,
the bleeding—that I miscarry as I speak.

[MS. BELATEDLY *enters, a child strapped to her chest in a sling. She
goes to a corner of the room and starts an inaudible conversation with
one of* THE MOB.]

MR. SOMEONE [*coming over to* MS. MISCARRYING *and* MS. CHILDLESS]
Would you like a drink ladies?

MS. MISCARRYING
Yes, a large one for me please.

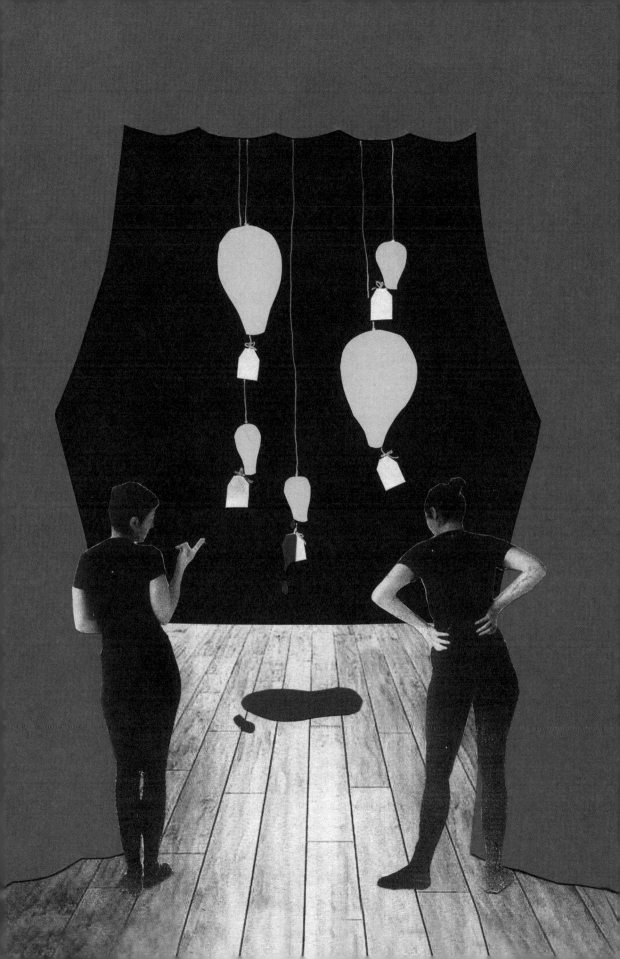

MR. SOMEONE
Ms. Childless?

MS. CHILDLESS
I'd better not. [*But looks enviously at the enormous and spilling glass of wine in* MS. MISCARRYING's *hand.*]

MR. SOMEONE
Driving?

[*Everyone ignores him.*]

MS. CHILDLESS
There's Ms. Belatedly.

MS. MISCARRYING
And the Belatedly babe.

MR. SOMEONE
Does it make you feel broody, ladies?

[MS. CHILDLESS *and* MS. MISCARRYING *stare at him until he goes away.* MS. MISCARRYING *laughs at his back.* MS. CHILDLESS *sighs and turns her attention back to* MS. BELATEDLY.]

MS. CHILDLESS
I can't believe it: a baby already. *And* she's also just had a promotion *and* been awarded a grant *and* won a prize.

MS. MISCARRYING
True.

MS. CHILDLESS
Some people just have it all. And others like me, who have done nothing to offend the gods, as far as I know, are so unlucky.

MS. MISCARRYING
Well, . . . I think Ms. Belatedly's baby was hard come by—indeed, quite belated. And I hear that the birth was brutal—her bowels, you know. Then her partner left her, of course—for her best friend. Although I don't know why any of that would help you feel any better.

MS. CHILDLESS
Yes, quite: she still has a baby.

MS. MISCARRYING
True.

[*Aside to the audience.*] And here I am, miscarrying. How did I end up in this ridiculous ranking of successes and failures? I must get out of this place.

MS. CHILDLESS
She had been with her partner for ages before she got up the duff.

MS. MISCARRYING
What are you saying?

MS. CHILDLESS
It's *just* a bit of a coincidence that she got pregnant *just* after I mentioned to her that I was trying myself, when she'd had years . . .

MS. MISCARRYING
So you thought of it first . . .

MS. CHILDLESS [*sadly*]
Yes.

MS. MISCARRYING
Trademarked it?

[**MS. CHILDLESS** *pretends not to hear. Enter* **MS. BLESSED**.]

[*Aside.*] Now I will be avenged.

Ms. Childless, have you met my friend Ms. Blessed? She has had a lot of success in exactly the area you aspire to work in. [*Calls out.*] Ms. Blessed.

MS. BLESSED [*turns, revealing an enormous pregnancy bump and a huge baby-on-board badge on her lapel*]
Hi, guys. Just made it. The babysitter was late.

MS. CHILDLESS [*with gritted teeth, eyes glued to* **MS. BLESSED**'s *bump*]
What a trial that must have been for you.

MS. MISCARRYING [*going*]
[*Aside to the audience*] I wonder how quickly she will find out that Ms. Blessed has three children as well as this new one on the way. Now, I must get home and attend to my miscarriage. [*As she puts on her coat, she can hear snatches of the conversation she's left.*]

MS. BLESSED
Would you believe it, *another* boy! Four boys. What have I done to deserve it? Bet you're pleased to be child-free, Ms. Childless. Oh, look: there's Ms. Belatedly with her newborn. Damn, I bet it's a girl.

[**MS. BELATEDLY** *comes over.*]

Aw, what a gorgeous baby Ms. Belatedly. [*She chucks it under the chin.*]

[*Exeunt omnes.*]

FINIS

Dressing Up

In her 1979 memoir, the novelist Naomi Mitchison writes about dressing up and its decline since the 1930s as collateral damage in the move to "the present idea that anything goes, so we can always and everywhere be in fancy dress."[5] It's mostly true now, too, that anything goes. You have to go all out at fancy-dress parties to make it clear you're dressed up.

Going all out, I once tried to go to a fancy-dress party as a Swan Vesta matchbox, wearing an elaborate cardboard contraption painted with a lot of time and effort. The party turned out to be on a roof that could be accessed only through a window too small to fit the matchbox. So I went to the party wearing the clothes I had on underneath the costume.

"What have you come as?"

"Um, as an invisible matchbox? Can't you see?"

It's true, lots of things "go" but still not quite everything. Mitchison overstates it. Haute couture catwalks couldn't show unwearable fashion if everything "went." It's mostly not acceptable to go about daily life dressed as a matchbox or wearing a bird's nest, rubbish, or lobster claws on one's head, even if it is designed by Dior. And for those who aren't pregnant, bump-baring maternity wear is currently unavailable. In the 1930s, Mitchison remembers, "pretty maternity dresses" ended up "in the acting box."[6] Yet even now, maternity wear is strictly for pregnancy or let's pretend.

There was one amazing year, though, 1793, when the pregnant look did "go" and anyone could wear it. You could buy a false bump called The Pad and wear it under a flouncy dress with a push-up cleavage. London's *Morning Herald* newspaper, notes that "*Pads* continue to be worn; and on account of these the dress is still a loose gown of white muslin flounced in front, appearing to be put on with the negligence permitted to the supposed situation of the wearers. A narrow sash ties it at the waist."[7] This wasn't quite the little white empire-line muslin dress familiar from Jane Austen costume dramas, but it was heading that way from the exoskeleton corsetry of the *ancienne régime*. You could put on this pregnant outfit and walk around the fashionable districts of town.

The twenty-first century has seen a trend for pads, fillers, and surgery to enlarge lips, breasts, and buttocks, but we don't yet have off-the-peg belly pads as they did in 1793. Celebrity gossip keeps a close eye on body fakery. Has she or hasn't she had her nose, breasts, bum done? The charge of feigning pregnancy has an edge which allegations of other cosmetic enhancement do not. Meghan Markle, Beyoncé Knowles, Katie Holmes, and others have been suspected of faking pregnancies. These duplicitous celebrities, so the rumour mill grinds, have hired mysterious surrogates to do their gestating work. Suspiciously, a dress folds in the wrong place, a bump is too low or high or slips down, a shadow looks photoshopped to hide the join of a prosthetic bump. The bloggers and columnists, clickbait news sites, and social media influencers promise forensic detail: the way clothes move, the anatomy of the pregnant body, the tone of her denials, the baby's resemblances. The fear is that celebrity women are winning fraudulent membership in the sacred motherhood club whilst holding on to the perfect bodies which real mothers are prepared to sacrifice on entry. Who is and isn't in the club is policed.

The eighteenth-century fashion for The Pad began at the point at which we stop, with the padded bum, being preceded by a much longer-lived fashion for the bustle. A cartoon from 1785 called *The Bum Shop* (historical figure 1) shows women buying petticoats with built-in bustlers (segmented pouf-like pads) to extend the dress at the back. Several pads hang on the walls, and others are piled on the floor. One woman sits grinning idiotically at a huge, puffed-up pillow on her lap. Others are being helped by two attentive salesmen. The bustles underpin the distinctive *chemise à la reine* that was popularised by fashion icon Marie Antoinette, with its cloud of white ruffles around a low neckline, sashed at the waist. A poodle, coifed to make pompoms of its torso and tail, stands on its hindlegs: puffed, ruffed and bum-padded, just like the ladies being fitted for bums.

But then, the bon ton, not content with padding only bums, moved the bustle round to the tummy at the front. And once it got there, it took on more meaning than it had as a bum pad because now it simulated pregnancy. Contemporary commentators are clear that that was the intent. A 1793 cartoon designed to imitate *The Bum Shop* called *The Cestina Warehouse or the Belly Piece Shop* (historical figure 2) shows two salesmen attending women who are shopping for tummy pads. The words at the bottom of the cartoon voice the assistants' sales patter in heavily accented French (all the silliest fashions come from France). Whilst Mr. Derriere (behind) is the assistant in *The Bum Shop*, Monsieur Devant (in front) presides in *The Belly Piece Shop*. The pads hanging on the wall or already strapped onto customers are marked up with gestational ages: two months, six months, or twins. One padded woman looks out grinning, enjoying the jest. Another is presumably padded, but her closed lips form a smug and knowing smile, a hand over her bump dotingly, as if to say, "Who knows?" Behind them, a slim figure reaches up on tiptoes, but the one-month pad is still out of her reach. I know the feeling.

Unbelted tents (systematic cover up) have been more usual in the history of Western maternity clothes. When corsetry was in,

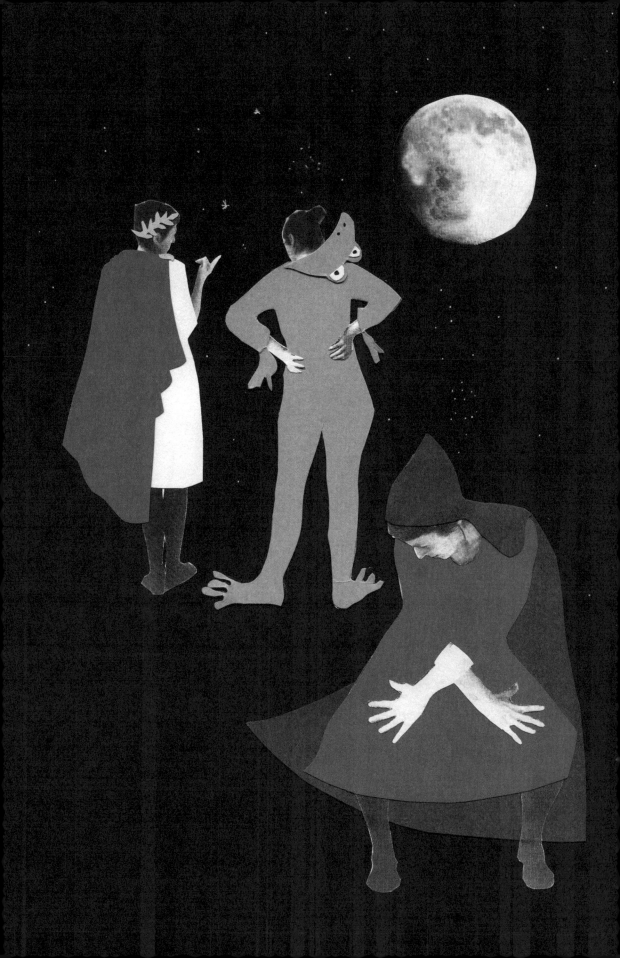

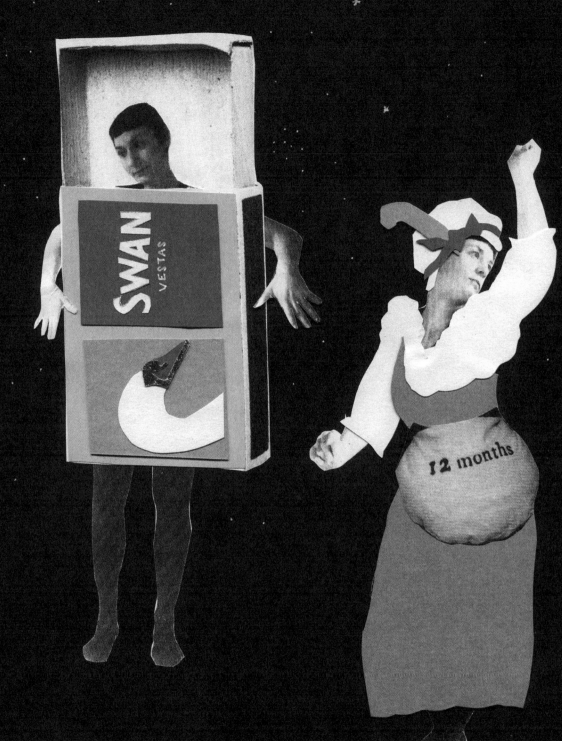

expander panels conceded space, but often pregnancy was too rude and ugly to be revealed with a defining belt or sash. The advice in *Vogue* in June 1930 is about how to pass as not pregnant:

> At first, complete concealment is easily effected by any woman with an eye for dress, but, after the figure is obviously changed, it is still possible to achieve, sometimes to the very end, the effect of a normal figure. Not one's own figure, to be sure, and thicker than one might wish. But, still, one may look to the casual observer like thousands of others that pass on the streets.[8]

Yet there are points in history when pregnancy gets a makeover and gathers enough cultural cachet that the bump can be flaunted. Indeed, The Pad demonstrates that there were times when the preference was effectively reversed: not only that the pregnant were happy to admit to it but that the not-pregnant sought to look pregnant, too.

Looking back to the padded-out pregnancy look of the late eighteenth century, the nineteenth-century physician Thomas Tanner (1824–1871) saw it as a political gesture that emerged in relation to the French Revolution:

> after the first French Revolution there was a great cry about patriotism, and the need of children for the Republic. Hence, those Parisian ladies who were fortunately *enceinte* [pregnant], made the greatest possible display of their condition; while such as were less happily situated, invented a style of dress which should at least give them the reputation of being as they vainly desired to be.[9]

Historian Leslie Tuttle has described a "pronatalism" dominating political and cultural ideology in early modern France, which brought with it a powerful emphasis on marriage, the family, and sex positivity.[10] Across the channel, an English ballad contemporary to The Pad also suggests that padded fashion victims pretended not just to pregnancy but also to patriotism:

> Had I really not known
> This odd taste of the town;
> I'd have thought ladies gone very far,
> And have laid any bet,
> All the women I met
> Were raising recruits for the war[11]

The war here is the Napoleonic war with France. Historian Lisa Forman Cody corroborates the idea that pregnancy was beautified as an English patriotic endeavour at the end of the eighteenth century: "patriots beat the drum most loudly for building a hearty population against the French menace."[12] Pregnancy was flag-waving, and padding up was a travesty. Some historians have suggested that The Pad fits with the fashion for natural, even eroticized motherhood, with an emphasis on the breast and maternal breastfeeding,[13] although in simulating pregnancy, it looks less about getting back to nature than being anarchic and playful with those trends.

The Pad was lambasted in the print-shop windows where caricaturists laid into all the ludicrous fashions: bums, breasts, bellies, skirts, hats, and hair. If, in 1793, you were going to visit the full-scale model of the guillotine exhibited at S. W. Fores's Piccadilly print shop, you could hardly miss these merciless cartoons. Marie Antoinette would be executed in October the same year; French fashion influence was a sign of an effete aristocracy that was potentially losing its grip. The satirical prints let you know that you might see The Pad worn in the fashionable streets of London's West End, modelled by the glitterati around the Prince of Wales near St. James's Palace and other celebrity hangouts.

A cartoon by Isaac Cruikshank, *Frailties of Fashion* (historical figure 3), shows just such a scene, with the prince arm in arm with his long-term mistress, Mrs. Fitzherbert, and the diminutive Duchess of York; both women are padded. In the middle are two young society beauties wearing the new clingy fashions with uncaricatured style, but amongst the mixed-sex groups that mill around them are gratuitously padded older women. Low necklines with floppy white collars plunge to rising abdomens. Several of the figures rest a self-satisfied hand at the apex of their bump. The bumps push out candy-striped and aproned gowns; they are exaggerated by belted waists, and one particularly protuberant tummy doubles as a perch for a parakeet.

The medieval belts I began this chapter with also managed a celebration of the pregnant silhouette, but devotion to Mary rather than patriotic "populationism" legitimised it. Mary, as an icon of virginity, broke a conceptual link between sex and conception, making it morally all right or even pious to sport a bump. That link has been severed for us, too, and pregnancy made less sexually suggestive than it was in the past by innovations in contraception and particularly the pill. Once sex could be enjoyed with less risk of pregnancy and once pregnancy could be more readily planned, sex that resulted in pregnancy took on a more pious character in moral opinion. This purification of pregnancy has seen maternity fashions exploit the full potential of spandex, belts, and bows to annunciate rather than conceal the baby bump. Even bridal wear can be in on the act, with pregnancies

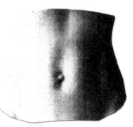

Table III

Fig 1.

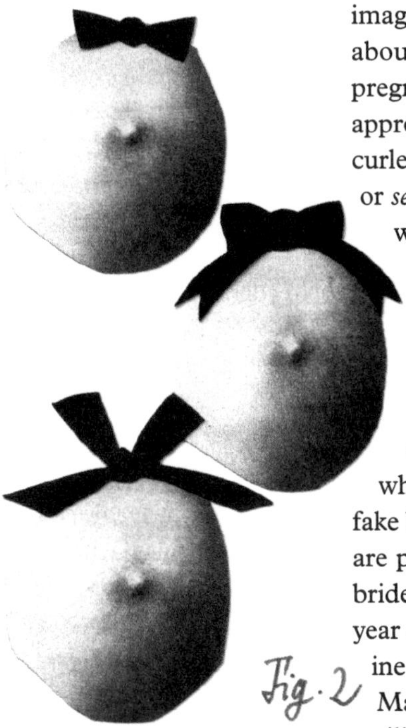

Fig. 2

she's padded

Fig. 3

"showcased even as women walk down the aisle."[14] Bridal-wear shops have moved from concealing sexual shame to articulating pregnant pride. Since Demi Moore's famous 1991 cover for *Vanity Fair* where she posed naked at seven months pregnant, we have steadily recovered from the shock at seeing the pregnant body celebrated in fashion shoots and celebrity images. The naked bump is the ultimate in maternity wear. Maternity wear is part of our wear-once fast-fashion culture, but nakedness pretends to timelessness. These are images which evoke nature as a force at apparent odds with fashion, holy versus unholy.

Pregnancy can be privatizing, and it is fitting that it registers in conspicuous consumption. *Conceited* and *smug* are words which look as if they were made for the pride brought on by pregnancy. *Conceit* has the same root as *conception*, a word with a dual role: a mental image or an idea and the beginning of pregnancy. Conceitedness about anything is being full of ideas of self, inflated with pride, pregnant or padded with it. Conceitedness about pregnancy is as appropriate a relationship between word and meaning as a foetus, all curled up, in the womb. *Smug*, as we use it as a synonym for *conceited* or *self-righteous*, emerged from its earlier sense of "neat and trim," which is exactly the ideal of a pert bump. Conceited? Smug? These are thought crimes, but they are discovered through dress, accessories, and gesture: a bow, belt, hand, or parakeet on a discrete and defined bump.

Memoirist Maggie Nelson describes shopping at something very like a twenty-first-century Belly Piece Shop, putting on a "gelatin strap-on" in a Motherhood Maternity store to see what a jumper with a bow on the bump would look like.[15] Yet a fake bump in a fitting room like this is intended for those who really are pregnant. Trying on prospective bridal wear is for prospective brides, and trying on maternity wear for mothers. Only in the crazy year of The Pad could everyone try on pregnancy for size. Imagine a flash-mob historical reenaction descending on Motherhood Maternity—dressed like the proto-punks of the 1790s in nipped-in military riding habits, big curly wigs, and feathered millinery—as they shoplift their gelatin strap-ons. Sacrilege.

Performing Pregnancy

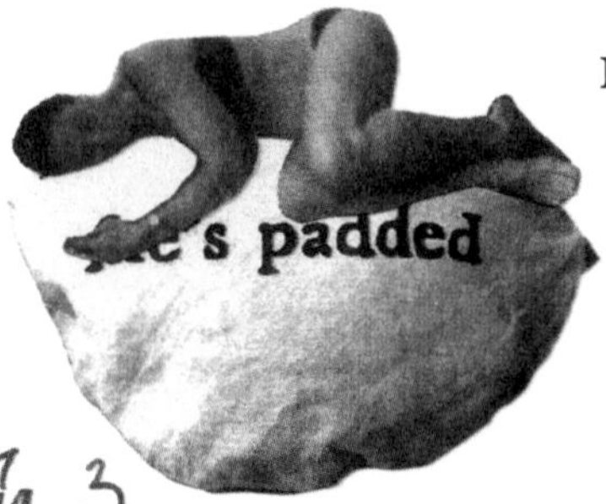

In 1793, you could watch a play called *The Pad, a Farce, in One Act* at the Theatre Royal (now the Royal Opera House) in London's Covent Garden.[16] A contemporary review gives a quick impression:

The whim which some ladies have lately taken of wearing a protuberance about the waist, called a pad, . . . is the subject of the above piece. A captain returned from a sea voyage, a young lover on the point of marriage, and an old baronet in want of an heir, with their wives and mistress, are the persons who are tormented by the appearances produced by the pad. The subject itself is slight, and the effect produced is feeble: but the satire and the moral are just.[17]

That's the main plot: three couples' relationships are temporarily disrupted by The Pad. This review leaves out the main character, Lovejoke, a prankster, as his name suggests, who orchestrates the play's action. His ambition is to bring couples closer together and to make the world more harmonious, but he also enjoys The Pad's anarchic force, its capacity to generate misconceptions. Its inventor, Lovejoke says, should be given a patent for the "sole making and vending" of The Pad as a reward for giving him such "excellent sport."[18]

As the review notes, the play is not high art, and it emerges from a period not particularly famed for its theatre. Even at the time, it was openly said that "modern dramas are the worst that ever appeared on the English stage."[19] The Pad is not a work that you should expect to see revived soon in a theatre near you. However, it at least had the advantage of being short, a one-act farce, so you could spend longer eating and drinking in the fashionable taverns and coffee houses round the theatre.

Surely another plus is that playgoers could go padded. I like to imagine they did, crossing the Italian-style cobbled piazza at Covent Garden with makeshift bumps strapped around their middles, squeezing with difficulty between the fruit stalls and tethered horses. When someone's Pad drops out from beneath crinolines, getting soaked in a puddle, raucous alcohol-fuelled shrieks ring out as it's tossed amongst the little group, a wet baby no one wants the responsibility of carrying.

In the auditorium, the actors' thick greasepaint is melting in the heat of the lamps and candelabra that light the stage, rouge on cheeks sliding down over a bright white base. For the time of the play, the audience is the whole world. The lights do not dim, and members of the audience do not go quiet; instead, they become public opinion and part of the action. When Lovejoke asks Captain Credulous about his plan to throw his wife out of the marital home, he appeals to the audience ("What will the world say?") while gesturing to the boxes and stalls.[20] It will "applaud me for my spirit," Credulous suggests and waves to raise that applause. "Hoot you for your cruelty," Lovejoke corrects him, giving the "world" its cue to hoot.

Despite this reproach, Lovejoke allows the Captain to believe both that his wife has been unfaithful to him whilst he has been off in a far-flung part of the British empire for fifteen months and that his unmarried niece, Nancy, has also betrayed her fiancé and fallen pregnant. In a slightly different storyline, Lovejoke plays a crueller trick on a third couple, Sir Simon and Lady Meagre. Theirs is a loveless marriage, brought to bitterness by failing to conceive an heir. Things have become so bad that Sir Simon tells Lovejoke that, like Captain Credulous, he is also thinking of throwing out his wife. Lovejoke again solicits public opinion ("Oh, fie, Sir Simon, what will the world say?") as he cues the audience for responses.[21] Sir Simon says, "Pho—the devil take the world," prompting booing from the stalls. "Did ever a Baronet care what the world said?" he asks, and the audience admits loudly that baronets never did. Lovejoke prevents the Meagres' separation by leading Sir Simon to believe that his wife is finally and miraculously pregnant, bringing a refreshing harmony to their stale marriage.

Meanwhile, the women don't seem to understand what's causing confusion. "What is the matter? . . . What do you mean?" Mrs. Credulous asks when her husband accuses her, completely oblivious to the fully accessorised enormous false stomach she must be wearing to make this scene work.[22] All the characters are brought together in a final showdown in which Lovejoke winds up his pranks: "This *(producing a pad),* this is the cause of all these mistakes," at which, according to the stage directions "the ladies shriek."[23] That is presumably the cue for members of the audience, too, to pull out any remaining Pads from under their clothes and shriek along in response or throw them as a parodic tribute onto the stage.

But before Lovejoke's revelation that the women are padded rather than pregnant, Sir Simon Meagre makes this touching speech:

> And though Providence for these twenty years last past,
> that we have been married, had withheld the blessing I have
> always prayed for on our union—yet at last my silent wishes
> have prevailed—(*Lady M. appears much distressed—The
> company scarce refrain from open laughter*).[24]

The audience, playing the part of the world looking on, is expected to join in with the actors' onstage laughter, knowing that Lady Meagre is not pregnant with Sir Simon's precious heir. The actors slated to play the Meagres in the *dramatis personae* were leading comic actors of the day: Mr. Quick and Mrs. Webb. The audience's laughter is sanctioned by Lovejoke's description of Sir Simon as a "childless curmudgeon" and his wife as "ill-natured and ugly" and by Sir

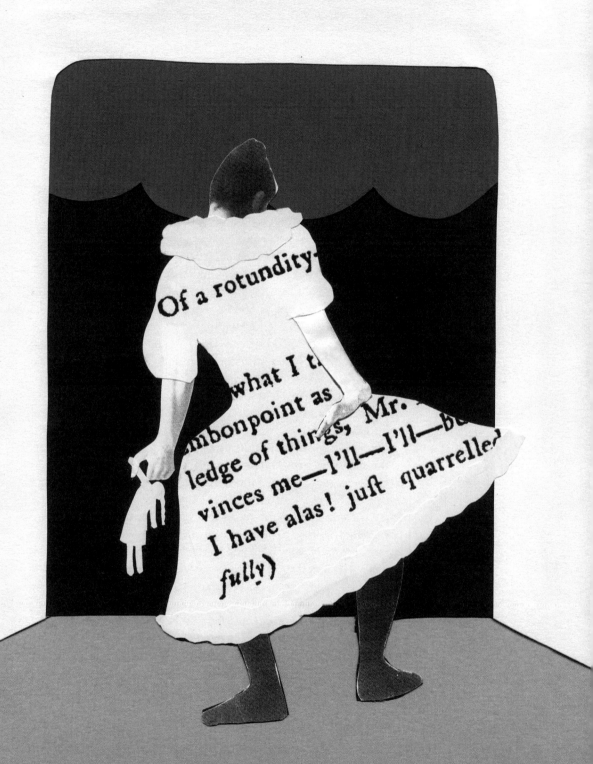

Simon's entitled dismissal of the world's opinion. If he doesn't care what the world says, then they can laugh as much as they like.[25]

There is an odd edge to the comedy. When Lovejoke delivers his moral message at the end of the play about what his tricks should teach the various characters—warning women against hazarding their reputations by wearing a Pad and Captain Credulous against cultivating groundless jealousies—Sir Simon responds with: "And what will it teach me?"[26] Lovejoke says that The Pad has brought happiness back into his childless marriage and, because of that, Lady Meagre alone of all women should be allowed to wear it. To that, Sir Simon responds, in a way that disrupts the play's comedy: "Poor comfort!—sad substitute for a Son and Heir!—I thought to have had a little baronet." So the play ends with the dashed hopes of a trying-to-conceive couple.[27]

Amongst the hooting and laughing audience, could there have been people disappointed like the Meagres, looking on with dismay, feeling sad for and sympathetic to them, despite their peevish characters? How much sympathy was available? The representation of Sir Simon Meagre, in particular, is striking from our historical vantage point. The involuntarily childless man longing for children is affecting. We tend not to see male grief at childlessness expressed like this or at least not as often as we do female grief.[28] If we take down from the shelf a female-authored comic play from the same year, Elizabeth Inchbald's *Every One Has His Fault* (1793), we find the character Mr. Solus, played by the same actor, Mr. Quick, who always imagined his life as being married with a clutch of children but is disappointed. The sad childless man was familiar enough to be a stock character; his regret was stageable, acknowledged, and culturally obvious.

Sir Simon Meagre presents us with the question of what exactly, in the staging of thwarted fatherhood, is being regretted: what does a child represent to him? Sir Simon's wistful "I thought to have had a little baronet" seems mostly to be about perpetuating his name and title, marks of social status and capital, ambitions which are not necessarily incompatible with loving and nurturing a child but are not precisely the same. His frustrated patriarchal desires write over his wife's, and the play stages little more than the failure of his family's investment in her as breeding stock. What does she think or feel? The play doesn't care; it is more interested in how men negotiate silly, simple, and misleading femininity. Lord and Lady Meagre, in a play where name signals character, are scanty, deficient, inadequate examples of their sex, because they are childless in a world in which parenthood very explicitly marks adulthood. But it also works the other way: they are childless because they are inadequate; the audience can rest assured that the Meagres deserve a punishment which is of their own making. The name Meagre also means thin, even emaciated; fittingly Lady Meagre's natural silhouette is very unpregnant.

By ending with this uncomfortable bite, the play turns The Pad into a badge of public humiliation for the involuntarily childless, for men as much as women. This really must have been a rebellious fashion if such heavy artillery had to be deployed to bring it down. In the end, Lady Meagre is given Lovejoke's permission to wear The Pad so that all self-determination, all resistance, all personal desire is removed from her; and The Pad's possibilities—for female play, resistance, solidarity—are negated. Addressing The Pad itself, Lovejoke tells us why it provokes this scathing conservative satire: "there is one thing I don't like you for—you are a Leveller—you are for making all alike."[29] Yet clearly it was levelling in one way only: not of wealth, social status, or even really looks but of sexual and reproductive status. Was she or wasn't she? The Pad so mashed things up that it was hard to tell. The Pad doesn't respect the cult of motherhood. If anyone can pad up, then there's no superiority in the pregnant silhouette.[30] From the moralists' point of view, that shocking insurrection needed quashing.

Maternal Age

The most frightening thought in 1793 seems to be that an older woman might put on a Pad. That nightmare is the subject of another of the satirical takes on The Pad. *A Vestal of '93 Trying on the Cestus of Venus* by James Gillray (1756–1815) (historical figure 4) purports to be an engraving of an ancient bas-relief, a fragment from antiquity, yet depicts the fashion of the moment. The subject is an old woman who is looking in a mirror while being dressed in a large saggy Pad by three cupids. This is one of several satirised caricatures of Lady Cecilia Johnston (1727–1817), although what she did to be such a target I leave other historians to discover. In the cartoon, she looks pleased with The Pad's effect, smiling and holding her hands up in delight. She has a copy of a work by Ovid in her pocket, whose title can't be read. It ought to be the *Ars amatoria* (The art of love), but perhaps *The Metamorphoses*, Ovid's catalogue of mythic shape-shifters, would be more fitting for an old woman who wants to pass as or even be young. One cupid carries a quiver, but in the act of tying The Pad round the woman's waist, he inadvertently spills his arrows. Whatever sex appeal the Vestal imagines The Pad confers, it disarms Love. There is no vitriol so acid as that hurled at the aging woman, and the most caustic of all is reserved for an aging woman pretending to fertility, wearing young women's clothes.

The quotation at the bottom of Gillray's image and the phrase in the cartoon's title, the Cestus of Venus, is from Alexander Pope's translation of Homer's *Iliad* (1715–1720). Gillray places his scene in bathetic contrast to the highest epic form. The cestus (or belt) of Venus had magical properties to inspire love and lust. In *The Iliad*, Hera borrows it to seduce Zeus so that during his postcoital slumber the Greeks can steal an advantage in the Trojan war. Here is the luxuriant description of Hera in her boudoir preparing for the seduction:

> Here first she bathes; and round her Body pours
> Soft Oils of Fragrance, and ambrosial Show'rs:
> The Winds perfum'd, the balmy Gale convey
> Thro' Heav'n, thro' Earth, and all th'aerial Way.[31]

Then she does her hair in a half up-do, the top in ringlets and the rest "wav'd like melted Gold" over her shoulders. Then she dresses: a flowing "heavenly" mantle with a gold clasp, pendant earrings with gems like stars, a dazzling white veil like "fall'n snow," and some "celestial Sandals." When a goddess gets dressed, the whole universe shifts on its axis. In contrast, Gillray's Vestal is ungainly, squatting to see in the mirror. Her wrinkled chin is jutting below a protuberant nose and concave cheeks with too much rouge, even for a period when rouge was the rage. Her grey hair is only just visible beneath an odd bonnet, with copious drapery flopping down to ugly bloomers and slippers. Homer's picture of great erotic power, a realignment of epic history, is punctured and deflated in Gillray's response.

She shouldn't be old. That's the point. Old women should not wear the cestus of Venus; nor, in fact, should Vestals, who are sacred priestesses of the goddess Vesta and dedicated to chastity. Vesta's temple was in the forum of ancient Rome, and the priestesses were entrusted with protecting the sacred flame on which the fortunes of the city were said to reside. In Gillray's engraving, the lamp has fallen on its side; its flame is still lit, but for how much longer? The world is upside-down. An old woman beautifying herself with a Pad, pretending to sexiness and, worse, fertility, is a category error that makes everything unsafe. The universe shifts, as it does in the boudoir scene from *The Iliad*, but for the worse, brought on by female self-delusion.

The issue of maternal age is like a grenade. Wait until it's reasonably apposite in discussion, pull out the pin, and throw it in. The abiding question is: how old is too old to become or try to become a mother? There isn't any neutral ground. Everyone has a view. A

Chapter 2

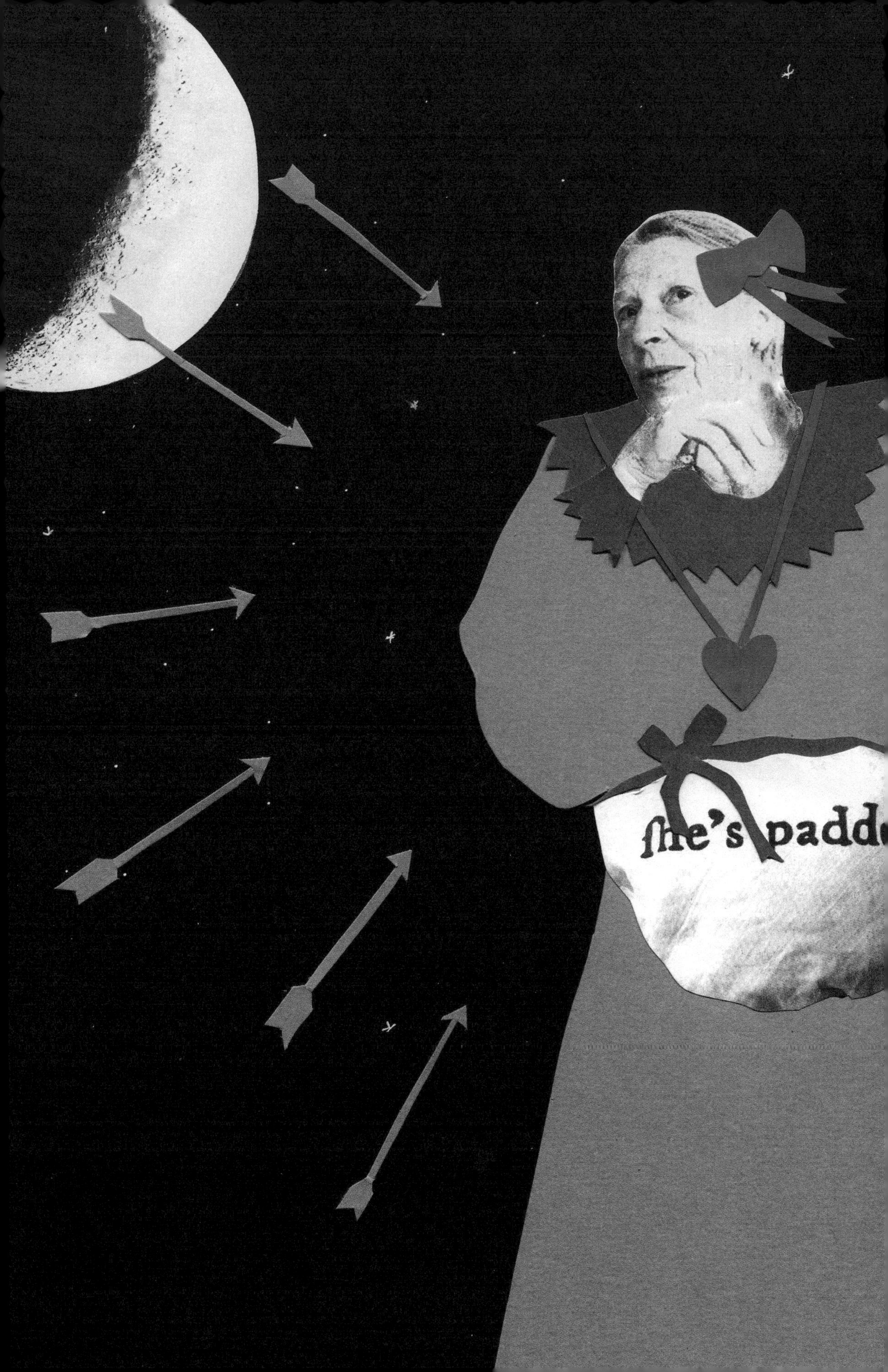
ſhe's padd

key flashpoint, for us now, emerges around the political and popular interpretation of medical messaging about pregnancy postponement.[32] Memoirist Cari Rosen, writing about coming to motherhood in her early forties, describes internalising a particular politicized line: "apparently it was *me* who the papers were shouting at." "I must be (among other things) a selfish workaholic who has given her best years to her career and now wants to have it all."[33] She identifies the print media as the source of criticism and the underlying point of contention, the advances women have made in the workplace. Feminism is the target, but medicine and nature are the weapons.

Fertility scientists, clinicians, and professional bodies are not always trumpeting breakthroughs and advances in fertility therapies. They also have a message about the limits of their powers. They particularly underscore maternal age as a powerful block for fertility medicine. As the rates of women like me having their first babies later continue to rise, specialists are increasingly insistently calling people to have their families at the optimum time physiologically.[34] The concern is that more and more people (again, like me) will experience fertility complications or unwanted childlessness.[35] The cliff is the image that is often evoked to identify thirty-five as the age at which women's fertility decline steepens. There are deniers and believers in the cliff, but it is hard to ignore the bodies at its foot.[36] The evidence for it is contemporary but also historical data drawn both from a time before birth-control technologies complicated the demographic picture and from religious communities that have deliberately rejected those technologies.[37] Beyond the limits of science, beyond the clinic and lab, the waves still erode the coast, and women's age is still the biggest determinant of fertility outcomes. Cliffs are natural features; you can't argue with a cliff.

History haunts the dispute about female fertility and age because the problem is perceived to be modern. It is a mistake, though, to think that people in history lived in a state of nature, having children from puberty to menopause and their first child universally early. Average maternal age fluctuates over time, social status, educational profile, and place, but in Western Europe it is often surprisingly late.[38] The key indicator for population historians is the average age at marriage, which was more indexed to maternal age in historical societies. Historians of population in England, for example, typically track a fall in the average age of women at marriage from 26.5 in the later seventeenth century to a low of 23.4 in the early nineteenth; with average age at first child tracking approximately 1.5 years above, from 28 years to 24.9.[39] Looking just across the course of the twentieth century, the figures don't trend only one way. In the UK, the average age at which women had their first child rose in 1946 to 26.2

(the women of my grandmother's generation were having their families around the impediment of World War II), fell to a low of 23.7 in 1970 (my mother's generation), but has since climbed to 29.1.[40] It is worth noting, in case we hold it out as some kind of "natural" or "norm," that the average age at first pregnancy in the late 1960s and early 1970s was a historical low.[41]

War is a good excuse for falling off a cliff. So the childless women of the war generations get some pity, albeit pity complicated by the suggestion that they were embittered battle-axes, getting their fair share of antifeminist Vestal-style slurs. The generations after mine get some sympathy because of the price of houses and their zero-hours contracts, a sympathy muddied by the suggestion that they would be on the housing ladder if they spent less money in hipster cafés. Generation X-ers like me—born in the 1970s—have fewer excuses; less sympathy leavens the backlash which holds us to blame for drinking too deeply at the fountain of feminism. We deliberately strode off the cliff in business suits, according to the conservative columnists. Yet it was "circumstance," "not choice," Cari Rosen notes, which delayed her bid for parenthood.[42] People do not come to their childbearing years in a vacuum; they traverse a complex social and economic landscape. Settling to family life in a gig economy and hustling for every opportunity and modicum of lived security: these are some of the things which delay those people who always wanted to be parents. How do they get from here to there?

Rosen, for example, wanted to parent in a companionate heterosexual partnership. Lots of people do. I caught an interview with Rosen on the radio one morning. Asked by the male interviewer why she hadn't had children sooner, she responded with something like: "What was I supposed to do? Jump the pizza delivery man?" Those, like Rosen, who have struggled to manoeuvre themselves into conducive circumstances, feel compelled to self-justify, often by differentiating themselves from the childless by choice. Increasingly, women are freezing their eggs or going alone to fertility clinics, becoming solo mothers as a plan A, deliberately divorcing their desire for children from the whole crappy dating app swamp.[43] Lesbian couples and trans men have extrafraught routes to pregnancy, negotiating clinical pathways on top of the added familial, social, and political pressures applied to their lives. The complaint about our new world is that it gives people too many choices, illegitimate choices that fly in the face of nature and history. But my generation and the ones coming after me are saying that *choice* might be the word for people who don't want to become parents—and why not?— but that social circumstance, not choice, delays pregnancy for those who are sure they want it.[44]

Generation X didn't face a global war and mass casualties, but (just to put in the requisite personal mitigation) a lot of men in the UK did inexplicably go missing. They were missing from the UK's 1991 census, which puzzled demographic statisticians into "correcting" the numbers.[45] They were missing again in 2001. Even though more boys are born than girls and immigrants are more likely to be working-age men, their numbers were down. Where were they? Perhaps they were less likely to fill out the census form or more likely to be itinerant and sofa-surfing. Perhaps they had gone out to staff the clubs in Ibiza or the coffee shops of Amsterdam when the Maastricht Treaty gave us freedom of movement. Whether or not they were fatherhood material no one could ascertain because they had up and vanished.

But at a considerable distance from the macrodemographics are the logistics of an individual life. When a man I imagined I would settle down with, let's call him Mr. Inconstant, left me, I headed to a Greek island and worked as a housekeeper. In the time that I spent working by myself—cleaning, ironing, shopping—I talked to him in my head, inventing my life not exactly as it was but in a much-improved version: a more glamorous job, a new love affair, fluent Greek, a perfect tan. But babies, a marriage? These were things I did not work into the fantasy because that narrative was not the best revenge. I had been accused by Mr. I., on his way out, of the "thing men think is the most insulting thing they can accuse you of" (according to that feminist prophet Nora Ephron)—"wanting to be married," a charge I strenuously denied.[46]

I wrote letters I never sent in which I told him that, instead of feeling broken, I had flown away into a better life. I spared him all the mundanity, missteps, and disconnections strewn about me like the pack of cards that Alice beat off as the looking-glass world came to its scattered end, inventing instead a life coming together, settling in some fortuitous new pattern in a beautiful land where the sun always shone. Each day, I gave the dreams new details and could sometimes forget that I was merely inventing rather than living this other more perfect life. Meanwhile, Mr. I. was a married father within a year or two of our split. Close shave.

For women, in amongst the chaos of living there is always the drone of the moralists upholding the double standard: women are too picky, demanding, ambitious; women are not doing this or that; women ought; women should. Women's defenders and detractors slog it out, as energetically as ever. Modern antifeminism holds out involuntary childlessness as a warning, the price exacted for women's successes outside of the domestic sphere. Women only have themselves to blame. Meanwhile, in amongst it all, people just live in the only way they can, dreaming of things they want for themselves and doing their best to get there.

When I found M.—a man who is good at filling out forms and so will have been counted—I did ask him where he had been and why he wasn't an attached father already. It turns out that, like me, he was looking for the right person, although with decidedly less urgency. I was right on the cliff edge, at thirty-four, and knew it. The conversation went a bit like this:

ME: When are we going to have children then?
M: We've only just met.
ME: You did tick the I-want-children box on your dating profile.
M: It's not a contract. I need time to think about it.
ME: OK.
[A few minutes pass]
So, have you thought about it?

On paper he might have been thirty-nine, but in his head, he felt like he was twenty and had time with which to play.

Play Time

Women want to know: where is the line of men queuing for early fatherhood? Systematic miscommunication of the message about the cliff edge sees it directed at women, as if it's information *only* for women. When I stepped out of my teenage years, my peers were not settling down for family life quickly or, as we'd more likely have expressed it, getting tied down. That was even more true of the men than it was of the women. My male peers yearned for the footloose life modelled by the beatnik generation. They channelled the spirit which was Jack Kerouac's *On the Road* (1955), dreamed of gunning the old Hudson across America with Sal Paradise and Dean Moriarty, saying goodbye to static domesticity and sobriety, living and loving as "broken-down heroes of the Western night."[47] Paradise (Kerouac's in-text avatar) rejects the thought of marriage with this endearing self-assessment: "I like too many things and get all confused and hung-up running from one falling star to another till I drop."[48] And why not? Why shouldn't the young pursue the stars? You can't want what you don't want.

When, as teens, my best friend and I read Carolyn Cassady's non-fictional counterblast to Kerouac's novel *Off the Road* (1990), which recounts her attempts to settle down with Neal Cassady (a.k.a. Dean Moriarty), we caught an early glimpse of something else: of the 1950s

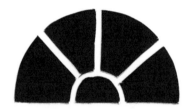

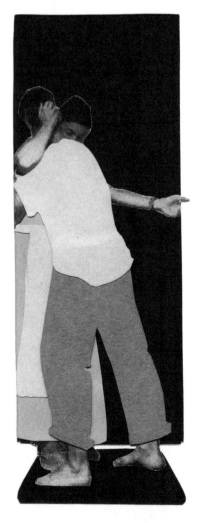

past but also potentially our future, where another kind of desire, for a family life, might creep in. Cassady's book was unsettling in that it builds its resistance out of convention and refuses to conform to beatnik rootlessness as much as to bourgeois stasis and mediocrity. The way she wrote it, the "in" things and the "out" things swapped clothing and lost identity. She wanted to live, to have a family with, to "tie down" a man she loved quite in the face of his unfaithful resistance and some truly bad sex. The beats' iconoclastic spontaneity didn't sound so liberating from her perspective.

She describes their early cohabitation as playful: "For a while Neal and I enjoyed playing house."[49] Even their emerging familiarity and shared humdrum challenges content her: "Despite debts, Neal's health problems and the unfortunate experience of his taking a short-lived job as an encyclopedia salesman, these were months of great happiness for me." But she writes of the turning point where the playacting started to get real: "they were about to come to an end. I missed a menstrual period."[50] That was a warning to shiver at, as was that phrase, "playing house": be careful that the doll doesn't wake; it'll want feeding.

In *The Argonauts*, Maggie Nelson describes receiving a barbed message from her partner's ex about her attempts to be an engaged stepmother: "Tell your girlfriend to find a different kid to play house with." Why, she wonders, does this dig "sting so bad?"[51] The accusation is of inauthenticity— that Nelson has betrayed her queer and feminist principles and her art, reconstituting a simplistic model of family to the exclusion of other wild and wonderful things. The barb stings because it accuses Nelson of betraying her side in a centuries long war for girls' education and full humanity. How do we live with a preoccupying desire for motherhood in the shadow of the dehumanising domestic trap that feminism has taught us to resist?

Mary Wollstonecraft, writing in the time of The Pad, was in the frontline of that war. Here we look in as she considers the girl's relationship to her doll and the way it fits her to wifehood within the house:

> As for Rousseau's remarks, . . . , that they [i.e., girls] have naturally, that is from their birth, independent of education, a fondness for dolls, dressing, and talking—they are so puerile as not to merit a serious refutation. That a girl, condemned to sit for hours together listening to the idle chat of weak nurses, or to attend at her mother's toilet, will endeavour to join the conversation, is, indeed, very natural; and that she will imitate her mother or aunts, and amuse herself by adorning her lifeless doll, as they do in dressing her, poor innocent babe! is undoubtedly a most natural consequence.[52]

Wollstonecraft here refutes Jean-Jacques Rousseau's argument that girls are naturally drawn to dolls and that dolls train them in fashion and childcare. In Wollstonecraft's view, the girl dresses the doll like the girl's mother dresses her, emulating the only model that she is given and cannot transcend because of the oppression of domestic time. But the doll is "lifeless" and threatens to deaden the child, preoccupying her with clothes rather than allowing her to exercise her body, cultivate her mind, or care for her soul. The danger is the one that Betty Friedan picks up in *The Feminine Mystique* (1963) in her discussion of dolls and dolls' houses: not that the girl would be confined forever to playing at house, never maturing to full adulthood, but that she would herself become a doll, a beautiful but lifeless toy.[53] Looking at the narrow image of the ideal housewife in the 1950s and early 1960s and kicking against the domestic drudgery and economic dependence sold as a package with motherhood, Friedan asked, "where is the world of thought and ideas, the life of the mind and spirit?"[54]

The Pad occupies an odd position in the political battles over the socialisation and education of girls. It is clearly an absurd fashion, a frippery of the kind that Wollstonecraft wishes didn't waylay women's energies; yet it is also not straightforwardly beautiful, disrupting an easy association between women's fashion and sexual objectification. Mr. Dighton's satirical bawdy ballad about The Pad urges women to take it off:

> Let no swellings appear,
> In the front or the rear,
> But that which sweet nature allows.[55]

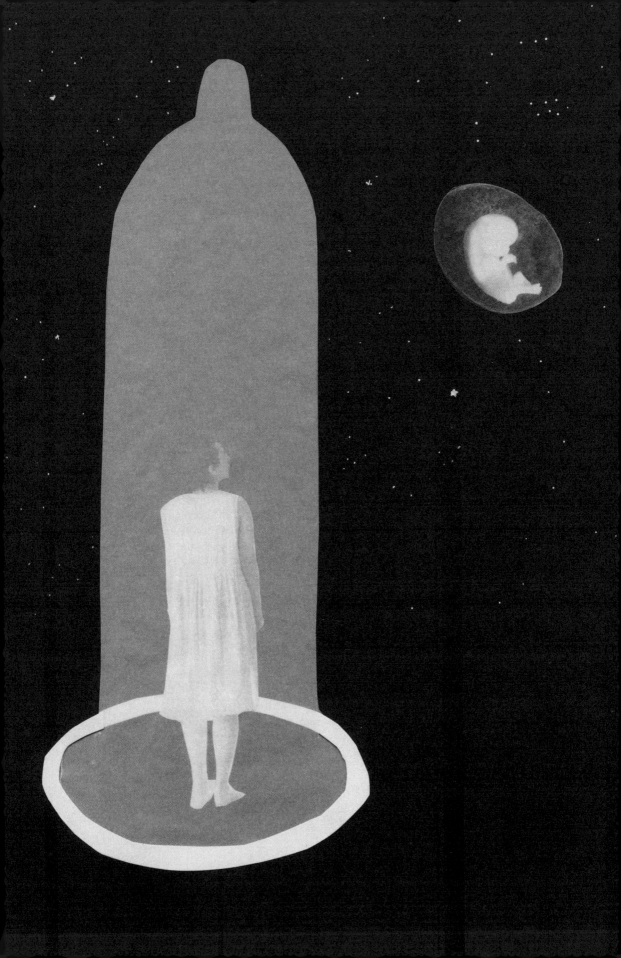

The single *entrendre* here is that the erect penis is the only swelling permitted in the population games. Looking in from the left edge of the scene depicted by *Frailties of Fashion* (see historical figure 3), the satirical print I discussed earlier, is a little girl, padded, holding a doll, also padded. She watches the padded adults playacting with studied seriousness, gathering a model of adulthood to herself. Put a cushion up your dress, and pretend to be heavy with child; hold your bump with one hand and the small of your back with the other; go into labour, and birth the cushion; swap it for a doll; wrap it in a towel, and cradle it—all with your tights still on. These are the things that children do when they are happy for motherhood to be a lifetime away. Let's-pretend pregnancies, the girl's sober look says, are silly for adults. The cartoon can't laugh with so it laughs at women sporting The Pad, spoiling, and neutralising their playful revolt.

THE PARENTHOOD CLUB

A one-act farce

SCENE: EVENING IN A STREET NEXT TO AN ENORMOUS CLOCK TOWER, SHOWING 10 O'CLOCK, WHOSE HANDS ARE VISIBLY MOVING.

[MR. INCONSTANT, MR. UNCONCERNED, *and* MR. CAN'T COMMIT *are queueing behind a sign for what they think is paintballing. A time-travelling tourist,* MR. TIME, *dressed in late eighteenth-century wig and costume, watches and listens in from stage left.*]

MR. CAN'T COMMIT
Women in their mid-thirties are so hard to date.

MR. TIME
[*Aside*] What is this . . . dating?

MR. INCONSTANT
Tell me about it. Dump them the moment they hit twenty-nine and three-quarters. That's the motto I learned in Inconstant School.

MR. CAN'T COMMIT
I really like this one, but she does seem to be in an unnatural hurry.

MR. UNCONCERNED
What? She wants to get married? What happened to the revolution, comrade?

MR. CAN'T COMMIT

I'm trying to keep the revolution alive, of course. But she's so on my wavelength. I don't know if she minds about marriage, but she wants to move in together and have kids . . . and soon.

MR. TIME

[*Aside*] What infernal reckonings are these? Outside of marriage?

MR. INCONSTANT

I can just imagine you pushing a buggy down the nappy aisle.

MR. CAN'T COMMIT

Don't . . .

MR. UNCONCERNED

Next thing you know, there'll be scatter cushions on your sofa and ambient lighting messing up the visuals on the Xbox.

MR. TIME

[*Aside*] What enormous children there are in this future time. Where is the honour in their name that they would not seek an heir?

MR. CAN'T COMMIT

I went to pick her up from her work the other day . . .

MR. TIME

Women at work. What upside-down world is this? When will they breed and nurture heirs?

MR. CAN'T COMMIT

. . . and she was on about her desk-share colleague who's sold her flat and bought a house *outside* of London . . . with a dishwasher!

MR. INCONSTANT

Don't they have Nandos in the provinces?

[**MR. TIME** *puts on a bouncer's uniform and sets up a purple stanchion. He turns around the Paintballing sign. Now they are queuing for* **THE PARENTHOOD CLUB.**]

MR. INCONSTANT, MR. CAN'T COMMIT, AND MR. UNCONCERNED
ARGGHGHGGHGHGHGHGHGHGGGGGGGGGGGGGGG.

[*Then follows an inset choreographed ballet:* **MR. INCONSTANT, MR. CAN'T COMMIT,** *and* **MR. UNCONCERNED** *try to turn around and leave but are prevented from doing so by* **THE CROWD** *entering stage left and moving towards them. In* **THE CROWD** *are couples (heterosexual and same-sex) and a few individuals.*

Two diversion signs are set up, one by **DOCTORS IN WHITE COATS** *marked "Assisted Reproduction" and another by* **OFFICE WORKERS** marked "Adoption." Different people (all the same-sex couples but also some of the heterosexual ones) in THE CROWD try to take those routes. Some couples and individuals get to THE PARENTHOOD CLUB entrance, are turned away, or go of their own volition, and they leave at different stage exits.

Couples and individuals go at different speeds. One in each partnership is often a bit ahead of the other, pulling. Some go straight over THE PARENTHOOD CLUB threshold. Others stop and move backwards and forwards over the line. Some retrace their steps to one of the diversions and then either move smoothly over or are held up, running on the spot or moving through the different routes sometimes walking backwards. MR. TIME pushes some of them over or bars others. Some look as if they're not going into THE PARENTHOOD CLUB but then stumble or fall over the threshold.

Some couples stand closely together, others are an arm's length apart, some remain as couples, and some separate after crossing or carry along a bit farther before dividing. Some individuals form couples with others who have divided off from their partners (or not) or with those who they help to scale the fence into THE PARENTHOOD CLUB. Some women and a few lone men are waiting at the entrance to the club, trying to grab others to form a couple.

Inside THE PARENTHOOD CLUB, all the women have absurdly large bumps and are handed belts, bows, or birds to accessorize them. One man is beating his chest with pride. Some women and a few men are visibly preening themselves.

MR. TIME looks at the clock in the tower, which is now nearly midnight, and begins to close the enormous doors of THE PARENTHOOD CLUB. This accelerates the dance as people try to move faster to get in. A few squeeze through the doors at the last minute, including a couple who are just passing and seem to think of entering only because they see the door about to shut. A woman appears and tries to grab MR. CAN'T COMMIT but, at the last second, gives up and catches MR. INCONSTANT unawares instead. They are the last through the doors, followed only by MR. TIME as the doors close.

MR. CAN'T COMMIT and MR. UNCONCERNED are left outside in the dark, quiet street. Others traipse around them. Some don't look bothered, but others are still trying to get into THE PARENTHOOD CLUB.]

MR. UNCONCERNED
Narrow escape man, narrow escape.

[MR. CAN'T COMMIT joins others who are banging on the door.]

But Sue, I love you. Come back. Sue?

FINIS

3 Broody Mary: Narrating the In-Between

Long before Kate [the Duchess of Cambridge]'s
big news was announced, the tabloids wanted
to look inside her to see if she was pregnant.
Historians are still trying to peer inside the Tudors.
Are they healthy, are they sick, can they breed?
—Hilary Mantel, "Royal Bodies" (2013)[1]

Unsettling Stories

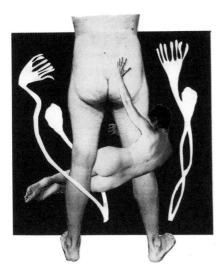

RE YOU, YOU KNOW, going to . . . ?"

This question comes at me, with a knowing nudge, from my husband's long-lost relative. We are at a gathering in a residential care home after a family funeral.

"Going to what?" I ask, assuming she means am I going to ask the staff for another sherry.

"You know . . . ," she says, a star of interest glinting in her eye.

I say I don't.

" . . . to have children?"

"What is this?" I say, looking around at the mourners gathered to pay their respects. "One in, one out?"

Many thirty-something women will have a story like this: a coy, only half articulated *sub voce* question, asked with intent desire from the questioner. In the moment, a dizzying range of possible responses fan out—caustic, dismissive, angry, light, sad, honest, a hard blink?

I'm beyond those inquiries now. No one looks at my forty-something face and wonders. Or at least, not in that way. But when such interrogations were prospects, they were unsettling rather than straightforwardly irritating, because they met a similar question mark in me. Every nosy, jealous, rude, well-meant, puzzled inquiry was directly mirrored by a similar interior preoccupation.

Childless women, at least those who still might have children, are unfinished stories. Will she? Won't she? Can she? Can't she? Is she?

Isn't she? If not now, when then? What is more, they are unfinished stories in a culture not used to waiting for narrative instalments: can't we stream and binge-watch the whole series at once?

What will happen in the end? Unsettling midpoints in stories drive readers to keep reading. But lots of fiction resists closure, forcing readers to do interpretative work. To achieve its discombobulating effects, inconclusive narrative forms still rely on readers' desires for finality, albeit only to thwart them. Childless women in their childbearing years present a readerly challenge, as do other people who defy easy categorisation—like the gender fluid, for example. Betwixt and between states test the limits of social tolerance. In this chapter, I consider life in the in-between, partly by focusing on those who live pregnancy ambiguity, so the ambiguous themselves (amphibians, perhaps, between two worlds). But I am also thinking about readers looking in from outside. I register those readers' discomfort and interpretative responses to ambiguous stories. At the core of this chapter is a famous story about the two false pregnancies of English Tudor queen, Mary I (1516–1558) in the middle of the sixteenth century. I suggest, though, that Mary has become an icon of pregnancy uncertainty rather as an effect of the way that her story has been recorded and retold by her Protestant enemies. Political animus, primarily, has narrated her conception confusions. A larger question here is why the maybe-pregnant body is and was so hard to get a fix on. I look at some historical midwifery writing to try to answer that question. As an amphibian myself, I have found it consoling to see that sane and intelligent people in the past found the trying-to-conceive body was not an open and immediately legible book.

Childless women are and always have been a conundrum. Sheila Heti writes in her autobiographical novel, *Motherhood*, of her indecision around starting a family:

> There is something threatening about a woman who is
> not occupied with children. There is something at-loose-
> ends feeling about such a woman. What is she going to do
> instead? What sort of trouble will she make?[2]

And historians have told us about the lives of the childless in the past, examining how and why people bucked the strong heteronormative reproductive narratives into which they were socialised. Historian Rachel Chrastil, for example, describing her upbringing in 1980s America, writes that "childlessness did not appear to be an option," yet her research shows how normal and multitudinous are the histories of childless people.[3] Like Heti, she finds that the childless have often fallen under suspicion, although every period applies its pressure to reproduce differently with varying intensities and divergent consequences.

In this chapter, I am moving in closer than Heti and Chrastil to those who look as if they are trying for pregnancy or who seem framed by a desire for children who aren't materialising. Look at this haunting little scrap from the church courts in the early sixteenth century (1518–1519):

John Phipes and Alice his wife are suspected of idolatry.
They have a cradle near their bed every night and it is used
as if there were an infant in it.[4]

This snippet is all there is, but it tells a huge story, which takes us back to the play houses and dolls that I was considering at the end of chapter 2. What happens when our fantasies and simulations extend into adulthood—when they begin to look like an ache rather than a game? The church courts read John and Alice's behaviour as heretical religious practice. That was the only narrative they could see that fitted: a perverse kind of worship. The saddest aspect of the story is less John and Alice's pretend parenting than the fact that neighbours or relatives must have reported them. How else did officialdom know about the cradle except through the neighbourhood watch?

When artist Tina Reid-Peršin took a mannequin of a child to a funfair on an English village green in 2012 as part of a photo shoot for her art project *Photos I'll Never Take*, she was accused not of idolatry but of "drawing a crowd and upsetting people," especially "families with children."[5] To create a fictional family album, she and her husband, Barry, took the mannequin, Katrin, to different places, photographing themselves sledging, sitting on the steps of a beach hut, and walking in the woods. The photographs are arresting, haunting, sad, but also playful. Art is like that: poised in the in-between. Dolls and idols are integral artists' props, standing at the threshold between animation and inanimation, exploring our fears and hopes about their readiness to quicken. Reid-Peršin's photo shoots in public spaces were mostly received with humour, cooperation, and interest. The ticket vendor at a historic castle joked that he should charge them for a third ticket; Santa and his elf gave Katrin a present at a Christmas grotto. But at the funfair, one onlooker told her, "We are horrified!" Reid-Peršin packed up her camera and mannequin and left. The funfair is already a celebration of the phantasmagorical and grotesque, already a kitsch fantasy, but evidently nothing could be more disturbing than attending with a doll. If there were still church courts in England, this case would be in their remit.

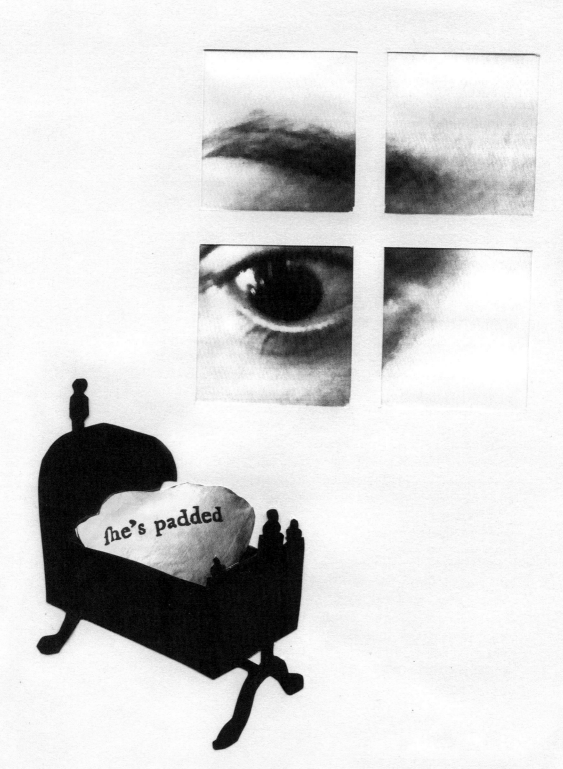

Let's return briefly to the two Grimms' fairytales with infertile beginnings that I began with in chapter 1: "The Juniper Tree" and "Briar Rose." Wished-for children always materialise in fairytales. But wishing never turns out well. Wishes are always fulfilled but in backhanded ways: by terrible means or with unforeseen consequences. In one way or another, the wish must be paid for. The story of "Briar Rose" you know: the child is born, but the father messes up the guest list for the christening and doesn't invite the right fairy, who then hexes the child out of pique. The wished-for child in "The Juniper Tree," on the other hand, so delights his mother that she dies of joy at his birth. Later, his stepmother decapitates him and cooks him up in a stew which is then fed to his father. There is a "happy" ending, though: the stepmother has her head crushed by a millstone. And the child, whose bones have been buried with his mother's beneath the juniper tree of the title and whose spirit has travelled through the tree and into a bird, is miraculously resurrected, and he and his stepsister live happily ever after with the father who once ate him. Not everything, however, can be recovered: the child's lost wishful mother never returns in "The Juniper Tree," and in "Briar Rose," the time lost to sleep cannot be regained.

The middles of stories are not wiped out by their ends. Outcomes do not cancel the in-between.

Lost and Found

A foundling is left in the crook of an ash tree, abandoned with identifying tokens—a gold ring tied to her arm with silk and an embroidered textile wrapped around her for warmth. Her name is Le Fraine (based on the Breton word for the ash tree, which bears no fruit).[6] Just as I always do when I hear about any abandoned, abused, or murdered children, I think: I could have cared for her, I had more love to give. But that could never have been: she's a textual figment and a medieval one at that. Registering the mismatches between desert, desire, and upshot has become a reflex, as if unwanted and undeserved babies are somehow going spare.

Instead, Le Fraine is fostered by the porter of a priory, breastfed by his wife, and then brought up by the good-hearted prioress. In time, she is courted by a high-born man, Sir Guroun, and becomes his mistress, but he must make a marriage of alliance. The girl chosen as his wife is Le Codre (the hazel tree, which does bear fruit), who, unbeknownst to all, is Le Fraine's twin sister. Le Fraine meekly dresses the bridal chamber with one of her two worldly possessions: the beautiful fabric in which she was swaddled when lost and found.

Le Fraine is reunited with her parents and sister, identified through her gift of the token with which she was abandoned. Another bridegroom is hastily found for Le Codre, and Le Fraine and Sir Guroun can marry after all.

Le Fraine's mother gave her up to save face in the fertility game. She is jealous about her neighbour's good fortune at giving birth to twin boys and so starts the rumour that twins are only conceived by women with two lovers. She spreads this bile despite the honour of being asked to be godmother. Several women overhear her and beseech God to bring down a "worse fortune" on her head if she ever has children herself. And she duly does: twin girls. "I have made my own fate," she cries, agreeing that her midwife should take one of the babies away before she is either accused of having two lovers herself or discovered to be a muckraker. The twist in Le Fraine's tale is that an excessive and jealous desire for children is best punished by a multiple birth.

At the final reunification and revelation, lots of things are forgiven and resolved—child neglect and abandonment, extramarital sex and concubinage, sexual betrayal and a bloodless arranged marriage—but the female jealousy which set the whole story off is not. The neighbour doesn't reappear for the final scenes; Sir Guroun and the second bridegroom do not turn out to be the neighbour's twin boys; the vicious defamatory claims are never retracted. Fertility rivalry is so extreme in this tale that a child must be given up as a punishment. Foundling children always create a problem in the stories they inhabit because, even if they are recovered, they missed time in their rightful home. An intolerable narrative section where a child is in jeopardy can never be erased.

The mistake made by Le Fraine's mother is to forget that she is a character in a story. She lives in an ordered universe authored by God. Imagining she is beyond narrative, she puts what happens to her down to unplotted luck—"hap." The parents of the twin boys, on the other hand, fully recognise God as author of their lives, thanking him four times for the safe delivery of their sons and preparing carefully for their baptisms. The midwife prays over Le Fraine as she leaves her in the tree hollow, and the reader is expected to recognise God's protective hand throughout Le Fraine's life, finding nurturing fosterage solutions. But God also looks capricious: why isn't the jealous woman's uncharitable attack on her fertile neighbour best punished by infertility rather than twins? God works in a mysterious way indeed if he sends healthy children as punishments. And whilst the story mostly works out, that doesn't erase the midpoint jeopardy, like the chilling point where the baby is carried through fields on a clear moonlit night and left alone in the tree just as dawn is breaking, the cocks starting to crow and the dogs to bark.

Despite the perversity of divine orchestration in this tale, its explicit evocation is to be expected in a medieval romance. In our own day, lots live explicitly religious lives in which God determines events and outcomes. Yet even the most toughened atheists struggle to live their lives as if they are governed purely by "hap." We cannot shake off the feeling that achieving pregnancy and parenthood is somehow divinely overseen and that there might be ritual habits we can observe to shift outcomes. The phrases we use imply some organising consciousness, even where their secular use has cut away God as author. "It was (or just wasn't) meant to be" suggests a mind to do the meaning that a pregnancy fulfills. In my trying years, I constantly caught myself imagining being subject not to a benign or just principle but to the sneakier type of operation found in stories like Le Fraine's: Sod's law rather than God's law. In this legal system, the surest way to find a lost item is to buy a pricey replacement. I would get pregnant, then, if I booked a holiday, took a role at work, or planned an activity which was incompatible. I would get pregnant if I precisely didn't do the things recommended for those trying to get pregnant. Maybe I should take up a fast-living approach and swap folic acid for some hallucinatory party acid.

Assuming that we are not characters in a great story book, why does progress or frustration in trying to conceive feel like reward or punishment? Why are we proud or ashamed if we "win" or "lose"—as if arbitrary outcomes disclose innate virtues or vices or as if the status that is conferred by becoming a parent really were a credit to us? Why does the humiliation of failure feel personally targeted, like a huge finger is pointing from the heavens and a disembodied voice is saying: "You? You didn't think you could join the club, did you? What overweening presumption left you thinking you could be a mother?" Even if the imagined divine organising principle is an abstract one like fortune or nature rather than an identifiable God from an established religion, people often, however unconsciously, live as if "seen" by and subjected to a regime in which some are chosen and favoured and others are not. And that impression extrudes into rivalries and schadenfreude, with fortune, nature, or God weighing in on one side or the other, arbitrating disputes, and dividing fortunes according to some logic, even if it is a twisted one.

Broody Mary

Symbolic mother figures abound. But who or what is the epitome of reproductive disappointment? And what should we call her? What is the right epithet—the Great Nearly Mother, the Never-Almost, the

Wish-I-Were-a, the Wannabe Mother? What is her story? Who could represent the unconceiving and rival the great mother goddesses—the Venus of Willendorf with cascading fat rolls; Demeter with her spilling horn of plenty; the Egyptians' frog-headed fertility goddess Heqet, celebrating the fecundity of the Nile; the Hindu deity Durga, a weapon in each of many arms, riding a lion, ready to defend her children with force; and Mary, in her guise as Madonna della misericordia, who spreads her motherhood cloak round her kneeling devotees? Where did the Nearly Mother icons go? There's Midrashic ladette Lilith, but she hasn't had the necessary brush with motherhood to qualify as a full Almost-Mother. Diana, ditto.

A good candidate for a, if not *the*, icon of the Great Not-Nearly Mother is Queen Mary I of England, Mary Tudor. Since her death, historians have been writing her story to make that bid. She achieved that unenviable position through European sectarian geopolitics and history. Mary and her husband, Philip of Spain, had two unreproductive pregnancy events. In 1554–1555 and again in 1557–1558, she and those around her thought she was pregnant, although she wasn't. The failure of those hopes had long and deep repercussions for British and global history. In this book, I haven't included all the well-known stories in the history of not conceiving, the stories of other candidates for the honorific. I haven't, for example, covered Mary Toft, Joanna Southcott, or Lady Flora Hastings, whose astonishing lives have been interestingly treated elsewhere.[7] I tell Mary's story, though, partly because it is the one that I am most often asked about but also because of the defining pressure it has applied to histories of reproduction, particularly pregnancy uncertainty: impoverishing and narrowing them. My concern is with how her storyline has been shaped by habits of history writing, which have kept us in the dark about the wider experience of pregnancy ambiguity.

Mary's story was scripted by people who understood that God authored the world and took sides in a polarised world. The suggestion put to Mary—that she was pregnant—must have been irresistible because it was part of the ritual choreography around her instatement as queen. Historians especially foreground Mary's spiritual advisor, Cardinal Reginald Pole (1500–1558), who returned radicalised from continental exile, part of an affirmation of Mary's holy destiny.[8] At their first meeting, he greeted her with Gabriel's words to the Virgin Mary at the annunciation—"blessed art thou among women"—and later she said she felt the child move within her. Mary Tudor was already thirty-seven, *geriatric primigravida* in today's terms, but she had already seen God take her side. She had survived her younger brother, Edward VI; raised an army; and won a civil war to take her throne from the Jane Gray faction. God was not impartial. He would realise Mary's providential hopes and

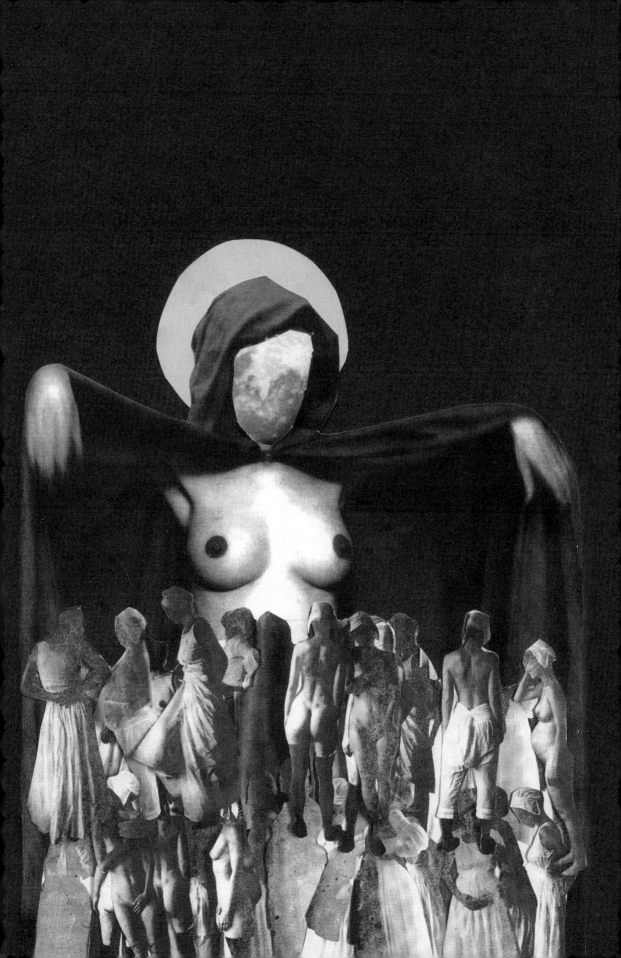

redraw the world map in her and her descendants' favour, however apparently unlikely in physiological terms. The end.

Whilst Mary was waiting to be delivered of the first child she wasn't carrying, her attendants and physicians were calculating and recalculating due dates, as each was successively missed. The am-I-aren't-I time was extended; it must have been excruciating. And then, somehow, someone announced that the birth had happened. Was something innocuous like "being considered" misheard for "the queen is delivered"? Was "dawn" misheard for "born" or "quince" for "prince" ("Delivered of a prince! Oh, happy day")? And did the news go viral before anyone could catch and correct it? Or it could be imagined this way: A man rides up to a gate inside the walls of London and needs to get out before the gates are locked at curfew, but the Bow bells are already tolling. He's too late but can't wait until sunrise because he needs to get somewhere in a hurry. Thinking on his feet, he says that he's come from the palace, carrying a message out about Queen Mary's delivery. The gate opens to let the news on its way. The queen is delivered! The message takes on its own life, passing about the streets and becoming knowledge. The queen's child is delivered! More bells toll. Fireworks are lit. The planned public celebrations kick off. The officials who organised them raise themselves from their beds. It is now. Their career-defining day has come.

The next day, May 1, 1555, the celebrations were abruptly halted: the news was premature; it turns out that the baby wasn't born . . . yet.[9] The streets were full of rumours. One woman, Alice Perwiche, was arrested for saying that the queen was never pregnant and that she planned to swap in another woman's baby. Alice was sentenced to be put in the stocks, have her ears cut off, be fined 100 pounds, and be given a three-month prison sentence (although from all of these she was eventually let off).[10] As spring gave way to summer, some people reported that royal agents were moving around London trying to buy baby boys.[11] By the end of August, the special prayers that for months had been said in every parish church in England for the queen's safe delivery also stopped. Eventually, to prove she was still alive, contrary to more rumours, Mary and her husband and King of England, Philip of Spain, took a miserable public ride in a horse-drawn litter, curtains open, to Temple Bar in London.[12] Two days later, humiliated, Philip left for Spain. God palpably did not weigh in. Philip and Mary's enemies crowed.

An invariable plot element in stories about lost or nonexistent pregnancies is all the baby stuff. Mary's is no exception. Looking around Mary's birthing chamber, we must imagine it busy with people and filled with material goods. Royal babies today generate costs and preparations, and you don't have to be royal to throw

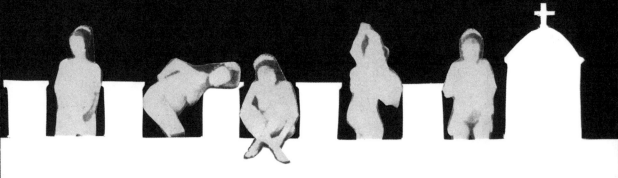

money at childbirth either. Some of today's parents are taking out payment plans to afford all the kit. A 1548 letter from Katherine Brandon, Duchess of Suffolk, describes the burden of looking after another queen's baby: Katherine Parr's baby, another Mary (named after our Mary). Baby Mary was foisted on Brandon's household after Parr's death from childbirth complications. In her letter, the duchess complains about the expenses she has had to bear both for things (expensive carpets, fine bed linen and bedcovers in crimson taffeta, gold cushions and matching upholstered chairs, hangings painted with scenes of the months, a lute, furniture, and silverware, especially spoons) and also attendants (a governess, maids, wet nurses, and others) who "daily call on me for their wages, whose voices my ears may hardly bear, but my coffers much worse."[13]

Did the crowd of Queen Mary's attendants slowly dwindle and drift away as doubts gradually rose? Or were they dismissed all in one go at a decisive moment, perhaps in early August when Philip and Mary retreated from Hampton Court to a quieter royal residence, Oatlands Palace, about eight miles west? What about the stuff? Did they send it into storage or parcel it out to expectant court ladies, their own bumps rising? No one was too good for a castoff in those days, especially not from the queen. Like rumour, material things constantly worked their way out from the bodies of monarchs and their intimate spaces to followers and clients and then to their followers and clients, cascading down.

Prominent amongst that stuff was an empty cradle:

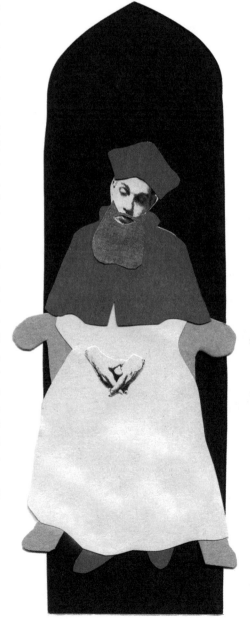

very sumptuously and gorgeously trimmed,
upon the which cradle for the child appointed,
these verses were written:

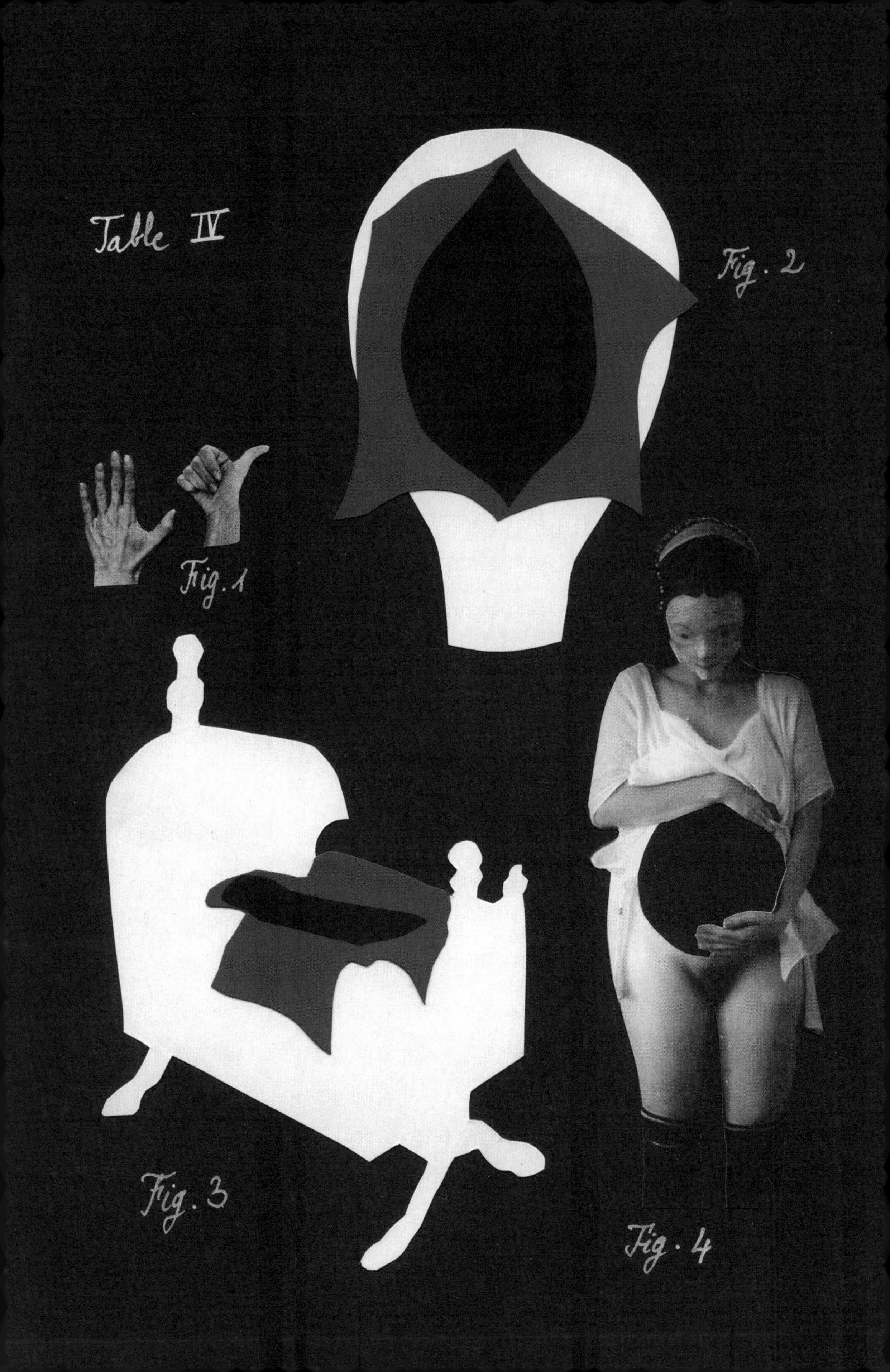

Table IV

Fig. 2

Fig. 1

Fig. 3

Fig. 4

The child which thou to Mary
O lord of might has sent
To England's joy in health
Preserve, keep and defend.[14]

This we hear from the Protestant historian John Foxe (1516–1587), writing in the reign of Mary's half sister, Elizabeth, a generation after Mary's death. If the cradle existed, he must have known about it from the viral news machine rather than firsthand. It is not a neutral description; Foxe was not on Mary's side. He tells his readers about the cradle not because he wants them to sympathize but to reveal how wrong those in Mary's faction were about whose side God had picked. Readers should see the presumption of the verse's "sent" rather than the poignancy of the little bed. Foxe invents a gloating response to the crib's inscription:

The child which thou to Mary
O Lord of might hast denied,
May Elizabeth bear by Thy auspices!

He wrote with hindsight but not quite enough. The story was not quite finished. Elizabeth wasn't going to have a child either. An odd effect of Foxe's answering verse is that it implies that Elizabeth's baby will be *the same one* that God denied Mary, as if a child exists somewhere and can be redirected by God to a mother with the right religious beliefs and laid in the same, redecorated crib. Taking aim at Catholic theology, Foxe asks why, if Catholic prayer can reach into purgatory and change the fortunes of people's souls in the afterlife, it can't reach into Mary's birthing chamber and help the queen to be delivered.[15]

The birthing room may have been intimate and so personally bespoke that Mary's name was painted onto the furniture, but it was not private. All the world was looking in. Wrapped up in any contemporary description of Mary and what she suffered are a bundle of other investments, which are plainly written into the surviving evidence. Much of that evidence comes from the despatches of European ambassadors. They, though, are not disinterested parties but are working for foreign powers. They are also keen to talk up their intimate access to the queen to their respective governments. Nonetheless, the snapshots of Mary have shaped how the story has been told and retold. This is the perspective of the Venetian ambassador, Giovanni Michiel, from June 1555, when a sliver of hope still remained: "I found and saw the most serene Queen . . . looking very well, for, placing herself at a small window, she chooses to see the procession pass."[16] He captures a sense of the pressured environment of court with its endless ritual

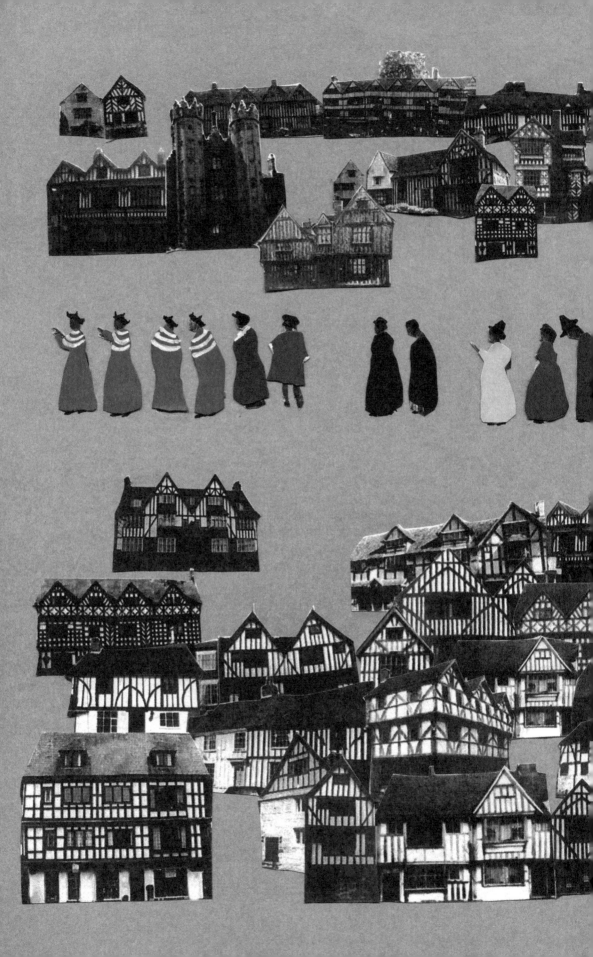

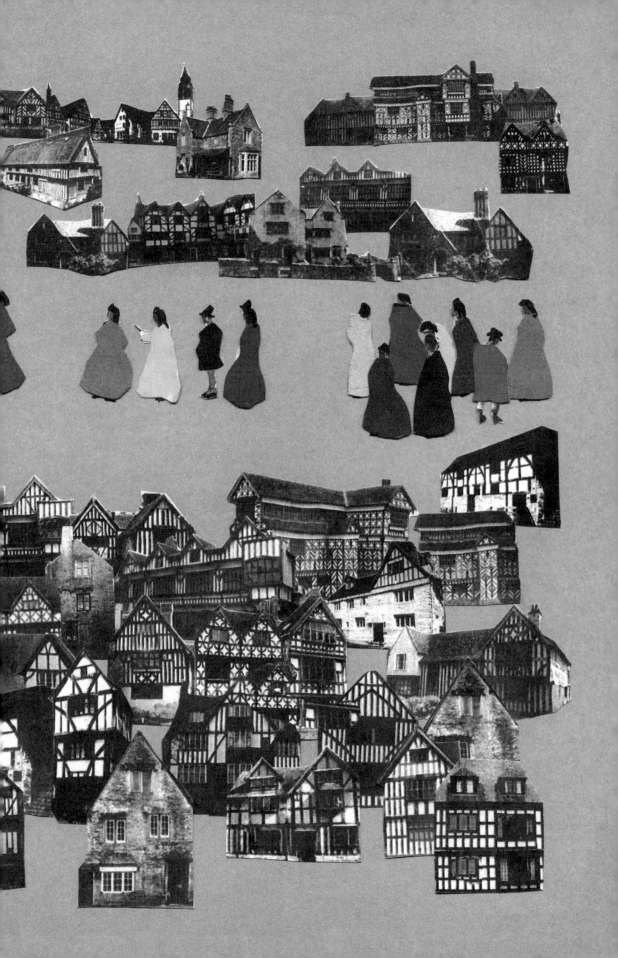

observations focussed on the queen's delivery. Later in the summer of 1555, when hope was ebbing away, the French ambassador, Antoine de Noailles, describes Mary sitting on a floor cushion, her head resting on her knees drawn up to her chest.[17] A lot has been made of this posture, which has been interpreted as a sign of depression and humiliation, a pose it would be hard to take up if heavily pregnant.

Everything that we know about this story is mediated, and so truths—what Mary really suffered from, what she really thought— are impossible to recover. Contemporaries were as undecided as we should be. Perhaps she was ill or miscarried or suffered from a psychosomatic condition. Perhaps, others suggested, she was bewitched and gave birth to an animal which leapt away. None of it is authored by the queen herself. The closest we come to her own account is a sheaf of letters with her signature penned in 1555 but never sent to a range of international heads of states and other VIPs in anticipation of the birth.[18] Blanks are left for the baby's date of birth, and enough space to change prince into princess. The letters themselves are written in officialese, some in English but most in Latin. The blanks are their most authentic and articulate part—physical traces of Mary's maternal disappointment.

The ambassadors broadcast across time as well as space, sending despatches to future historians. Mary's case of nonpregnancy is familiar to historians and has also filtered through to popular knowledge of Tudor history, an ever-present cultural obsession. Indeed, it has eclipsed other examples of ambiguous pregnancy and negative reproductive experiences: other women's names that historians plough up get buried again under the weight of Mary's story. A recent UK exhibition on the history of pregnant portraiture, *Portraying Pregnancy: From Holbein to Social Media*, included a famous portrait of Mary from 1554 by painter Anthonis Mor; it stood amongst the many other images of the securely pregnant.[19] Mary stared out of her frame at an embroidery of the visitation, showing the other, biblical Mary with her cousin Elizabeth, their hands on each other's swelling bumps. Mary Tudor's anomalous inclusion testifies to the status she has garnered as the iconic could-have-been mother. Mary was and is the often solitary reminder that not all historical "pregnancies" went to plan.

Mary's isolation as a spectacular case is largely the effect of politicized history writing, of *how* her story was written. Here is another picture of Mary in her room, drawn four hundred years after her death by the nineteenth-century historian J. A. Froude (1818–94):

the collapse of the inflated imaginations which had surrounded her supposed pregnancy . . . affected her sanity. Those forlorn hours when she would sit on the ground with her knees drawn to her face; those restless days and nights when, like a ghost, she would wander about the palace galleries, rousing herself only to write tear-blotted letters to her husband; those bursts of fury over the libels dropped in her way; or the marchings in procession behind the host in the London streets—these are all symptoms of hysterical derangement.[20]

The images of Mary with knees drawn up and of the formal processions clearly borrow from contemporary ambassadorial accounts. But Froude was also a writer of fiction, and his novelist's touch is evident: Mary is imagined "like a ghost." In Froude's version, Mary's tummy rises and falls in response to the fantasies of Spanish courtiers and evil counsellors. Froude offers a psychological diagnosis, "hysteria," imagining Mary unmoored from daily routines or official duties, weeping, and wandering through the palace. Froude makes Mary into a character like those in Gothic novels from his own time, narratives rendered atmospheric by the architecture and Catholicism of the late Middle Ages. His word "galleries" looks historically accurate: a technical architectural term which comes into English with the adoption of Italian styles, like those showcased at Hampton Court. Yet it is also a tell. In a defining novel in the Gothic mode, Anne Radcliffe's *Mysteries of Udolpho* (1794), galleries are sites of psychological unsettlement, where distant footsteps can be heard and veiled portraits hang: "These dismal galleries and halls are fit for nothing but ghosts to live in," a servant tells the novel's heroine, Emily St. Aubert.[21] Froude's galleries and his spectral Mary are similarly haunted and haunting.

Froude was not alone but part of a pile-on by Protestant historians concerned to justify and defend the Reformation, which has had a knock-on effect on histories of dashed pregnancy hopes. Mary's pregnancy problems were usefully symbolic in a narrative of larger regime failure. The reign and the attempt to reinstall Catholicism were panned as "sterile."[22] Mary's burning of some 280 Protestant subjects was also linked to her fertility frustrations. Froude, for example, understood the burnings to be Mary's spiritual purification strategy for securing a future healthy delivery. Yet early modern queens did not need to experience reproductive failure to pursue violent purges. Catherine de Medici (1519–1589), for example, had ten children yet presided over the St. Bartholomew's Day Massacre in 1572: a week of killings in which anywhere between 5,000 and 30,000 French Protestants (called Huguenots) were slaughtered. In the 1930s, the satirical *1066 and All That* dubbed Mary "Broody Mary," taking aim at partisan Protestant histories making spurious

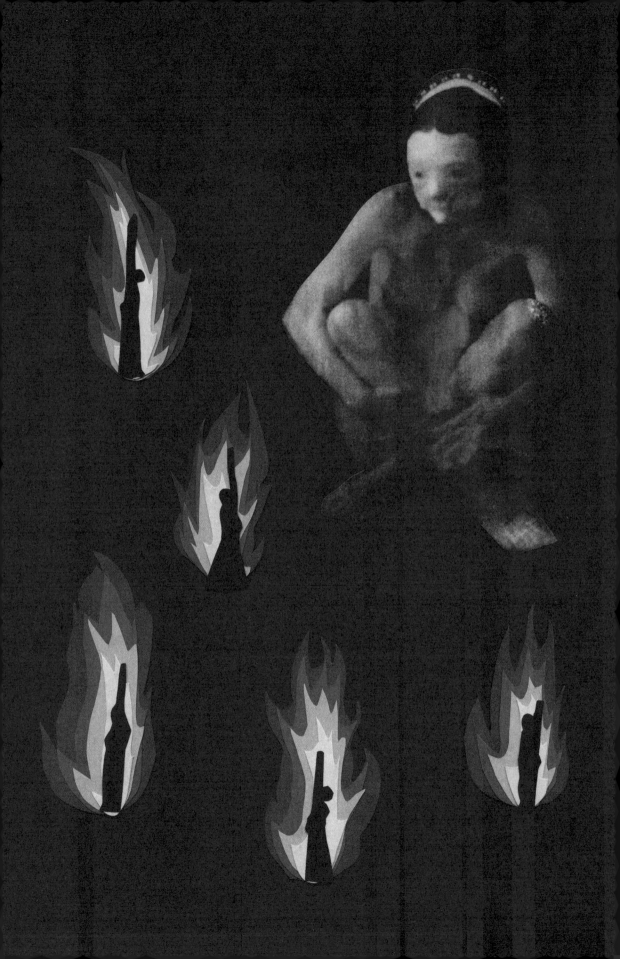

links; the persecutory burnings and the not-conceiving had ludicrously become the same thing by historiographical habit.[23]

More recent historians and biographers, whose ranks now notably number more women like Linda Porter, Judith M. Richards, and Anna Whitelock, have tried to break these associations and remove the dark gothic patina that the story of Mary's reproductive failures has acquired.[24] We don't know what caused those failures, and it is far from certain that Mary suffered from a psychological condition specifically. According to these newer narratives, in casting Mary and her violent counterreformation as hysterical, Protestant history writing overstepped the available evidence. What is more, revisionists note, false pregnancies (whatever their cause, physical or psychological) in a time before pregnancy testing were reasonably common rather than abnormal and mad. The historical record has turned up the names of other women who experienced unclear pregnancies, and there are more in this book.[25] There is no logic to reading the "pregnancies" as further evidence of wider regime failure or dysfunction. Yet the royal biographers' task is to single out their subject, and the wider history of false or failed pregnancy is not their central interest, so their discussions are necessarily defensive, dismissing tired old allegations swiftly because they have a whole reign to assess. The withering away of Protestant sectarian interests in national history writing allows for a reassessment of the reign of England's first queen but understandably—because this is not their point—leaves little clearer in terms of revising the history of trying but not conceiving.

Before these historiographical correctives could be issued, though, easy assessments of Mary's unreproductive events had already percolated into medical literature. The assumption that Mary suffered from a psychological condition of some kind ("hysteria," in Froude's estimation) has been important. So that when the much later construction of diagnostic categories was under way in the nineteenth century and typologies and classes of psychiatric disorders were created and refined, Mary's spectacular case was already in mind. The modern diagnosis *pseudocyesis* (which I discuss in more detail in chapter 7) emerged in the mid-nineteenth century and was increasingly narrowed to refer to psychosomatic pregnancy. It has been associated with Mary and also has been shaped to accommodate the partisan version of Mary's case. "One of the early well-known cases," reports the American textbook *Pseudocyesis* from 1937,

is that of Mary Tudor, Queen of England (1553–1558). Mary, finding herself without her expected baby, imagined herself deserted by God, all because she had been too easy on the heretics. As a result, many deaths followed. During the time of her supposed pregnancy . . . her favorite amusement, other than attending Mass, was counting on her fingers the number of months "she was gone."[26]

There is no doubt in this shorthand version that Mary suffered from pseudocyesis, a psychiatric condition; all other possibilities have melted away. The scene resembles the snapshots in the ambassadors' despatches, with new fictitious detail which channels the tone of triumph in British national history writing. Violent sixteenth-century religious contests, which were also the contests within a few interlocked royal families, have muscled their way into much more recent medical understandings of not achieving motherhood. Queens are always anomalies. Mary's reproductive ill fortunes have been singled out to the impoverishment of a wider history of pregnancy inconclusiveness.

In the In-Between

The first month we tried, I got pregnant. It was M.'s half term (he's a history teacher), and we went to Riga, Latvia, for a few days. The day before we flew, my breasts were so sore that I bought a new bra without underwires. I contemplated but didn't get around to buying a pregnancy test. On the plane there, I felt tired, emotional, but happy. The weather was cold, and the sun glinted off the three stars held aloft by the female figure on the top of the Latvian national memorial. I felt stunned; I had steeled myself for a wait. M. and I held gloved hands and kicked up autumn leaves along the river path. It turns out that I'm one of those people who just "falls" pregnant, straight off.

I swallowed hard in our hotel bed on waking from vivid dreams. This is it, then, I thought. I felt ambushed by the resistance I felt even to something that I wanted: the dead of night fear of an undoable action. You've really done it now, I told myself. Happy now? The whole of the winter telescoped away, and I imagined holding a baby on a warm summer's day.

M. and I agreed that my breasts were larger. "Not on the top," he says, "but underneath and round the outside edge," saying exactly what I thought, too, without my telling him. This is not like him. Usually when I ask him direct questions about my appearance, he deflects it with a question of his own:

"Do you think I've put on weight?" I might say.

"This is a trick, isn't it?" he'll respond.

"Let's test when we get home," he said. I understood his desire for objective proofs, though I felt no need because I already knew. But by the time we arrived at the airport, I had started to bleed. Even though I mostly bled monthly, I had not expected it. Gunshot victims in films have the same confusion, touching the blood leaking from their side, looking amazed into the eyes of the killer they have known all their lives, too surprised even to express pain: "You?" they mouth. In the rush of takeoff, I looked at M. "What's going on?" he asked, as baffled as me. By the time we got home, I had convinced myself I had had an early miscarriage. But there is no knowing.

A few months later, it happened again, and then, months later, again. One month, a great tick appeared on my basal temperature chart midmonth. Everything seemed right. Day fourteen, day sixteen, day eighteen. But a pregnancy test showed negative . . . again. "Might it still be possible?" I allowed myself to think for two more long days before my uncharacteristically late period. As so many others describe doing in trying-to-conceive web forums, I disrobed my test sticks, holding the blotting parchment to the light to get a better view, hoping for a barely perceptible line rather than the blank white space that stared back. I kept up a hope of the false negative. "Why don't you trust the test?" asked M., but the next day, he fell into the trap himself, wondering whether its "reach" was too short. I got so used to feeling pregnancy symptoms that I learned to recognise and dismiss them as imaginary. So that in the months when I was pregnant, I missed it. I bled in every pregnancy: the ones I lost and the one that resulted in the birth of my son. Even some scans were inconclusive—or at least the sonographer said so to spare our feelings through another wait to confirm a miscarriage. There was rarely an objective clarity, an alignment of symptoms with a test which matched an inner conviction.

This is not peculiar to me. I am no anomalous Mary. Fertility memoirists often report on smudgy symptoms which come and go, appearing and disappearing signs, even ambiguous test results and scans. Writer and activist Jessica Hepburn, for example, describes "feeling cheated" by an inconclusive pregnancy test taken in the very sanctum of modern fertility science, the IVF clinic: "I had naively thought that, whatever happened, it would be a straightforward 'pregnant' or 'not pregnant.' I wasn't prepared for a situation where it seemed to be both 'pregnant' *and* 'not pregnant.'"[27] Yet pregnancy tests are not actually a test for pregnancy. They test not for the presence of a viable embryo but rather for the presence and concentration of a hormone which is present in pregnancy but does not instantly evaporate on loss.

Maggie O'Farrell describes the opposite confusion, writing about giving all her "baby blankets, Moses baskets, maternity clothes"

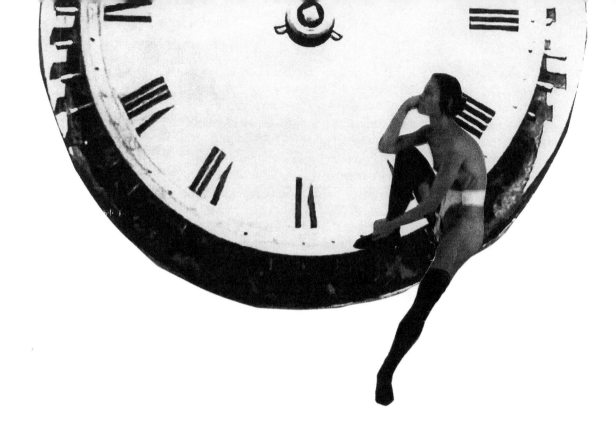

to charity shops after an apparently failed round of IVF. "There would," she decided, "be no more fertility treatments, no more trying; there would be no more babies in our house."[28] Only to find, after a scan some weeks later, that she was pregnant after all. Her baby was due in just six short months:

> The doctor gasped. The nurses covered their mouths, then began fluttering anxiously through my file. How had this happened? They asked. How had this embryo held on, despite no signs of pregnancy, despite the heavy bleeding, despite the loss of its twin, despite the negative blood test, despite all the evidence that the embryos had left, departed, drifted loose?

She concludes: "It was a brand of magic. Of this I am certain." What a thing of which to be certain!

Hepburn's expectation of a simple binary is widely shared. I was also surprised to live so often with so much doubt. Waiting for results is always going to be an in-between time; yet those who are trying to conceive live that time repetitively and not in health crisis and illness but as part of their ordinary lives. Now that technological solutions like home tests and sonography are available, any confusion of symptoms and signs that proliferate beyond their aegis is forgotten, repressed (another thing we don't learn about in school) until we live with them. In the midst of it, I turned to historical writing on pregnancy diagnosis as a way of channelling my curiosity. I could not discover what I wanted to know about my own body and future, but I could look at how similar curiosities had been worked through in the past. There was consolation in discovering that the problem was not just mine and that I wasn't alone; the same thing had confused others in the past. The historical practitioner is an effective analogue for a layperson like me. We are both, in different ways, outside of the high-technology world of twenty-first-century clinical medicine, excluded from its esoteric language, and we have a similar range of tools—clock, thermometer, calendar, and our own senses—with which to work. The historical literature on pregnancy diagnosis is vast and, although not now useful for its first purpose, fascinating as a record of efforts to establish a secure epistemological framework within radically ambiguous ground.

A particularly anxious edge emerges in discussions of diagnosis in the nineteenth century, which is much more explicit than earlier writing about some of the perplexities. Jane Sharp, in the late seventeenth century, matter-of-factly gives fourteen "common rules" and instructions for two urine tests to mitigate against women's ignorance: "Young women especially of their first Child, are so ignorant commonly, that they cannot tell whether they have conceived or not, and not one of twenty almost keeps a just account."[29] The fourteen rules stretch from the quality of the sexual act itself, to observable physical changes—periods, breasts, complexion, veins. She has this to say about their fallibility: "The rules are too general to be certainly provided in all women, yet some of them seldom fail in any." They are generally but not infallibly accurate, but she says so with little unease. Sharp feels untroubled by the inexact nature of some of her work, expecting that not everything "can be certainly determined by us who are not of Natures Cabinet counsel."[30]

Sharp hopes that women will have some idea about their own conditions but gives professionals guidance for making a judgement if they don't. She does, though, expect practitioners to diagnose the harder cases which closely resemble but which aren't pregnancy; "false conception," she cautions "hath many signes whereby it personates and shews like a true Conception."[31] A false conception could be many things, which before sonography were hard, even impossible to disambiguate: molar or ectopic pregnancies, conditions that resembled pregnancies, or a psychological impression. Before "delivery," if it ever came, diagnosis could be elusive:

To distinguish then false conceptions from true, but if there
be both true and false at once that is very hard to know.[32]

Disambiguating "true" and "false"—whether false is imagined here
as a material mola or a less material cause—is impossible before
delivery. This statement is a riddle: only if a conception is true and
false at once, can the diagnosis be accurate. The tone is not worried;
there seems a resignation to, even humour in, the fact of not being
certain, a shrug.

The nineteenth-century work on diagnosis, on the other hand,
articulates more anxiety. How could ignorance persist in such modern times? Irish obstetrician William Montgomery, for example,
turns to the past to think the problem through, citing cautionary
words from Dutch physician Gerard Van Sweiten (1700–1772), writing a hundred years earlier, words which, in turn, invoke yet older
authorities:

> The reputation of a physician is perhaps never more in
> danger than when determining pregnancy: everywhere
> frauds are perpetrated, and traps laid for the unwary.
> All who have written about the signs of pregnancy, who
> are historically celebrated in the art of midwifery, are
> unanimous in admitting that, in the first important months,
> the signs of pregnancy are quite uncertain.[33]

Here is the Frankenstein reflex again: where present ignorance provokes a return to old books. And the glance back soothingly confirms
that people have been in the same quandary before. According to
this caveat quotation, the first and most profound truth of pregnancy diagnosis is its initial difficulty, a truth which is historically
invariable and still putting practitioners at reputational risk. This
heightened hazard emerges because of the potential consequences
of pregnancy misdiagnosis.

I single out Montgomery because pregnancy diagnosis is his
whole subject rather than an introductory consideration, as in
most historical midwifery textbooks. Montgomery's work is full of
cases of women who thought they were pregnant when they weren't,
sometimes for extended periods of time, sometimes repetitively.
Sometimes a cause was identified, and sometimes not. Mary really
was not by any measure anomalous. And yet pregnancy must have
been one of the most common, routine matters on which medics
were consulted—a bread-and-butter task and yet one of the potentially trickiest and most exposing. Just as I do, Montgomery finds
consolation in the fact that at least others have been there before
us and felt just as stupid.

I also find compensatory pleasure in reading about the confusions and reputational fear of those historical male practitioners who, by their own admission, were often pitched against, rather than working wholly in, the interests of women in their care. In the quotation above, for example, the feared frauds and traps might be set by the unconscious operations of the female body, but Montgomery, via Van Sweiten, really is alleging that women are often silly or unscrupulous: gold-digging fakers, sexually immoral deniers, or deluded fools. The oppositional politics of diagnosis are not peculiar to Reformation in-fighting. Reaching for a diagnosis of a woman's condition—is she or isn't she?—is not always to wish her well. Montgomery comes to the topic of pregnancy diagnosis via medical jurisprudence rather than the care of women exactly and is describing how to gather forensic evidence in the face of female noncooperation. Montgomery's work coincides with the emergence of detective fiction as a genre, and he plays with similar motifs: the technical skill and knowledge of the investigator ranged against a cast of liars, criminals, and patsies; the got-'em moment; the restoration of justice.

He lists both early pregnancy signs and symptoms and also later ones up to and including childbirth. The birth of a child is, after all, one of the few sure signs. Whilst Montgomery says he can spot when a "deep asseveration of unspotted purity" is a lie, he warns others of the bare-faced persistence of female dishonesty:

> I was once called to see an unmarried patient, whom I found in labor, and even when the feet of the child were beyond the external parts, she resolutely denied that she was pregnant.[34]

I gather heart from being a resistant reader, cheering on not only the women covering, pretending, and resisting but also those in Montgomery's moralising anecdotes who are trying to have a moderately good time, doing things of which he disapproves: "indulging too freely in frequenting balls and late parties," "dancing, especially in a crowded and overheated ball-room," and "riding on horseback."[35] I particularly like the woman Montgomery was called to see who, finding herself newly affluent after years of paid employment, "spent her whole day lying on a sofa at the fireside, or with her feet on the fender, reading novels, eating and drinking heartily."[36]

Eventually, after all his different expressions of bewilderment, Montgomery comes to tabulating symptoms, where the implicit narrative is that he is mastering the problem and sorting women into categories and that, with his book as a guide, his professional male readers can do the same. Montgomery's book swells and swells

Table V

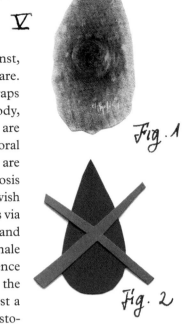

Fig. 1

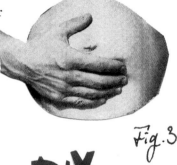

Fig. 2

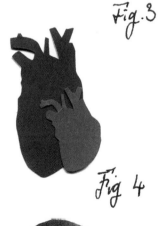

Fig. 3

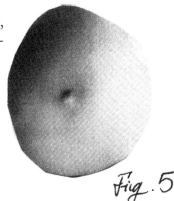

Fig. 4

Fig. 5

through new editions. What started as a forty-two-page encyclopaedia entry ended as a 600-page book twenty years and three editions
later, parsing every niggle and nobble, assessing its usefulness for diagnosis. Montgomery's own original contribution was on the appearance of the breast at different points of gestation and particularly
the tubercules named for him which become increasingly prominent
on the areola as pregnancy advances.[37] The first edition of the book
went out with several beautiful colour plates detailing the tubercles
as well as other changes of skin colour and texture: the deepening
blue venous web stretching out beneath the surface of the breast.

Montgomery was by no means alone in identifying, listing, and
ranking pregnancy signs and symptoms. Taxonomy was one of the
central endeavours of nineteenth-century science: the comprehensive naming and sorting of things like languages, animals, plants,
minerals, diseases, and races. List making was not new but was newly
systematised and turned to sociolegal functions. In pregnancy diagnosis, this meant that women's health was only one issue amongst
others at stake:

> On the correctness of his [i.e., the medical examiner's]
> opinion frequently depend the claim to fair fame, virtue,
> and honour;—the succession to property, and the rights of
> legitimacy;—the judicious treatment of disease;—and, in
> criminal cases, the preservation or destruction of the unborn
> innocent.[38]

The attempt to standardize and to develop an agreed set of universal diagnostic principles was a matter of effective law and
state. But the push to generalise left the problem of the individual
whose peculiar circumstances invariably threw up exceptions and
contradictions.

The ever-expanding trend within Montgomery's work demonstrates the attempt to manage but also the unmanageable nature
of the problem, giving us a sense of why and how, exactly, it was so
knotty: a problem that could hardly fit into a book. Without imaging
technologies, there was no chance of categorising, as we do, by cause;
and without our imaging technologies to cap them, potential alter-
natives remained live for an extended period. An enormous range
of signs and symptoms might be considered, anything from sex to
delivery, across the whole body and mind: dryness, dreams, aches,
and agues. Sometimes these might be intense and unavoidably obvious, and other times for other individuals, completely escape notice.
Those who are trying to conceive will know from experience the

bewildering myriad possibilities: any and every twinge or fainting feeling might be IT.

Montgomery begins by grouping symptoms into three: presumptive, possible and unequivocal, narrowing the latter down to three:

- Active movements of the child, unequivocally felt by another;
- Its presence in utero ascertained by ballottement [that is, through vaginal examination];
- The pulsations of the foetal heart.[39]

On these three, many writers were agreed. Thomas Tanner had the same three and puts them into a handy table along with some of the presumptive and possible.[40]

A TABLE OF THE SYMPTOMS AND SIGNS OF PREGNANCY.										
TERM OF PREGNANCY.	Morning Sickness.	Suppression of the Menses.	Mammary Areola.	Enlargement of Abdomen.	Foetal Movements.	Shortening of Cervix.	Ballottement.	Uterine Souffle.	Foetal Heart.	Dusky hue of Vagina.
End of First Month,	+	+	...	...	...	...	...	...	...	...
" Second "	+	+	?	...	...	...	...	...	...	...
" Third "	+	+	+	?	...	...	...	?	...	?
" Fourth "	?	+	+	+	?	...	+	+	?	+
" Fifth "	...	+	+	+	+	...	+	+	+	+
" Sixth "	...	+	+	+	+	...	+	+	+	+
" Seventh "	...	+	+	+	+	...	+	+	+	+
" Eighth "	...	+	+	+	+	...	?	+	+	+
" Ninth "	...	+	+	+	+	+	?	+	+	+

The very earliest signs—morning sickness and the stopping of the menstrual flow—were the most distrusted and gather copious caveats in the obstetrical literature. Although interruption of the menstrual cycle was and is the first rule-of-thumb sign, the problem with menstruation was its intrinsic flux, being "liable to very many exceptions and deviations."[41] Importantly for the legal frameworks which Montgomery is establishing, it is a particularly untrustworthy sign for women in prison, who are both physically and emotionally tested in ways that might affect menstruation.[42] Yet the cycle is so easily disrupted—whilst breast-feeding, for example—or for no discernible reason at all. In Mary Tudor's case, one of the other bits of intimate information from the intrusive ambassadors' despatches is that she had consulted at least one doctor on her menstrual health in her teens.[43] Bleeding also carries the obvious drawback of not being in the physician's immediate view. Montgomery describes a case of a woman concealing her pregnancy who "deceived those about her by staining her linen at the usual periods of menstruation."[44] Montgomery's list has a preference, then, for signs over symptoms, for his own objective observation over a patient's subjective narrative: foetal movement, for example, must be "unequivocally felt by another."

The three unequivocals are not all present until the fifth month, well into the second trimester. For us, foetal movements and heartbeat are perceived less as signs of pregnancy and more as foetal monitoring, and the shortening of the cervix as a sign of impending labour. Whilst these *are* signs and symptoms of pregnancy, it is extraordinary to see them in play for specifically diagnostic purposes, giving some sense of the potential extremities of the outlying cases. Montgomery adds this disclaimer beneath his list:

> If any one of these be ascertained beyond doubt, it settles the question; but then, we must remember, that they are decisive only on the positive, or affirmative side; if certainly recognized, pregnancy is indisputably proved, but their absence, or rather our not being able to discover them, would be no proof that pregnancy did not exist.[45]

Montgomery's discomfort can be read in the tangled negatives at the end here. Pregnancies could present straightforwardly: a case looked like a pregnancy, and often it was. The test was not whether practitioners could diagnose a positive pregnancy but whether they could appropriately and reliably rule it out. What the historical textbooks tell us is that, in the early days, a woman's own subjective best guess was really all there was. It wasn't the case that historical people had special methods which we've put away with the advent of home testing and sonography. When we rifle through the possible twinges, we do what historical observers do: marvel at their multitude and variation.

■

Sonography has changed the world forever, moving us from "wait and see" to "see." As social historian Barbara Duden writes, "there is no way back to what pregnancy was."[46] Duden's argument is that modern imaging techniques have atrophied physicians' skills in palpation, eroded women's haptic knowledge of their own bodies, and degraded their sociolegal position in relation to a newly visible and individualised foetus. The pregnant woman, Duden writes, has become "a participant in her own skinning, in the dissolution of the historical frontier between inside and outside."[47] We can see the desire to police female reproduction with Montgomery, and sonography supplied a new surveillance kit. The law already compromised healthcare for women, and the sonographic visibility of the foetus added pressure. Journalist Randi Hutter Epstein describes a similar effect: "In the beginning, the pregnant woman was housing an unknown, invisible creature. She alone was the patient."[48] The legal borders between mother and foetus have been redrawn by *in utero* imaging. I only add a reminder that the care of the female patient was not always practitioners' sole priority in the time before ultrasound.

Women's self-knowledge may well have been a more sophisticated sense prior to sonography, but it surely must also have been variable, dependent on an individual's personality and circumstances. And intuition must particularly have been tested in harder negative cases, where doubt could be protracted. Anyway, with no routes back to the past, we are left to make the best of it, to remember that women often want antenatal ultrasound and actively sign up to it.[49] And even in our new time, self-knowledge could still be fostered; we could reclaim it, for instance, by putting fertility awareness on school syllabi. The negative cases, where sonography does mitigate, can get forgotten in the discussion about foetal imaging and its revolutionary sociolegal impact. I was grateful for a sight of the single-pixel heartbeat flicking rhythmically on and off after a bleed in my positive pregnancy, but even more so for the knowledge I was given in the pregnancies I lost. Absorbing the reality of a miscarriage in the sepulchral side room set up for bad news—a sofa, leaflets, pictures of daisies—at least M. and I knew what kind of machine we were in: what might happen next in our stories. In that moment, there was a truth, an end, and we could know it. Yet that vision was vanishingly rare. Nearly mothers usually inhabit the in-between, not exactly in the same way as those of the past but enough to be kept company by them. And we are a company, not anomalous lonely examples; not just one queen but a whole load of us.

■

In the chemist one day, the preconception vitamins I went to buy were on special offer: three for the price of two; you could mix and match them with vitamins for pregnancy or postnatal breast-feeding. The boxes were arranged on a specially constructed stand-alone

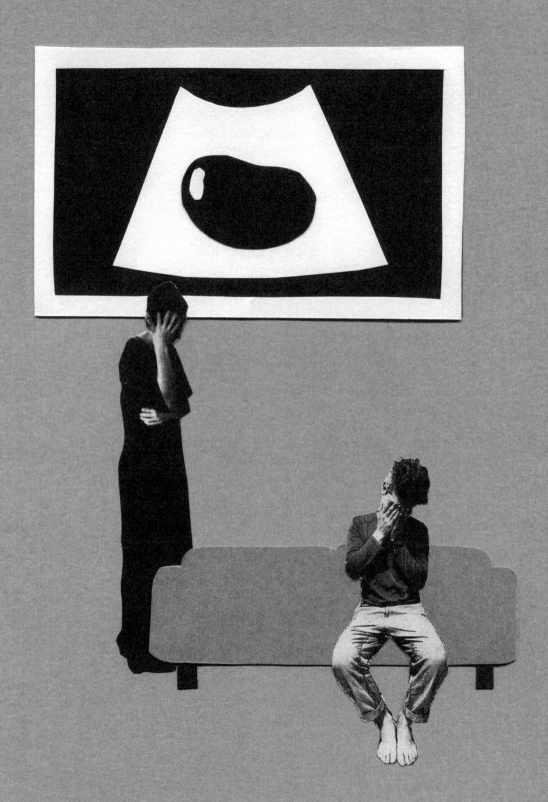

display. On the top was a bank of preconception vitamins, with a young couple, head to head and looking knowing, her whole body replaced by an enormous basketball-sized egg, being nibbled by a solitary sperm. On the shelf below, the pregnancy supplements: with a similar woman resting her hand on her heavily pregnant abdomen in the annunciation pose. He, on the other hand, is nowhere to be seen. He was there for the sex and then, alakazam, gone. Below them, on the third shelf, the boxes showed yet another woman with a child at her obscured breast. Here was a straightforward narrative progression from conception to breast-feeding, from top to bottom shelf, with no hold-ups, no uncertainty. Beginning. Middle. End.

The pregnant and the breast-feeding mothers know what to do with this deal. I, on the other hand, had a wider choice: a complete spectrum of combinations opened up. I stood and wondered about the authors of the display. Not one of them can have reflected on the profound unknowability of the human body. They must, I decided, be just mindlessly working to contract, dead now to any metaphysical reflection. Not one of them can have considered that a fellow human being, at a low point, would have to face this stand and feel defeated by its story-board logic. M. dealt with my frustration with his own, picking up one box (only) and marching to the counter. I sloped around making the automatic doors open and close, feeling the cold from the street and the heat of the shop, while he paid the inflated price which "discounts" vitamin tablets for the fertile. Pregnant women, I thought: they've got all the babies, the seats on the tube, and a discount on their vitamin supplements.

4 Wind and Waves: How to Self-Help

Lastly, There is Barrenness by Inchantment, when a Man cannot lie with his Wife by reason of some Charm that hath disabled him; the French in such a Case advise a Man to thread the Needle *Nouer O'eguilliette*, as much as to say, to piss through his Wifes Wedding Ring and not to spill a Drop, and then he shall be perfectly cured. Let him try it that pleaseth.
—Jane Sharp, *The Midwives Book* (1671)[1]

In general we may conclude, whenever we read of Virgins got with Child by Rivers, by Dragons, by golden Showers, &c. &c. that it was Wind, nothing in the World but Wind, only for want of knowing the real Cause, they were glad to assign imaginary ones.
—John Hill, *Lucina sine concubitu* (1750)[2]

How Men Can Be Helped

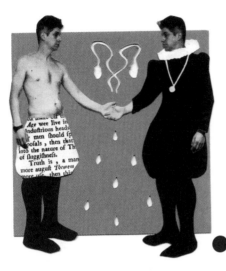

AND I GET some initial medical test results: normal. M. is disappointed. He wanted his sperm singled out for special praise, as if they were already children. When he collects the printout, there is a fuller breakdown. His sperm have been counted and tested for motility, and their morphology evaluated. The count looks good and so does the motility, but only (let's say) x percent of the sample has a normal morphology. M., who has never got anything so low in a test, says, "I could have done better, but the pot put me off," and then, after a pause, "Are you going to put my disappointingly 'normal' sperm morphology in your book?"

It turns out that M.'s low normal morphology result really is "normal." In the Alice in Wonderland world of clinical andrology, the majority of most men's sperm is abnormal: struggling with two tails or heads, dented, kinked, concertinaed, coiled, or giant.[3] So "normal" here means conforming to a beauty standard—of symmetry, straightness, style—rather than to what is typical or most common. How exactly the percentage of morphologically abnormal sperm in a sample relates to conception, infertility, or subfertility seems not to be known. "Let him try it who pleaseth," writes Jane Sharp after the folkloric remedy for "Barrenness by Inchantment" in the epigraph above, which seems to be something that men suffer from, by which I think she means: you might as well try something obviously useless as nothing at all.

In contrast, in my home reference books, there is some silence and haziness on the topic of what men can practically do to increase their fertility. Miriam Stoppard's *Conception, Pregnancy and Birth: The Childbirth Bible for Today's Parents* gathers some thoughts under the heading "How Men Can Be Helped," reassuring men with indifferent sperm test results that they can still be good lovers and men with erectile dysfunction that they can still father children, before going on to mention that environmental pollutants can negatively affect male fertility. None of these thoughts detail how men can be helped, breaking the heading's promise. Stoppard concludes:

> At one time, much more was known about female infertility than male, but fertility clinics now deal just as much with male problems and diseases. There's a greater chance than ever before that men who have low fertility or are infertile can be helped to achieve natural fatherhood.[4]

Although readers still get no clarity on how men can be helped, Stoppard reassures them we can nonetheless still legitimately think of ourselves as modern. Whilst "at one time" the topic of male infertility trailed that of female, now we live in a time of "greater chance than *ever before* that men . . . can be helped"—but by what? "Much can be done to enable men to father children naturally or with assisted conception," says Zita West's *Plan to Get Pregnant: Ten Steps to Maximum Pregnancy*, underscoring it with a shaded inset with **emboldened** assurance: "Zita's tip: **Don't give up hope** if you get poor sperm test results—there will be **lots that can be done** to help."[5] There is no direct statement about exactly what. The emphasis is upon reassuring men against the fear that there is no help and that nothing can be done, which would feel like being stuck in the past.

This coy passive voice fudges the question of who or what, exactly, will be doing the helping. The issue left unstated is that there isn't a specific treatment that can boost sperm parameters—no drug you can take, no surgical fix, no laser to zap you better. What gets said only obliquely is that lots of what can be done must be done to women (insemination, egg collection, and embryo transfer) or to the sperm themselves (which can be selected, be washed, have their tails cut off, and be pushed head first into eggs)—none of which is the same as improving the count, motility, or percentage of morphologically beautiful sperm.

The low-tech thing that can be done to optimise gamete health— for both men and women—is lifestyle improvement: things like stopping smoking and drinking, minimizing exposure to toxins and

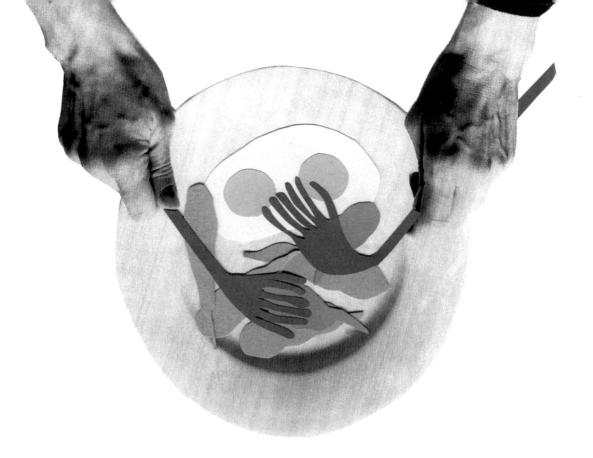

pollutants, enhancing nutrition, exercising, and wearing the right underpants. Men can't be helped there: they must do that themselves, self-help. Everyone knows that there is no straightforward justice here. Gallingly, people who have indulged in every sort of vice might be and often are hyperfertile. But shelving my envy, we cannot say that the past has been exceeded on lifestyle and that by instituting a new daily health regimen we have a "greater chance than ever before" of changing our reproductive fortunes. Health is variable across time, place, and social conditions. Yet unlike our historical counterparts, we are facing a climate catastrophe with wide implications for fertility health, both ours and that of the creatures with whom we share our earth. In this chapter, I think more about the history of this aspect of "trying": of taking active steps to conceive by rethinking the relationship between the human body and the environment. How much do our lifestyles matter? Is there anything we can do to improve them to optimise our fertility health? How do our mundane habits—breathing, eating, drinking, having sex—connect us to the wider world? Who or what is in control: are we, is our biology, or is nature? These topics also allow me to follow up on the aftermath of Mary Tudor's story, looking at some of the fallout in the next generations.

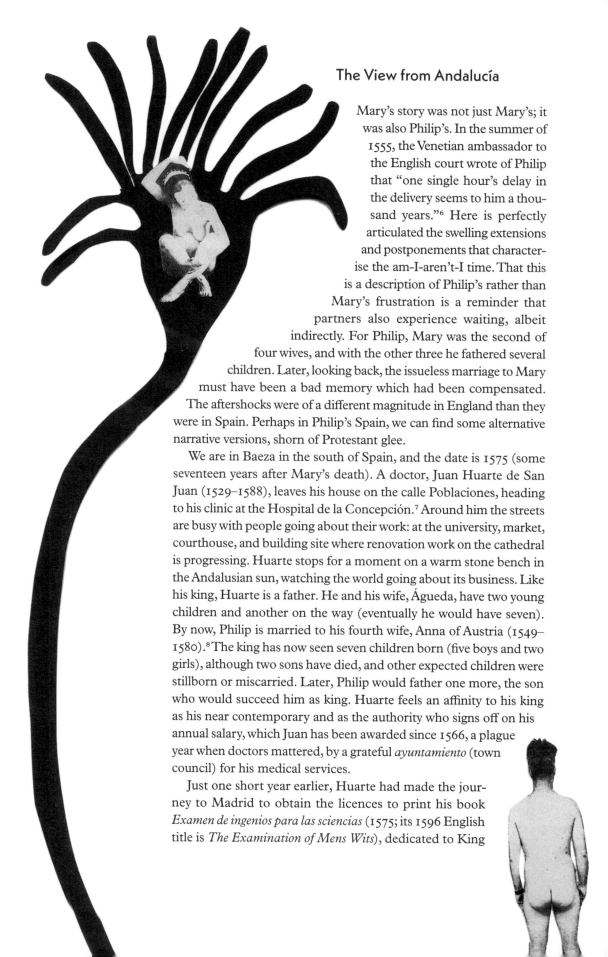

The View from Andalucía

Mary's story was not just Mary's; it was also Philip's. In the summer of 1555, the Venetian ambassador to the English court wrote of Philip that "one single hour's delay in the delivery seems to him a thousand years."[6] Here is perfectly articulated the swelling extensions and postponements that characterise the am-I-aren't-I time. That this is a description of Philip's rather than Mary's frustration is a reminder that partners also experience waiting, albeit indirectly. For Philip, Mary was the second of four wives, and with the other three he fathered several children. Later, looking back, the issueless marriage to Mary must have been a bad memory which had been compensated.

The aftershocks were of a different magnitude in England than they were in Spain. Perhaps in Philip's Spain, we can find some alternative narrative versions, shorn of Protestant glee.

We are in Baeza in the south of Spain, and the date is 1575 (some seventeen years after Mary's death). A doctor, Juan Huarte de San Juan (1529–1588), leaves his house on the calle Poblaciones, heading to his clinic at the Hospital de la Concepción.[7] Around him the streets are busy with people going about their work: at the university, market, courthouse, and building site where renovation work on the cathedral is progressing. Huarte stops for a moment on a warm stone bench in the Andalusian sun, watching the world going about its business. Like his king, Huarte is a father. He and his wife, Águeda, have two young children and another on the way (eventually he would have seven). By now, Philip is married to his fourth wife, Anna of Austria (1549–1580).[8] The king has now seen seven children born (five boys and two girls), although two sons have died, and other expected children were stillborn or miscarried. Later, Philip would father one more, the son who would succeed him as king. Huarte feels an affinity to his king as his near contemporary and as the authority who signs off on his annual salary, which Juan has been awarded since 1566, a plague year when doctors mattered, by a grateful *ayuntamiento* (town council) for his medical services.

Just one short year earlier, Huarte had made the journey to Madrid to obtain the licences to print his book *Examen de ingenios para las sciencias* (1575; its 1596 English title is *The Examination of Mens Wits*), dedicated to King

Philip himself, which proved an international success, going into multiple editions in all the main European languages.[9] In his book, Huarte thought about how to construct the perfect commonwealth by ensuring that people were fitted for their public roles, selected by aptitude, and educated in the right way; it is utopian fiction. All too clearly, the real world was imperfect, particularly because so many people were in jobs for which they were demonstrably unsuited.

However, the *Examen* did not stop at educational and organisational psychology. It also offered proto-eugenicist advice on how to conceive children who were suitable for positions in the perfect commonwealth in the first place. How could readers conceive children (sons, really) of wit and intelligence who were ready to rule? Huarte's treatise is not only about how to school but also how to breed native intelligence. His *Examen* is at least as much about fertility as it is about psychology and governance. The whole of the final fifteenth chapter is taken up with the question about how "parents may beget wise children, and of a wit fit for learning," and that chapter takes up about a quarter of the book.[10] "Fathers in the time of procreation" can make sure, he wrote, that "all their children shall prove wise, and none otherwise."[11] Huarte was himself a "father in the time of procreation," and so was Philip, the book's dedicatee. The author addresses himself to the male reader and King Philip, in particular, and is concerned particularly with male reproduction. As a self-help book on conception, with one eye on Philip's life story, the work gives us a potential lead on contemporary assessments of what happened in Philip's case.

Given that Huarte has Philip in mind, much of his advice is impolitic. Huarte's topic is wise children, and yet he dedicated his book to a man who personally arrested and imprisoned his first-born son and heir, Carlos (1545–1568), because he was so mentally unwell, indeed was by now dead. In the fourteenth chapter, on kingship, Huarte spells out the obvious, telling Philip that fertility is crucial for kings and that having healthy heirs forestalls civil wars.[12] The author warns, as if it were necessary, that a king might "take a barraine woman to wife, with whom he shall be combred all daies of his life, without hope of issue." During Philip's four years of marriage to Mary, that must have been a very real fear. Twenty years had passed since the first of Mary's false pregnancies. Now that Philip was a father to so many children, his English marriage adventure had perhaps diminished in significance. Yet he cannot have forgotten it, as Huarte seems to have done. Whilst there was a tradition of writing advice to princes which covered rulers' virtues and vices and offered sometimes intimate instruction on, say, the ethics of love and the virtue of chastity, Huarte found himself offering his king probably unwanted advice on raw topics and even sex guidance.

Although Huarte steers clear of the topic of false pregnancy, his advice is haunted by the spectre of failure: of not being able to conceive or of having children who disappoint and are unfitted for high office. After Huarte extensively praises Philip's wisdom and establishes wisdom as a key quality for a king, he bumbles on in the final chapter about how wise men are too dry to be optimally fertile and too inhibited by sexual shame to attend to "certain diligences" during sex, meaning they don't take enough pleasure in the act.[13] Because of this, the children of wise men are more likely to be engendered by the mother's seed, which can never result in a child of great intelligence because women are cold and moist, a humoral complexion which makes them "fruitfull and apt for childbirth, but [an] enemy to knowledge."[14] In Huarte's misogynist take on prevailing medical theory, there is an anxiety about male subfertility. He describes an unfortunate inverse relationship between wisdom (a male attribute only) and fertility, and so there is a potential instability, a fertility problem, at the centre of the good commonwealth. How can a well-governed polity be reproduced if its king naturally begets foolish sons?

The solution, according to Huarte, is for readers to attend to the practical advice in his book. In the first instance, he counsels, marry the right person. Fertility problems are rarely the fault of one partner, he says, more usually being the combination of both. On this account, he recommends that marriages should be brokered, as does Plato in his *Republic*, securing the political future by making the right humoral matches. Perhaps to that end or while such a Platonic brokerage system is being devised, Huarte sets out a handy crib so that readers can make an evaluation of the degree of coldness and moisture in a potential bride and the degree of heat and dryness in a groom, based on seven physical tokens—wit and ability, manners, voice (big or small), flesh (much or little), colour, hair, fairness or foulness—and learn how to match these humoral profiles to ensure the issue of "wise children" rather than "fooles and do-noughts."[15] Huarte is thinking about the population in general but also wades into the topic of royal marriage matches. Bearing in mind that royal marriages were painstakingly brokered, Huarte was again in sensitive territory.

In Galenic terms, humoral profile matching was about spotting the fixed parameters of the innate or the so-called naturals. However, Huarte also offers a fertility health regimen in relation to the six "non-naturals." The non-naturals were environmental or incidental factors which were potentially manipulable—air, food and drink, exercise and rest, excretion, retention (where sex is often included), sleep and wakefulness, and the emotions. Conceiving well is a matter not of fortune, Huarte says, but of the right knowledge and the sense to act on it. Given that girls can't be wise, his main piece of advice for prospective parents is about "what diligence ought to be used, that children male and not female be borne."[16] He sets out a program that favours boys as much as fertility more generally.

The advice is detailed, such as on the optimum temperature for drinking water; on types of food and on the preparing, seasoning, and preserving of it; and on the preparation for and timing of sex. For example, a woman who is trying to conceive should drink goat's milk six or seven days before sex, eating it with honey to prevent its corruption. She should have a warm bath to alter her temperature and increase her moisture level, preparing her flesh like soil is prepared before seeds are sown.[17] Both should take plenty of exercise and eat moderately, having sex about five or six days before a period is expected and after a period of abstinence. Huarte recommends the woman go to the loo before sex so that she has "no cause to rise" straight afterwards.[18] Instead, she should lie on her right side (male foetuses were thought to inhabit the right-hand compartments of the womb) "with her head downe and her heeles up," staying in bed for a day or two.[19] It sounds like a tricky position to hold. Maybe you prop your lower body with pillows . . . but for two days! Poor Águeda.

The English translation of Huarte's treatise is curious, particularly because the margins are dotted with sly planned-for-print
annotations. The annotator is particularly
exercised by Huarte's praise of Philip.
For example, when Huarte suggests that
men with auburn hair and medium stat-
ure must "necessarily be verie wise, and
endowed with a wit requisit for the scep-
ter royall," the annotator, noticing that
Philip looks like this, writes in the margin,
    "And such a one if you mistake
       not, is your king Philip."[20]
       The other point that this
        wry glossator pounces on

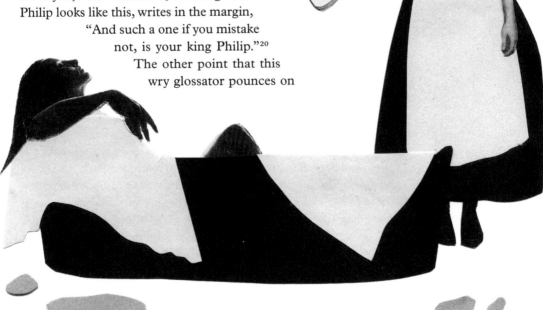

concerns the first "non-natural"—air and place—and its importance for promoting wisdom and fertility. Huarte notes that Spain is like ancient Greece: hot and dry, a climate conducive to philosophy.[21] Wisdom, he says, is the "ordinarie wit" in Spain. The problem is that a colder wetter climate is more fertile, both in arable agricultural terms but also for humans. Again, there's an incompatibility between wisdom and fertility. Places like "England, Flanders and Alamaine," Huarte maintains, have rich soil making for an "abundance of all the fruits." And in such places,

> no married woman was ever childlesse; neither can they there tell, what barrennesse meaneth, but all are fruitfull, and breed children through their abundance of coldnesse and moisture.[22]

Beside this comment, the English translator leaves a bald but pointed marginal note: "you are much mistaken."

The View from Cornwall

Let's fly over the Bay of Biscay and a decade and a half later meet the translator whose characterful comments engage so sceptically with Huarte's book. We land in the library of Francis Godolphin (ca. 1534–1608) in his manor house in Helston, Cornwall, sometime around 1590. He is with his younger friend, Richard Carew (1555–1620), who takes down an Italian translation of Juan Huarte de San Juan's *Examen de ingenios, para las sciencias* from the shelf and becomes intrigued, especially by the book's dedication to King Philip of Spain. Here is a book from the heart of enemy territory. Both Carew and Godolphin were involved in the war effort against the Spaniards, a war in which the English county of Cornwall was a central battleground. Carew would return the book to the Helston Manor library in 1594, along with the gift of his English translation, inscribed with a personal dedication to Godolphin. Using a tailoring metaphor, he describes the book as now "clad in a Cornish gabardine," which accounts for the colour of the marginal comments as much as the dialectical cut of the prose.

Carew was also a "father in the time of procreation."[23] His wife, Juliana, had given birth to some but not yet all of the ten children they would eventually have. His comment about Huarte's mistakenness comes not from a personal experience of struggling to become a parent but rather of living in Elizabethan Cornwall. When Carew picked up the *Examen*, Mary's half-sister Elizabeth was queen, England's second childless queen in succession, and both were tied up in different ways with Philip, the book's dedicatee. In Mary's case, he was the father of the children she was supposed to have but didn't. In Elizabeth's, his was the offer of marriage she rejected in favour of a childless unmarried life, and now the two were at war. Married northern European women, Carew read in Huarte's book, are never childless, and he laughed because Mary Tudor herself was surely evidence to the contrary, and her childlessness had wide implications for Carew's historical moment, especially as it was experienced in Cornwall. On July 29, 1588, for example, the ships in Philip's Armada were first sighted off Cornwall's Lizard Point, and from there beacons were lit along the English coast, alerting the navy at Plymouth to an anticipated land invasion by an army thirty thousand strong.[24]

Not conceiving and the Anglo-Spanish war are bound together for Richard Carew. We know this from another of Carew's works, a long poem from 1598, *A Herrings Tayle*, which is at once an allegory about the war and a reflection on the mythic roots of England's inveterate infertility.[25] By the time Carew came to write *A Herrings Tayle*, the Spanish had staged other attacks on England, including a land invasion of Cornwall in 1595, of which episode Carew happens to be the main chronicler. In his 1602 *Survey of Cornwall*, Carew tells us about how some four hundred Spanish infantrymen disembarked from galleons in Mousehole bay, spent two days burning Cornish towns and villages, and, just as shockingly, held a Catholic mass in Penzance. According to Carew's account, the Spanish were met by Godolphin, standing bravely at the head of an ill-disciplined and cowardly local militia.[26] Whilst *The Survey of Cornwall* tells the Spanish invasion story straight, *The Herrings Tayle* transforms it into a comic Ovidian beast fable, concerned with nonconception as well as war, unifying them through an engagement with Huarte's medical theory on conception, which Carew had translated and caustically annotated as *The Examination of Mens Wits*.

Richard Carew's *Herrings Tayle* starts with this Virgilian opening:

> I sing the strange adventures of the hardy Snail,
> Who durst (unlikely match) the weathercock assayle:
> A bold attempt, at first by fortune flattered
> With boote, but at the last to bale abandoned.[27]

And that is the story in a nutshell: a snail, Lymazon, climbs the tower of Tintagel Castle in Cornwall to do battle with a weathercock, Alectravemos, who is fixed there by one spurred foot. At first it looks as if Lymazon has the advantage because he is mobile:

> Swift move, but not remove could Alectravemos,
> Slow pac'd was Lymazon, but where he list he goes,[28]

[Alectravemos could move fast but could not move away.
Lymazon was slow but could go where he liked.]

In the end, Lymazon fails and is dashed from the tower by the wind. As a beekeeper, Carew was interested in invertebrate life, really looking at his snail and luxuriating in extended descriptions of its slow ascent—"no blood but in his lieu a liquide Christall cold."[29] Yet he is also thinking about watching an invader coming over the horizon—as Alectravemos does from the top of his tower—and the military mismatch between a force which is pinned in place, in Cornwall, suffering attack from a moving opportunist force able

> to exchange his neighbourhood at will,
> And still to bear, and still to use his shelly cave
> For house, for fort, for clothes, for bed, and for his grave.[30]

Ships are shell-like in this respect: forts and graves, if not precisely clothes and beds. The association between Lymazon and an over-stretched navy beset by the weather is continually underscored by naval and military metaphors. For example, his perilous climb is reminiscent of other unspecified foolhardy missions—"in quest of fleeting gain" "on the traytor sea, and mid the mutive [mutable] windes"—which are eventually aborted, the aggressors either killed or forced "homeward."

The interest in conception in *A Herrings Tayle* emerges in Alec-travemos's backstory, for which Carew found windy inspiration in the story of another shipwrecked fleet. In *The Aeneid*, the king of the winds, Aeolus, agrees to smash Aeneas's armada as a favour to Juno, and in return, she will give him the nymph Deiopeia, the guardian of her sacred peacocks, as a "bride." Aeolus, in Carew's version, transforms himself into a peacock—so that "untold, you would have sworne that he a peacock weare"—and takes up the place of another peacock abducted from Juno's sacred aviary by his henchmen, Zeph-yrus and Boreas, the west and north winds, respectively.[31] In this guise, he gains access to Deiopeia's bedchamber, forcing himself upon and impregnating her.

At the moment of the story where Deiopeia lays an egg, which hatches into a chick, which grows into a bird, Carew stops his tale to offer a scientific rationale: "Strange this may seeme, yet true, and reason naturall avowes such chances may befall."[32] The source for his perfectly natural explanation is Huarte's *Examen*.[33] Huarte relates "authenticall histories" in which women give birth to "per-fect men" conceived through copulation with animals—dogs, bears, and, in one case, a fish which "came out of the water, and begat . . . with child" an unsuspecting passer-by. These stories might be hard for the uneducated to credit, Huarte says, but they can be true, he

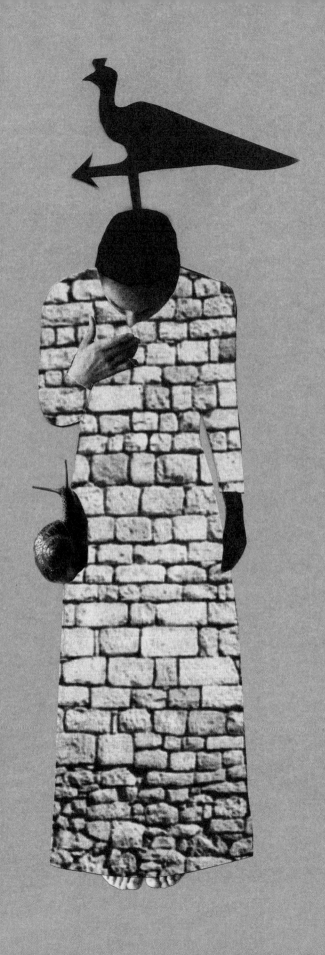

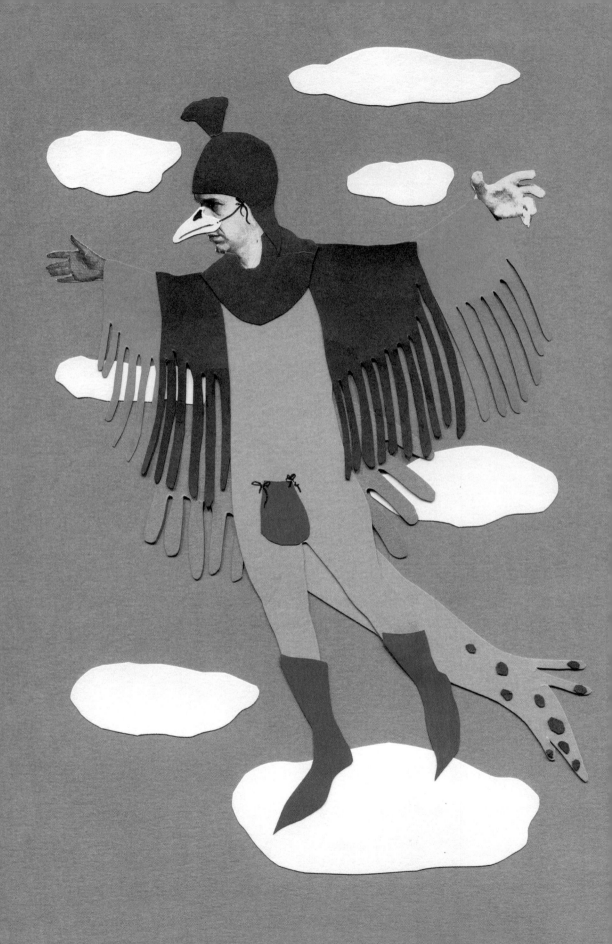

explains, because the female seed, in these cases, was the "greater in force," whereas "the seed of the brute beast (as not equall in strength) served for aliment [food], & for nothing els." Conversely, in Carew's comic take, the seed of Aeolus as peacock was stronger than the nymph's, so Alectravemos, a weathercock, hatches from an egg rather than being a more humanoid creature birthed viviparously.

Carew was not as optimistic as Huarte on what could be done actively to affect fertility or indeed future outcomes of any kind. The non-natural that Carew focussed on was not, say, food or the timing of sex, both of which were within human control, but instead air and place. You lived where you lived, in Carew's view; the way the local weather shaped your fortunes was non-negotiable. The English climate, especially as it was experienced by coastal counties like Cornwall, was very unlike that of Andalucía, especially in its most notable feature: the wind.[34] Huarte's advice to prospective parents on this aspect of climate had been that a west wind is better than a southwest wind for them "in the time of generation," "for the same is grosse, and moistneth the seed, so as a female and not a male is begotten."[35] However, he offers no sense of how to act on this guidance: Do you have to have sex when the wind blows from the optimum direction? Do you eat the local foods, which are also subject to the same weather conditions? What he observes here, though, is a very old and readily acknowledged link between the wind and conception through Greek humoral medicine and carried into classical literary traditions. The west wind, Zephyrus in classical myth, was the fructifying wind that blew in springtime, making all of nature, including people, fruitful. And the fertile influence of the wind was readily translated into Muslim Arabic and Christian medical writing where, as God's breath, it inspired and animated all foetuses at quickening.[36]

Whilst in good weather the wind disperses seed, in bad, it flattens the crops. In human reproductive health, wind was not only animating; it could equally cause and be a symptom of physiological derangement and morbidity. Pregnancy was most usually muddled up with windy dropsy or tympany, trapped wind inside the body, which could be suffered with varying levels of severity: it might be a trivial and temporary embarrassment, just farting, or a symptom of a much more serious, even potentially fatal condition.[37] The body was a microcosm of the larger atmosphere, so air movements could be experienced as anything on the spectrum from a cleansing ventilation to a more gaseous turbulence; it could be breath or flatulence. The wind's involvement in good or ill abdominal health enabled a convenient agnosticism about whether a pregnancy was "true" or "false," whether there were a viable foetus or some other intestinal

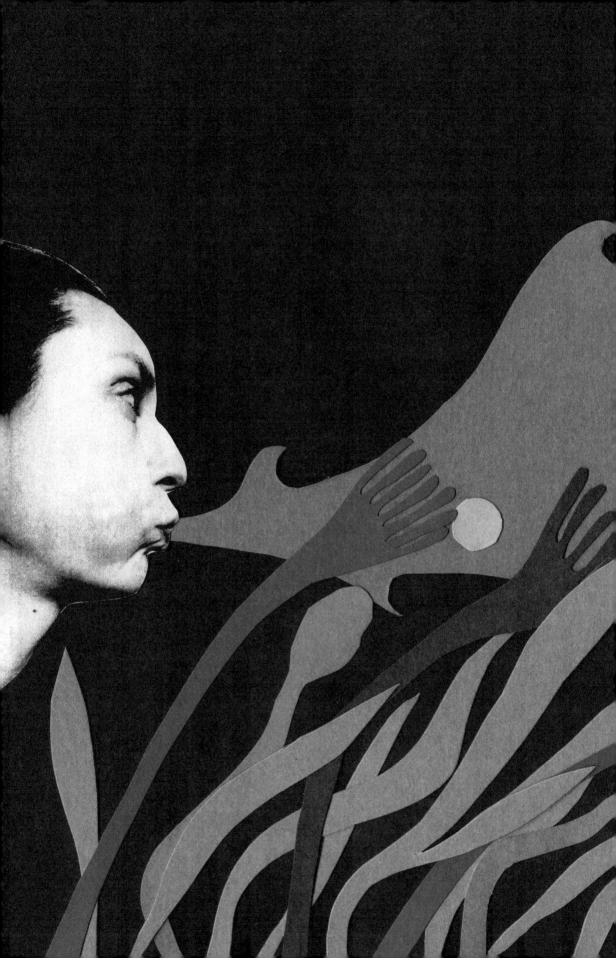

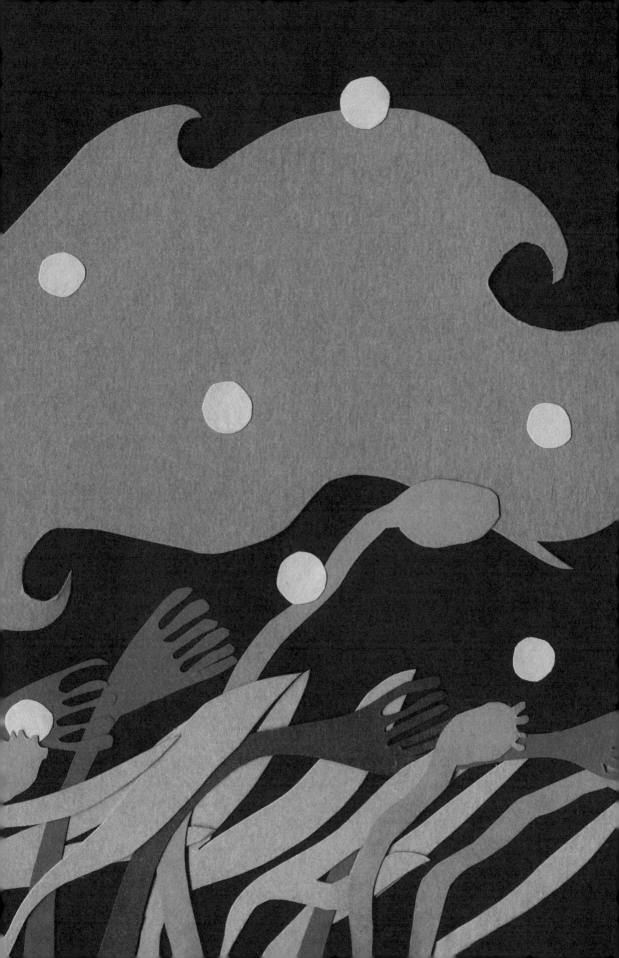

imbalance. What did it mean for English wombs and tummies, fertility and intestinal health, to be so beset by wind?

That the wind was savage round the coast of the British Isles was something that the Spanish were to find out during all their naval raids in the Anglo-Spanish war. Famously, in 1588 the armada was defeated as much by the wind as the English navy. Less than half the 130 ships that sailed for England in July returned; the rest foundered in inclement weather further north, smashed by the wind off the coast of Ireland.[38] Two further Spanish armadas also were scattered or wrecked by storms: in 1596 before the fleet had even left Spanish waters and in 1597 off the coasts of Cornwall, Wales, and the Isles of Scilly.[39] The weather was also decisive in the Spanish invasion of Cornwall in 1595. Just as reinforcements finally arrived to support Godolphin's stand, the wind turned, and the Spanish were able to evade an English ambush:

> within one houre after the arrival of these Captaines, the winde, which was until then strong at Southeast, with mist and rayne, to have impeached the Gallies returne, suddenly changed into the Northwest, with very fayre and cleare weather, as if God had a purpose to preserve these his rods for a longer time. The winde no sooner came good, but away pack the Gallies with all the haste they could.[40]

That the wind blew the Spanish ships away was not, by any means, an English military triumph, Carew admits; God preserved the Spanish fleet as a "rod" for England's future punishment. He does not claim God's straightforward intervention on the English side, as others did, crediting him with facilitating a Spanish escape from an English counteroffensive.

Carew does not write a great heroic past for England in *A Herrings Tayle*. His Arthurian history is magical but also disgraceful, bound up with sexual depravity. Alectravemos is the child of a rape, as was Arthur, begotten on Igraine by Uther, transformed by Merlin's magic into the form of Igraine's husband. Tintagel is the site of Igraine's rape and now Alectravamos's home, too. The battle with Lymazon is also not a triumph of courage and military stratagem. Instead, Aeolus, seeing that his son is about to lose the fight with Lymazon, calls a parliament of the winds and commissions them to protect and avenge his offspring. In the expressive Cornish dialect in which *A Herrings Tayle* is written, we learn that "the windes wedge wise in driue / Their blasts, and stitch by stitch his clibbie belly riue" (the winds drive their blasts in wedge-wise and bit by bit pull away his gooey body). Alectravamos is proud of himself but with no right; the victory is not his but his father's:

A Burgesse him he deem'd of the imperiall skie;
His glittering vesture pure gold he imagineth,
Imagines fond, for all not gold that glistereth.[41]

Alectravemos is a strangely animate and inanimate creature. Is he alive or dead? He can see, think, hear, and fight but only under the influence of his father, the wind, round and round in a circle. Deiopeia lays an egg, but is it a properly prolifical egg? It hatches into a chick which grows into a bird, but the creature has no agency of its own, being made of steel. That wind-child is taken by Merlin to ancient Britain where it is fixed to the tower at Tintagel. In the *Examen*, Huarte had connected Spain to ancient Athenian culture through their good weather, which gave their children an innate humoral proclivity to philosophy. Carew, on the other hand, connects Cornwall and the classical Mediterranean through their bad weather, their reputation for wrecking ships, and the strange metamorphic progeny conceived in their myths. England is founded on a violent windiness and the royal children that never were, the hybrid agent-offspring of the wind: nonentities with influence but no life or breath.

Queen of the Winds

Whilst Carew was not able to celebrate this great and terrible English windiness, others were. The three famous Armada propaganda portraits (ca. 1588) of Queen Elizabeth are pictures of her as Queen of the Winds (historical figure 5).[42] She is shown in front of two windows. In one can be seen the English navy in clement weather with full sails and orderly battle lines; in the other, the Spanish fleet is breaking up in storms. In her left hand, the queen holds a fan of puffy white feathers, as if she personally generates the winds that favour English over Spanish ships. This goes further even than the commemorative Armada medals which put the wind down to God's intervention on the English side, struck with the legend "Flavit et dissipati sunt" (He blew and they were scattered), featuring a storm cloud blasting the Spanish fleet and labelled with the Hebrew tetragrammaton יהוה (Jehovah).[43]

Other historians commenting on this portrait have noticed that it articulates a desire for empire (the queen has her hand resting on a globe turned to show the New World) and have also identified its paradoxical celebration of virginal fertility (the pearls and finial are egg-shaped, and the ovarian bow poised over the queen's groin is as voluble as a male codpiece).[44] But the connections between its wind and fertility motifs have not been noticed. The globe under

Elizabeth's palm is cut across with the rhumb lines which marked out the wind routes for shipping on sixteenth-century sea charts, or portolan maps. The portrait's composition is modelled on one of those sea maps, comprising a circle of circular shapes which quote the wind roses that structured these maritime maps (historical figure 6).[45] Rhumb lines, suggested by the folds in the queen's costume and strings of pearls, connect the circles, radiating from Elizabeth's head and a lower-than-centre point near her groin. If you resize the example in historical figure 6, a sixteenth-century portolan map made for Philip II, and lay a transparency of it over the Armada portrait, you will see this compositional cartography. The compositions match. Wind roses or compasses were synonyms in a period where the winds were directions, roads for ships, and they are explicitly celebrated in the portraits' textiles—in the queen's lace cuffs and ruff. And the mermaid, which other scholars have seen as a figure of unruly aqueous female sexuality showing up Elizabeth's virginity by contrast, is exactly what you would expect on a portolan map, at least on a library copy for display rather than one on active service onboard a ship.[46]

The wind puffs things out and made them round: sails, cheeks, tummies, the earth. Round things depend on the wind for their spherical form. A Renaissance drawing guide explains that the "winds must be drawn with puffed and blowne cheekes." Compasses, wind roses, and maps added the blowing heads of the winds as extra rounded-out points of design.[47] In the Armada portrait, the feathers in the queen's fan and on her head are symbols of the birds' mastery of the air, but they also resemble the puffs blown out by wind heads. In classical origin myths as retold by Hesiod, Ovid, and Virgil, the earth was round because it had once been pregnant with the squabbling sibling winds, raging for release, which the god-king Aeolus liberates by plunging a spear into the ground. In the *Herrings Tayle* version, Aeolus threatens the winds that if they fail to avenge Alectravemos, he will return them to their prison, the "void wombe" of the earth and there,

> . . . bounsing, and rumbelling,
> For issue, so her [i.e., the earth's] vaulted entrailes tosse and teare,
> That she new childing groanes with paine, and quakes for feare[48]

The winds are earth's children and derangements of her digestive system. There is no difference when the winds are your children. In her three Armada portraits, Elizabeth looks not like a woman with her "entrailes" tossing and tearing but rather a picture of personal possession. Her hand resting on the globe presents her as a female Aeolus, able to release and imprison the winds at will, directing them on her missions. More than just weathering storms, she commands them; the winds emanate from her.

The difference between Mary and Elizabeth on the question of childlessness and, by extension, windiness is that Elizabeth didn't "try." If you don't *try* to conceive, then you or your public relations team, if you usefully have one, can try to shape the childless narrative: it becomes about choice and control. The way Elizabeth wore it, childlessness was purity, a pearly virginal strength with its own potency, fertile but in an unconventional unreproductive way. In the portrait, all those pearls and the wooden egg-shaped finial capping the furniture may well be fertility symbols, but they are made of shiny resistant materials: pearl and varnished wood. Pearls are the traditional emblem of virginity, and they are particularly apposite for maritime propaganda: inaccessible and expensive jewels from the deep. Elizabeth's bow is not on a bump and proud of pregnancy, like those I look at in chapter 2, but a bow as a fastener, which locks out suitors and takes pride instead in virginal exclusivity.

The globe turned to the New World shows the viewer another theatre for the Anglo-Spanish war, other than the seas where the armada foundered. Yet England was a long way from rivalling, let alone outcompeting Spanish achievements in the Americas. Whilst Spain and Portugal had established large extractive global empires, Newfoundland, England's first New World colony, yielded up a lot of fish but little else, and those who attempted to settle the second, at Roanoke, were to vanish into thin air.[49] Further settlement was hampered by the ongoing war, which sucked resources from the English colonial endeavour. All the while, New World wealth flowed across the Atlantic to Spain and Portugal. The Armada, the largest fleet that had ever been seen at sea, was funded by the proceeds of mines in New Spain, such as Potosí in modern-day Bolivia.[50] The best that Elizabeth could do to try to monetise transatlantic shipping routes was to disrupt, licensing privateers to intercept or block treasure vessels, stealing from other empires rather than building her own. The way to control that somewhat cut-price narrative was to emphasise potential and expectation: fertility. The English colonial not-yet was an alternative kind of pregnancy, full and round but not yet delivered, and it relied for its maritime ventures on the generative operation of the wind, just as ordinary pregnancies did.

But let's look at the wish and imagine for a moment the queen herself speaking it. "What if I had a wind which I could control," she might say, "one private to me, unavailable to my enemies? If I had such a wind, I would not have to wait. I could launch a fleet at once or crush my foes at will. I would no longer be subject to the wind's caprice. *Then* who would have command of the Atlantic?"

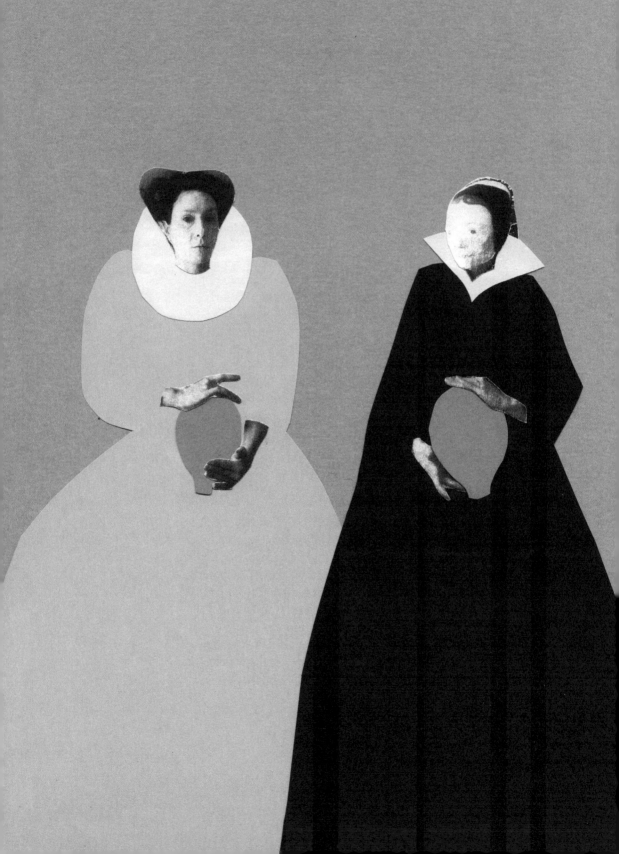

The three Armada portraits dream of freedom from the winds long before the invention of the internal combustion engine and the mass extraction of fossil fuels. They dream of the future Anthropocene.

Nature in Her Forge

What was—indeed, what *is*—the human relationship to nature? The ambition articulated in the Armada portraits is for nature as well as the human world to come under the auspices of royal rule. Let's turn to a book where the relations between nature and human desire and ambition were under ethical review, one which was available in all the sixteenth-century European royal libraries: the landmark, late thirteenth-century poem, *The Romance of the Rose*. There, nature is presented as a working woman in a smithy, wearing a leather apron, bashing out new babies, beasts, and birds with a hammer on an anvil (historical figure 7). Whilst she works, she vociferously and frequently complains about human desire: that people (clink)— paradoxically, the only creatures afforded a rational soul (clink) and so the power of reason (clink)—are the only animals whose sexual habits and desires are completely unreasonable (clink). Why can't they just couple up seasonally and reproduce like all the other animals, driven by marvellous instinct, to do what was necessary to continue their lines (clink)? According to Nature, the other animals don't have erotic imaginations, don't consume porn, and don't have sex with no reproductive purpose. They are unhindered by the whole unnecessary aesthetic and philosophical architecture of human love: they aren't obsessed with the wrong person and don't suffer from lovesickness or sexual jealousy. Why couldn't people be more like that? The way that Nature put it, she was daily offended by the extravagance of human lust. The puzzle or joke here is that Nature herself made human nature, so if there were a fault, it was hers. We are nature. Another way to depict "Nature in her forge" was as two lovers in a bed, banging out babies using a different kind of "hammer" and "anvil," by nature passing to their offspring their unnaturalness, their capacity to offend Nature herself, along with their eye colour.[51]

In this conceit, nature was God's delegated representative: God made the policy but didn't carry it out. There were other ways to imagine the relations between God, nature, and humans. This was a very separatist one, and it explained nature's copying errors: congenital disabilities but also the immoderation in the reproductive process, the subcontracting of jobs to Venus. God had set up the forge but left nature in charge. Speed of production in the forge is preset by death, sometimes depicted as a skeleton with a sword, or as the fate, Atropos, snipping the threads of life. Nature understandably made mistakes, working fast by hand in the heat and smoke from the furnace, reproducing children from the template of their parents.

Nature in her forge was a conceit which mashed up culture and nature, organic and manufactured things, but she also frames a sophisticated conundrum about the ethics of desire and human exceptionalism.[52] The push of our desires to know, to have, and to enjoy and the pull of high cultural, aesthetic, and scientific achievements set us apart and give us an apparently outside perspective on the workings of the natural world. To the question "Are we in or out of nature?" the answer was always, "We're in." But the question of exactly what levels of separation there were between people, animals, nature, and God was up for discussion. And at the end of it is another question: who or what is in charge? Do people have dominion over nature, in the way that Adam was given stewardship of the animals in the Judeo-Christian origin story? Or are we in nature's grip, as powerless to alter our desires or reproductive outcomes as we are the tides or storms? Human reason gives us the impression of control, of conscious charge over our bodies and environments, but why did reason not govern the passions, and why were the reasonless animals so much better at sex and generation, at moderation?

In fertility health, we all want to know how much is fixed and how much subject to our own will and habits. When I read these words in my trying-to-conceive years from the beginning of Rebecca Fett's best-selling guide, *It Starts with the Egg: How the Science of Egg Quality Can Help You Get Pregnant Naturally, Prevent Miscarriage, and Improve Your Odds in IVF*, I felt an enormous wash of relief: "This book will explain the simple things you can do to have the best possible chance of getting pregnant and bringing home a healthy baby."[53] Am I helpless? Is trying hopeless? Can I help myself, can I be helped, can human endeavour get an edge on nature? *Can* I "try"? Fett argues against the "conventional thinking" that "women are born with all the eggs they will ever have" and that "there is little they can do to improve egg quality." An ovum takes three months to mature before release, and those months open a window for change in an otherwise fixed frame. Fett is the Huarte of our day: she lays out what to eat, what to avoid, what to do. And, as far as I could, I did it. Trying is an expression of hope: hope that nothing and especially not our biology—dynamic, shifting, growing, reproducing, metabolising—is fixed.

One of the main topics in Fett's advice and other self-help writing for fertility is about reducing exposure to toxins. She mainly concentrates on two chemical compounds, the "everyday-everywhere-chemicals" bisphenol A (BPA) and phthalates, both by-products of plastic production.[54] BPA is an ingredient in hard plastics, and phthalates in soft. Both are described as "endocrine disruptors." BPA is even known as a "synthetic estrogen," interfering in the fertility processes reliant on hormone activity.[55] Both are ubiquitous, a component not just of plastics but also cosmetics, cleaning products, and pesticides, and from there they have leached into food, water, plants, animals, and, it turns out, people. Fett is concerned with minimising their influence—buying, heating, and consuming food in nonplastic containers, for example—rather than eliminating them, which she describes as an impossible task. She says minimising is enough or at least all we can do to optimise fertility health.

Yet what does it mean that these composites are not just outside of us but inside too? Fett writes, "these chemicals can be found in the bloodstream of the vast majority of people tested in the United States, Europe, and Asia."[56] I can stop painting my nails, but I am already partly plasticated. Plastic is being ingested, absorbed, inhaled like air "everyday-everywhere," as if it were a new element. The distinction that we have understood between things that are made and things that have grown seems harder to draw, as in nature's forge. My body is enfolded in a manmade disaster which reaches from the stomachs of whales in the deep oceans to the honeycomb of bees in hives and hollows.[57] Is it such a dystopian stretch to imagine a future in which the materials that plastic was created to imitate—ivory, tortoiseshell, silk, pearl—become so contaminated by plastic as to be indistinguishable from them?

Most plastics are made from petrochemicals. Their production is closely interlocked with hazardous air pollutants from burning fossil fuels. So we are still up against the wind, but now it has a special extra anthropogenic boost. Scientific consensus on our planetary emergency prioritises twin needs to reduce both the extraction and consumption of fossil fuels and

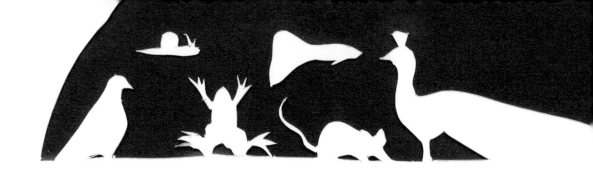

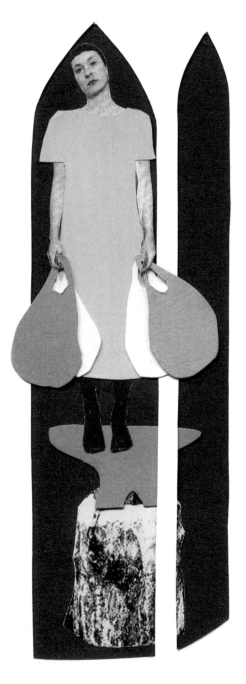

damaging industrialised farming practices. "The Anthropocene is the age of flatulence," writes anthropologist Radhinka Govindrajan.[58] She means that, in this new phase in which geological time is running at the speed of human culture, emissions from the burning of fossil fuels and the literal farts of factory-farmed animals are a great gaseous belching. If Fett is the new Huarte, I feel as overawed as Carew reading Huarte in windswept Cornwall.

Our collective environmental crises are understood like this: I pick up a book which is new to me to find out about how to manage my immediate circumstances right now. In it, I learn about my personal responsibilities: for instance, why I should use paper, glass, ceramic—anything rather than plastic. But I also learn that we are living with irreversible historical contamination: that the invention and mass production of synthetic materials, made possible by the processing of fossil fuels, has pushed us all over a natural boundary long ago. Philosopher Bruno Latour asks:

> How can we simultaneously be part of such a long history, have such an important influence, and yet be so late in realizing what has happened and so utterly impotent in our attempts to fix it?[59]

I do what I can as an individual, buy organic carrots loose, because each tiny act of fertility self-care turns out to be intricately enlaced but also ludicrously dwarfed by the scale of a tragedy which is already upon us. And my fertility health is the least part of it, as we watch the collapsing "distance between two calendars": geological time and human history.[60]

Nature was right to complain about the collective immoderation of human desire. Her forge has closed now, and she works instead in a plastic injection moulding factory on a poverty wage. And the premodern debates that have concerned me in this chapter—about how separate human beings are from the natural world; how far our fortunes are tied into the climates, places, and times in which we live; and who, humans or nature, is master of whom—turn out to be more relevant than ever.

The desire for influence over nature on display in the Armada portraits would come to be satisfied for some. Global expansion and mineral exploitation enriched European empires and gave them a political, cultural, and economic dominance, which would accelerate later with industrialisation. We could describe the terrible consequences of that desire as inadvertent—influence does not mean control—except there are still people individually enriching themselves and improving their private lot; making life increasingly unliveable, especially for the poorest, most historically exploited parts of our planet; generating and riding the increasingly destructive winds.

■

Amongst our many lifestyle adjustments, M. and I bought conception-enhancing vitamin pills. The ingredients listed in M.'s multivitamin included things you would expect, like vitamins B, C, and D but also more exotic elements: Peruvian maca extract, Siberian ginseng extract, and pine bark extract. Peruvian maca extract is, in fact, the largest ingredient. I look it up on the internet and tell M. that it is known as the "natural Viagra."

"What website was that?" he says. "The Peruvian maca marketing board?"

His tablets offer the quintessence of manliness, harvested from the great rainforests and desert steppes at the world's farthest reaches, flown or shipped from both East and West and distilled into tablet form. I like the sound of the mythic vistas these ingredients suggest and the primitive natural forces that they purport to command. They resemble the innumerable historical fertility recipes for men which involve the medicinal preparations of animals' testicles—weasels, otters, bulls, rams—based on the rationale of sympathy: that it takes one to cure one. M. hasn't got time to go on great journeys to other worlds to imbibe the manliness of special bark. Luckily, vitamin manufacturers have done it for him, scouring the earth, mincing, and confecting these primal essences into tablets at his blister-packed convenience (plastic, of course).

M. takes his first dose, which is a manly but unnatural aubergine colour and, as it goes down, waggles his head as if he is feeling the hit of a magical shape-shifting potion: "ROOOAAAAR!" he says. "I'm a tiger."

5 Credit: How the Money Rolls Out

And your final outcome card is . . . Seven of
Pentacles! That's a good outcome card! It
means, *I'm starting over with something great
and new.* Look at what you're going to produce!
Glowing, beautiful pieces of fruit—or whatever
those things are. And the light is shining through
them. That pink light is gorgeous, just *gorgeous*!
Maybe there can be something beautiful that
happens with the bleeding out.
—Sheila Heti, *Motherhood* (2018)[1]

Wednesday's Child

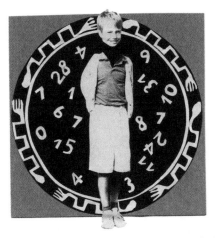

F YOU TELL my friend's son (let's call him Ben) your birthdate, he will tell you, without much hesitation, the day of the week on which you were born. Reverse forecasting is more doable than predicting the future, yet it is still an astonishing trick. If I look up the calculation, I see it is hard to do instantly, instinctively; there is a formula to run. Yet Ben, who has autism, seems able to hold the calendar in mind, consulting it without thought with access to some deeper knowledge. It seems more magic than maths. Folkloric but factual.

"You were born on a . . ." and he leaves a mere beat of a pause before settling on "Wednesday."

Full of woe, according to the old fortune-telling rhyme.

Ben speaks in a special kind of poetry, reciting information about the public lifts in his city: their makes, the weights they will carry, the number of floors they serve. Then he spools through lists of brand names, shops, and loyalty cards that connect his household's economy to the wider commercial world—all the minute literal parts which make up a whole whose edges are never seen or invoked. I let his words wash over me like music.

Once, putting his hand gently on my son's head and pausing the flow of his usual interests, Ben said: "And you will have another baby." I moved onto high alert.

"Yes?"

After a pause, he added: "A girl baby."

"Yes?" I said, desire blindsiding my scepticism of annunciations. Ben was uncharacteristically silent. His eyes were glassy, as if he saw something very far away. He has an angelic face.

"You will call her . . ."

"Yes?"

"Ruth."

With apologies to all the lovely people called Ruth, this is very far from a name I would pick. Ruth is a name from the Hebrew Bible but has long operated in English as a virtue name: compassion, pity. At a formative juncture of my life, I knew a Ruth whose nature did not match her name. The Ruth who most occupies that name for me was terrifying. She was an anti-allegory, embodying everything that was entirely un-Ruth-y.

"You've lost me now, Ben," I said, snapping out of it, pulling back my projected romantic fantasies of the child savant able to tap into some deep truth flowing under the surface of rational life.

Ben's mother says about his superpowers, "He can do the date thing, and that's it."

∎

At the limits of knowledge, at the point where conventional medicine and science draw blanks, is a point of raw vulnerability, a point at which we are ready to fall in with whomever if it will help. Operating at those limits are a range of institutions and individuals with their own agendas which are different from ours and are often commercial and not wholly trained on care. Some of those are bad actors who get dressed in special clothes, adopt technical languages and curious aesthetic forms, and science-wash their grift. Because we cannot check the full workings and credentials of all the expertise that is offered to us, laypeople must rely on trust. Within the trust landscape, we are tasked with distinguishing legitimate from illegitimate authority, true expertise from false claims, good from bad science.

Facing the edge of knowledge foregrounds the question of history. Historical ideas hold out the prospect of forgotten but ancient and extensively tried methods of calculation, detection, and treatment. Has some good knowledge, some part of our legitimate inheritance, been lost or overlooked? What has been lain aside in the privileging of certain kinds of authority? On the other hand, looking at the horizon ahead: what about the technologies of the future which are not yet fully with us? Legitimate new insights and technologies must begin with hypotheses which, in development phases, might have little or no evidenced worth . . . yet. Can we hazard anything on those not fully fathomed conjectural techniques and possibilities? We are asked to trust but only so far: don't raise modern biomedical services or products beyond their competence; withdraw our consent from excessively experimental practice. When does research become charlatanry? At what point do we refuse to pay for techniques and services, despite their promise?

Because of the difficulty of evaluating truth claims, clinical services come to us pre-endorsed by regulatory structures which operate on our behalf. But do we always want or trust regulatory protection? What if regulation limits our access to the therapies that could work? What if the priorities of regulators (frequently value for money) are not the same as ours—a throw of the dice, a chance, however slim. What if I want to blow a fortune on risky, magical, experimental treatments? Regulation *also* requires trust. Is the regulator any good? What if it fails us? What if it's in hock?

Although we want to tell ourselves that people were more vulnerable to faith frauds in the past than they are today, the never wider gap between lay and scientific language and knowledge makes us uniquely historically vulnerable to spurious or expensive services. Credulity does not steadily diminish over time. Desire switches on our capacity for faith, and then we look for things to believe. The aesthetics of scientific knowledge—the look of numbers, computational process, visual data—co-opt our desire by stressing insight, certainty, and settlement just as surely as the magical and religious practitioners who are still doing excellent trade.

Piss Prophets

Here we are in a pregnancy and parenting internet forum, in which a self-confessed addict of the site initiates a new thread on pregnancy and urine in the customary abbreviated code:

> Good morning ladies! I have a question and figured this
> forum would be a great place to ask! I am 11 spo and have had
> cloudy pee the last couple of days. I am not having any pain
> while peeing etc and seriously doubt its a UTI. Im just curious
> as to whether any of you had cloudy pee before your bfp[2]

Note: An spo is a typo for dpo, which means "days past ovulation." UTI means "urinary tract infection." A bfp is a "big fat positive" (a positive pregnancy result).

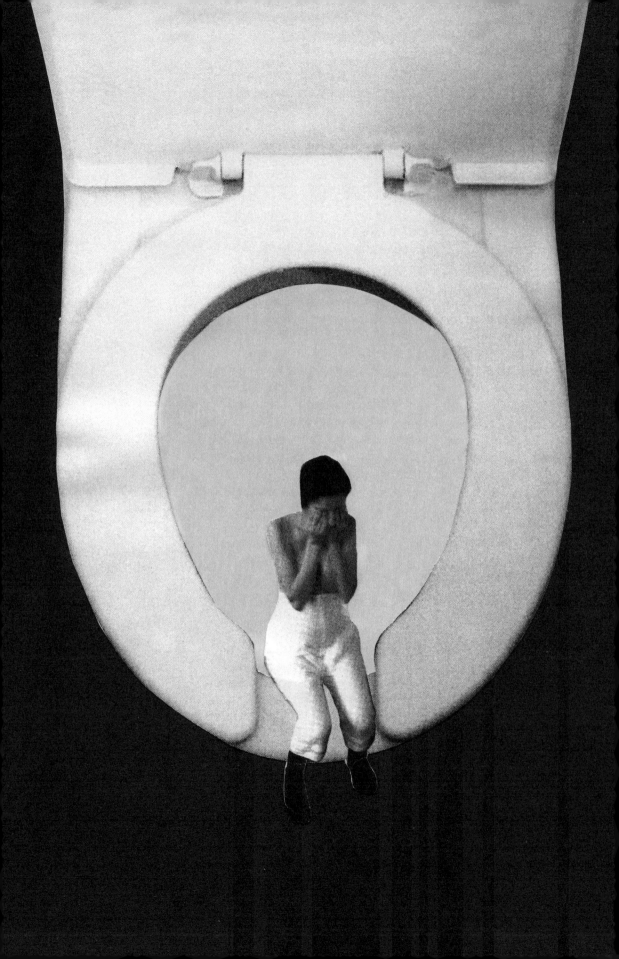

Various respondents chip in. They also observed this cloudiness in their pregnancies. One asked a nurse about it. Is it a sign, they wonder, or a symptom? One asks: "OK. This might sound like a weird question but can you describe what 'cloudy pee' looks like or is noticed by? Sorry." This induces some puzzlement for the original inquirer: "Ummm. Just cloudy. Not clear. Not sure how else to describe it." Another contributor helps: "maybe like cloudy apple juice but yellow?!!."

This is an attempt, however unofficial, to think scientifically. Am I pregnant (an ontological fact), and how can I know (epistemology)? These women know that this observation is likely to be inconclusive and divide it off from professional scientific practice or ways of really knowing. The comment about asking the nurse defers to professional authority. To come to this question, the original enquirer is deploying home technologies to pinpoint ovulation: thermometer, clock, calendar, ovulation detector devices. She is likely lining up a commercial pregnancy test kit. She may well have subscribed to a fertility app with calculators and so may be contributing her data to the commercial development of future fertility technologies. The internet interface which brings her into the forum is another technology again. Yet all the technology with which she is engaged is insufficient and cannot answer her question.

Her post is hosted by a web platform which contextualises speculative forum posts like these with sensible, static, school-shoe advice: in this case, you can't diagnose pregnancy by looking at urine with the naked eye. Official advice does not indulge the desire to puzzle-solve in a knowledge vacuum. The forums, on the other hand, offer an intricate and ever-changing supplement to approved advice which tells of more possibilities, of all the anomalies, of the variety and alteration found in every human body, and of ways to know first, in advance of qualified medical practitioners. They are a great living oracle of which you can ask any question, like: is piss cloudy in pregnancy?

At the same time, the forum hosts often monetize speculation. Throughout these chats, certain words can become automatically hyperlinked by the advertisements which ride them, selling different private medical services, literally underscoring the difference between lay speculation and the qualified medical opinions these women could buy. Words like *signs*, *symptoms*, *pain*, and *nurse* all work like this as portals to professional practitioners. Signs need trained readers. If forum users mention that they spoke to a doctor in their real world, then a doorway opens to a virtual marketplace ready to replace current sources of advice and care. At time of writing,

UK regulators are reviewing fertility and period-tracking apps, concerned with how they handle users' personal data. In an initial poll at the outset of that review, over half of app users "noticed an increase in baby or fertility-related adverts since signing up."[3] Resources that are or that look like sources of support have a business model based on feeding menstrual data to increasingly sophisticated, algorithmically targeted marketing machines.

It probably isn't surprising to know that there are people on the internet studying their own wee. All sorts of wonders are appearing in cyberculture, proliferating much faster than the ethnographic scholarship that might interpret it for us. The clear sight of such speculative terrain feels new. But unwittingly, these women are engaging in a practice of macroscopic urine inspection, which historians call *uroscopy* and which has a very long history. There is no explicit reference in the forum post to historical practice, although perhaps if they were pushed, these women might recall that people have historically thought about or tried urine inspection for pregnancy diagnosis; a buried memory spurs them to their speculation. Here, again, is that Frankenstein reflex: a curiosity about and resort to older ideas to address contemporary ignorance.

The broad history of uroscopy goes like this. It emerges in the ancient Greek medical writings of Hippocrates (ca. 460–375 BCE) and can be tracked through the works of landmark medical writer Galen (ca. 130–210 CE), into Byzantine and Arabic writings, and, through them, to the Latin West in the late medieval period. Its fullest articulation is to be found in the late Middle Ages in the circulation of extraordinarily beautiful illuminated uroscopy manuals, with characteristic colour wheels and tables.[4] Its continued practice has been charted throughout the early modern period and well into the nineteenth century, when it declines and dies.[5] Yet the internet uroscopers show us something else: that there is a continuing curiosity about and even attachment to historical forms of knowledge long after they have gone out of currency. Might there be forgotten ways of knowing, the speculating mind asks?

A central question for historians is: why did trust in uroscopy run so high for so long?[6] That question betrays a scepticism at the claims uroscopy made that all sorts of different conditions, including pregnancy, could be diagnosed by looking at a flask of urine with the naked eye. The answers that historians have arrived at for the persistence and depth of patient trust are good ones for considering our own potential susceptibilities: What promises are most likely to draw us in? What stratagems solicit and gain our trust and, with it, our money?

The most obvious advertisement for the macroscopic inspection of urine was the promise of a convenient answer to an intractable problem. And the mechanism of achieving that answer seemed self-evident. In the Middle Ages, bodily fluids were thought to be essentially the same thing—blood—in different states. Urine was blood that had been sieved. This sieving function separated out impurities and left behind urine, a translucent liquid, now with its base colour revealed. Both blood and urine were compendiums of the body, but, unlike blood, urine could be collected without pain. The fourteenth-century English medical writer Henri Daniel insists "id est [it is] a demonstracioun, a shewinge." *Id est* is our "i.e.," a technical phrase which breaks down the barriers between analogous things: they were the same rather than just similar.[7] Daniel uses it to stress the very direct access that urine gave to truth. Whilst the body might itself be opaque, urine had very recently been a part of it. Urine, captured in a flask, was an unmediated sight of the body it had just left.

Historians are sceptical of exactly the thing that made uroscopy appealing: its total view. The illuminations in uroscopy manuscripts often depict urine flasks in a complete rainbow. Urine schema were fitted into others—the elements, the zodiac, the movement of time—and, to learn about all of this, you could start with your eyes and a flask of urine. These grand schemes can be seen in a fifteenth-century manuscript now in the Wellcome Collection in London, the so-called *Wellcome Apocalypse*.[8] This encyclopedic compendium includes a treatise on uroscopy, with an image of a wheel of urine flasks which grow from a tree, each branch signalling a different category of diagnosis (historical figure 8). This work takes up codex space with other medical material (on phlebotomy, anatomy, and gynecology), an apocalypse of St. John, penitential materials (for example, writing on the vices and virtues, another complete system, and a treatise on how to die well), and works on astrology, meteorology, and the seasons. Urine fitted into the encyclopedic imagination: a comprehensive system fitted into other comprehensive systems.

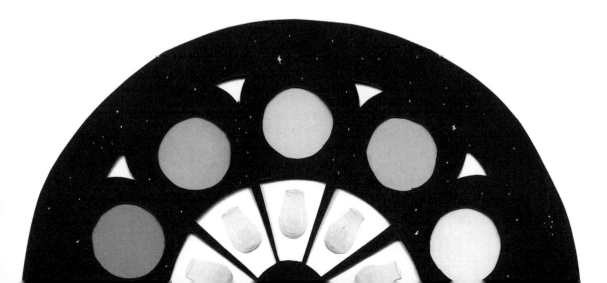

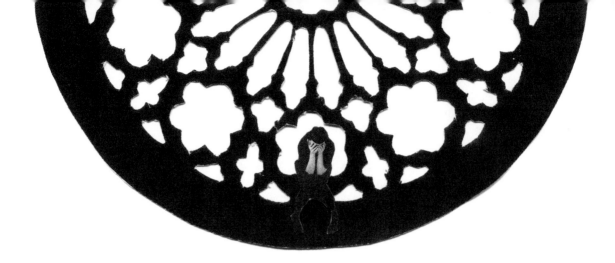

The human body was connected to everything else by a deep natural logic. One answer to the question of why we should trust in uroscopy is given in the satisfying total distanced view, an apparently objective and scientific rather than immersed perspective.

Running alongside this grand scientific vista, uroscopy also effectively domesticated diagnosis. The internet uroscoper's statement ("like cloudy apple juice, but yellow") does what the medieval uroscopy texts do: articulate colour and clarity in relation to other familiar, often domestic things. Medieval urine inspection worked through a mnemonic set of chromatic and qualitative analogies. This is the way that one Middle English uroscopy list begins:

> xix colorse haue vrense;
> Eche fro oþer haue defferense.
> One ys lyke to golde fyne.
> And þe toþer is not so fyne.
> And anoþer is as good rede blode.[9]

> [Urine has nineteen colours.
> Each is different from another.
> One is like fine gold.
> And the other (i.e., its pair) is not so fine.
> And another is like good red blood.]

The verse goes on to compare urine to a universe of other mundane things: firelight, liver, wine, lead, water, horn, whey, camel's skin (familiar presumably from scenes of John the Baptist), underboiled broth, boiled fish, and a fox, ranging through all the reds, greys, pinks, yellows, and cream colours. Other versions went through the blue and green colour spectrum, too. You might visit a doctor who practised uroscopy in his clinic, but the system also enabled a home diagnosis, because all sorts of ordinary objects and substances offered a key against which the glass flask could be held.

The medieval historian Laurence Moulinier-Brogi has noted the way that these chromatic schemata exceeded practical use: there are so many more colours than can have been possible; the textual descriptions change in different languages to maintain the rhyme; early printed versions, before colour printing was common, were for customers to colour in themselves.[10] Because of that excess, she says, we must ask not only how were they used (which they clearly were) but also what made up for their limitations. For Moulinier-Brogi, their offer is aesthetic: these are abstracted and beautiful and beyond any purely instrumental reading. She suggests that we read them as an expression of the curious gaze before a resistant substance, comparing the uroscoper's task to the modern historian's, trying to read the wonderful but obscure effusions of the medieval archive.[11] One response to the inscrutable body and urine, its opaque record, is an aesthetic one: to tabulate and admire its many signs as forms of expression, regardless of whether those expressions can be fully read. In Moulinier-Brogi's view, in uroscopy we are looking at conjectural epistemologies aestheticized, a cover for the inadequacies of the science itself. Trust was generated by a special scientific look.

Yet trust wasn't the only response to uroscopers and their work. Delightful urine-gazing monkeys are ubiquitous in the art of the Middle Ages, holding up their urinals for view and appearing in some surprisingly high-status and culturally sanctioned places. For example, some sit in the border of a prominent stained-glass window in the nave of York Minster—images of coloured glass urinals in coloured glass—and many others appear in the margins of expensive illuminated manuscripts. It is hard to know what the monkeys precisely represent: Are they signs of scepticism, warning us of the foolishness of doctors and uroscopers? Or do they indicate that the theory of urine analysis came, like pet monkeys, from foreign and perhaps suspect places, travelling West along trade routes in Arabic medical writing? Monkeys ape us, a fact that points to the

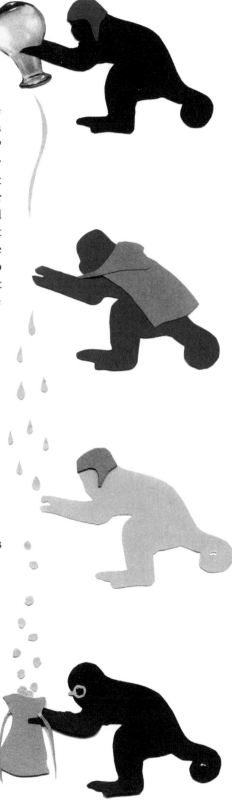

reflective qualities of the urinal, which shows us ourselves as if in a mirror. They look comical, fancifully interrupting the graver holier scenes that they border. The monkeys don't quite uphold the sense that there was universal trust in uroscopy; they look too irreverent.

Trust must have been patchy. Scepticism and trust always coexist, and paying patients may even be aware that they are paying for a speculative service. Even in the period usually characterised as the zenith of credulity, there was a mixed range of views from belief to disbelief. There was a medieval "bad science" brigade, just as there is today, which was prepared to call out spurious practice. Here is the fifteenth-century friar Girolamo Mercurio's take on uroscopy for pregnancy diagnosis:

> As to the signs that some people think they see in urine, this is such a false lie that it belongs more to charlatans than to physicians because the moon has more to do with shrimp than with urine in showing whether or not a woman is pregnant.[12]

Neatly, Mercurio registers his scepticism in an analogy like those that structured the practice of uroscopy (like gold, like blood, like apple juice): is the moon like a shrimp? This kind of evidence gives a dappled picture of trust, reminding us that the past is like the present, with as many kinds of beliefs as there are people, some more trusting and others more sceptical.

Mercurio's statement sounds so rational, and, yet, as it turns out, it is so wrong. Urine *has* come to be key to accurate and reliable pregnancy testing. At the very least, we can credit uroscopy with the idea that urine might be legible, at least in the case of pregnancy, as it has proved. Technologies must be imagined before they can be realised. Urine was waiting for good readers. The historians' question about why uroscopy maintained its hold presupposes that it was far-fetched and made impossible claims. Yet if we look at the special case of pregnancy, which was always the priority diagnosis for uroscopy, the idea that it was wholly an empty con looks less clear.[13] Whilst the universal diagnostic claims are doubtful, individual conditions and illnesses can sometimes be identified through the macroscopic inspection of urine. The internet uroscopers remind us that cloudiness can be a sign of a urinary tract infection. General practitioners today might take such cloudiness as a sign to investigate further. They might use a dipstick treated with a reagent, holding it against a chromatic wheel—a technology conjectured by the uroscopers' colour-wheel illuminations—to get a quick and early indication to

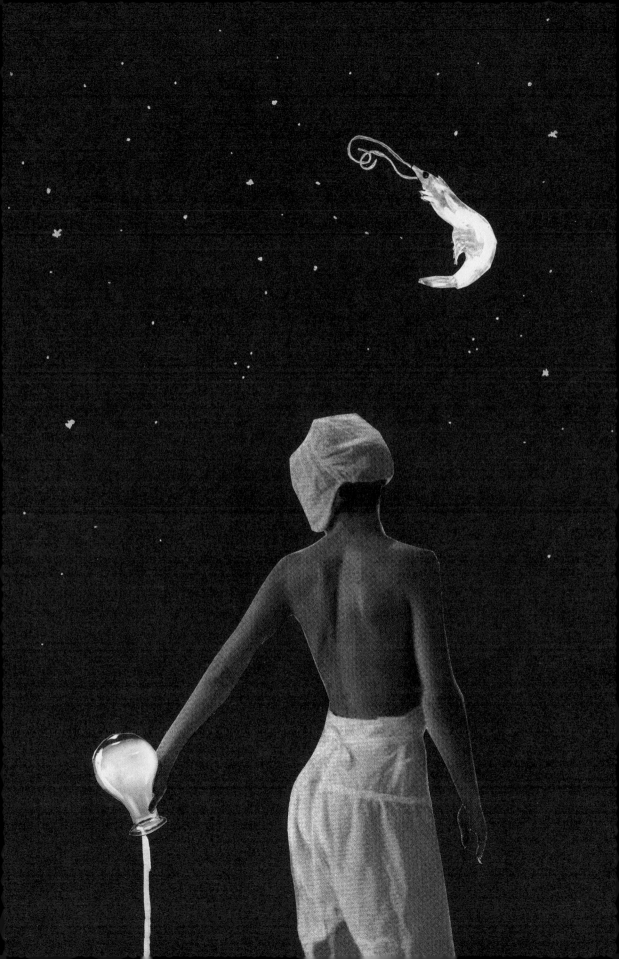

inform a prescription before more detailed results arrive from a pathology lab.

Uroscopy was a service that many medical practitioners felt they had to offer to meet customer demand and expectations. If they didn't, they would lose out to competitors who did.[14] Women wanted to know whether they were pregnant, whether they should still go riding, whether they should alter their diets or get linen and a crib. These customers distrusted the service which their medics really could offer: advice based on their clinical experience. Instead, they wanted an objective test free of the contaminating influence of patient-practitioner dialogue and subjective impressions. That dialogue, however, was likely the thing which made uroscopy "work." A good view emerges from the sceptical tradition, for example, from Thomas Brian's *The Pisse-Prophet, or Certain Pisse-Pot Lectures* (1655), a mid-seventeenth-century coney-catching treatise, purporting to be the anonymous death-bed confessions of a fraudulent uroscoper. The preface to the book states unequivocally that

> Urine is a Harlot, or a lyer, and that there is no certain
> knowledge of any disease to be gathered from urine alone,
> nor any safe judgement to be exhibited by the same.[15]

Yet the rest of the book takes a somewhat different tack, describing how pregnancy could, in fact, be diagnosed. Rather than offering a humbler confession, the dying uroscoper proudly insists that, whatever the truth claims of his competitors, *his* pregnancy diagnoses were always correct. The trick relies on the fact that the piss pot comes by messenger and clever questioning will extract information. So whilst he is waving the flask around, the uroscoper asks: When did your mistress have her last child? Is she still breast feeding? When did her periods stop? Brian's uroscoper tells how he affected to look into the flask to make the job look properly authentic: "I take the Urinal in my hand again and fall to peering into it (as though I looked for some little child there)," treating the flask as if it were the patient's body itself.[16] Brian's piss prophet also describes a pressure technique he uses to produce that patient dialogue. Aware that some clients may try to test him by refusing to speak, he arranges the piss messengers in a queue starting with the most talkative. The ones made to wait out at the gate are hopefully impatient enough to talk by the time they finally get into their consultation.[17]

What Brian's uroscoper hints at with his queuing system is the scepticism even of people who consulted uroscopers. Folktales with uroscopy plots also suggest that customers were liable to put practitioners' claims to the test. Comic narratives about urine samples dropped and swapped centre on the question of whether uroscopers could do what they said they could. For all their irreverent comedy, though, the wish-fulfilment fantasy is for uroscopy's claims to be credible. The story typically goes like this: a maid, who unbeknownst to all is pregnant, spills her master's urine on the way to the uroscoper and, being too lazy or frightened to go back, swaps in her own. The maid's am-I-aren't-I time generates the comedy in which her master is diagnosed as pregnant. Eventually, these stories reveal the maid's indiscretions and true condition but not before enjoying some anxieties about male pregnancy. Some of these male characters appear to give birth: a beetle climbs out of one man's bum, another man falls into a hare's nest and is relieved to see all the leverets he thinks he has birthed running away: "thank goodness I won't have to look after them," he says with relief, "but, look," he adds, shedding a paternal tear, "they have my ears."[18] In one of the most famous stories, recorded in the life of the ninth-century saint Notker the Stammerer, a duke decides to test the saint's medical skills by sending him a urine sample from his supposedly virginal female servant as if it were his own. "The lord is going to perform an unheard-of miracle. A man is going to have a baby!" Notker declares.[19]

Only intention distinguishes an out-and-out con from a flawed but sincere attempt to make a new idea work. We know from our own interests in scam stories, relayed to us in true-crime books and podcasts, that disambiguating fantasists, experimental scientists, and grifters is not straightforward. If we ever feel superior to the customers lining up at the uroscoper's gate, the case that should give us pause is Theranos, a company which falsely claimed to be able to diagnose hundreds of conditions and diseases from just a few pricks of blood in its "miniLabs" and "nanotainers."[20] If made to work, technology which brought phlebotomy practice and analysis down to a manageable size and painless process would have wide appeal and applications, not least in field hospitals attempting to contain disease outbreaks or in military combat zones. Some of the same fantasies are in play in the flourishing uroscopy practices of the past: a desire to master the diagnostic range through a single, mobile, and potentially at-home method.

By the time Theranos CEO and founder Elizabeth Holmes came to trial in 2021, the company's devices were in operation in Walgreen stores and elsewhere across the US, and over $700 million had been invested and lost. Well-known celebrities and politicians were caught up in the hype that slated Holmes as the next big Silicon Valley start-up success story. Theranos testing units did have some

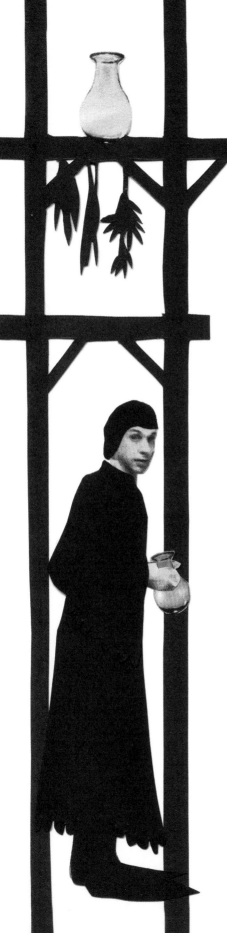

capabilities, but those capabilities weren't as extensive as claimed. Many of the tests supposedly run on Theranos units were actually run on standard third-party devices, using samples delivered by courier. When investors were shown them working, apparently in real time, a recorded result was fraudulently presented to them at the end of the demo.[21] For all that, Holmes's fraud trial was not as clear-cut as one might expect. She was found guilty but maintained that, for all its limitations, the technology was a sincere endeavour and could return valid test results, some of which were correct. Her own testimony was clouded by her seeming continuing belief in her concept. Between con and cure, there is a fudgy intersection where tests and treatments have partial efficacy and where those who vend them believe, rightly or wrongly, in their value.

Whilst Brian's *Pisse-Prophet* is clear that uroscopy is a fake science, that was not the position of all uroscopers or uroscopy manuals, which present with all sincerity, particularly in their specialism of pregnancy diagnostics. I wonder if it would interest these women in the internet forum to know that the cloudiness they think they observe is also what people in the past saw in pregnant urine. Historical descriptions of the urine of pregnant women always describe it as cloudy; if you shake it, it is said to develop even a woolly or web-like appearance.[22] This is one description from a Middle English translation of *De urinis*, a work of the late Middle Ages:

> Uryne of a whomon þt ys wt chylde here watyr schal haue clere styrpys þe moyst parte schal be trobyl
>
> [The urine of a woman that is with child, her water shall have clear stripes (or stirrups) mostly it will be troubled (or cloudy).][23]

The urine of the pregnant was not just opaque; it was also reflective:

ʒyf þu see þy face yn womanys watyr and sche be wtoute
feuyrys hyt be tokynyʒt þt sche ys wt chylde

[If you see your face in a woman's water and she is not
feverish, it means that she is with child.]

Just like the internet uroscopers, this treatise distinguishes between
urinary tract infection and pregnancy, a crucial capability within the
uroscopers' claimed expertise.

Urine inspection for pregnancy testing came with the stamp
of ancient authority. The information that pregnant urine can be
cloudy came to be extracted from comprehensive uroscopy manuals and bundled up with other so-called secrets of generation which
ended up in that popular tome *Aristotle's Masterpiece*, which I discuss in chapter 1.[24] Uroscopy for pregnancy diagnosis found its way
into its compendium of purple passages and boudoir vignettes, a
lush celebration of sexual pleasure, including female pleasure. Urine
analysis offers the technical cover for this kind of pornography, but
it is also of a piece with it: satisfying the desires to see and to know.
Desire for science, for knowledge, and for the beauty of scientific
media pulled in readers.

In *Aristotle's Masterpiece*, urine clouds took on a powerful mete-
orological character:

The best Clerks do affirm that the Urine of a Woman
with Child is white, and hath little Motes, like those in the
Sun-beams, ascending and descending in it, and a Cloud
swimming aloft of an Opal Colour; the Sediment being
divided by shaking of the Urine, appears like carded Wool.[25]

This quotation reads as if it were a direct forum post beneath the
internet uroscopers' speculation: "is pee cloudy in pregnancy?"
A reply from the past looks back to the past itself, nodding to the
authority of the clerical writers of uroscopy manuals as "the best
Clerks." The old aesthetic emphases are reproduced: of light, glass,
and jewels, along with domestic analogy (here, with carded wool).
Carded wool is not something we are particularly familiar with
now, but before mass clothing production, when most households
had to engage in small-scale textile production, the soft puffs created by teasing fleece with stiff brushes would have been a very
familiar sight.

These woolly clouds in the urine of pregnant women were eventually named and given a new technical identity by French scientist

Jacques Louis Nauche in 1831 as *kyestein* (spelled variously as *kystein* or *kyestine*).[26] This neologism was created by taking the Greek for conception, κύησις (kyesis) and adding the technical inflexion "-ine," which was being used to name the elements and other substances in a new nineteenth-century chemical lexicon (like chlorine, bromine, and so on). The mid-nineteenth century sees an agitated debate about kyestein and whether it could be used diagnostically in pregnancy. Technically, kyestein was understood to be a pellicle or skin that formed on the surface of the urine of pregnant women that had been allowed to stand for days. Obstetrical writer William Fetherstone Montgomery, whom we met in chapter 3, gives a full survey of the state of kyestein studies as they stood in the 1850s, suggesting in summary that "we should be very slow to place any confidence in such a sign" but that, "when well marked," it may have "some value as a 'corroborative indication.'"[27] Looking at different samples himself, however, he is stumped: "I confess I could not discriminate between them." The difficulty for determining whether uroscopers could diagnose pregnancy is that it wholly depended on the skill of individual readers. A self-confessedly inept reader of urine, Montgomery rules it neither out nor in.

One of the names that appears in Montgomery's survey is Elisha Kent Kane (1820–1857), who performed a series of experiments on kyestein, the results of which he wrote up as assessed work for his medical training in 1842.[28] Kane was an extraordinary figure: the chief medical officer on two expeditions to recover John Franklin on his doomed search for a Northwest Passage in the 1850s.[29] Back in the 1840s, though, he was engaged in another search: for kyestein in urine to see if he could diagnose pregnancy in contested cases. In addition to the urine of possibly pregnant and pregnant women, he also worked with urine samples taken from women who had recently had their babies and were still lactating, and he checked his results against control groups of patients with different pathological conditions. Although he develops a modern experimental method, using different groups of test subjects, he nonetheless credits the works of medieval medical writers like Avicenna (980–1037) and al-Rhazi (854–925), which, he concedes, described these clouds hundreds of years before him. Kane understood himself to be part of a very long tradition with a medieval highpoint.

Kane adopts the familiar aesthetic hallmarks of uroscopy writing, defining kyestein as

a continuous scum of an opaline white or creamy appearance, with a slight tinge of yellow, which gradually becomes deeper and more decided. The uniformity of this colour, however, is generally broken by granulated spots of a clearer white, giving it a dotted or roughened aspect. The crystals of the forming stage now appear like shining points, and I have sometimes found numerous small brownish specks, sprinkled over the surface, not unlike the gratings of nutmeg.[30]

Whilst he uses the word "crystals" here in its technical sense, referring to the process of crystallization, it also evokes, as with his use of "opaline," the preoccupation with light and precious stones in earlier literature. His final analogy is also new—"the gratings of nutmeg"—and responds to the cheapening of nutmeg in the nineteenth century.[31] Despite these renewals, there is still an attachment to the lucidity of urine and its ready comparison to a universe of domestic things, just as in the old books.

Kane presented his results in comprehensive tables, confirming whether a pellicle could be detected and, if so, after how many days. Kane's tables are a fascinating mass of information about pregnancies discovered and lost, infant death and survival, with some brief details of the circumstances of the women who found themselves caught up in his data collection. In addition to his tables, Kane also gives longer narrative histories of nine women who presented as hard cases.[32] We are sometimes given the names and ages of these women; we are often told in which ward of the hospital they were being treated. In some cases, we know that these women were Black or white, because hospital wards were colour segregated. Some of them have had many children and are already mothers. The list includes women who were deliberately pretending to be or not to be pregnant, and others who were mistaken about their own conditions. In some cases, Kane is just sorting those who were pregnant from those who weren't, with little comment about what the women themselves thought, believed, or tried to pretend. His testing technique is particularly useful for achieving those more elusive negative results.

The details of these women's lives rip vividly across time, but we have no way of finding out about how they felt either about being pregnant (or not) or winding up as a test subject in Kane's experiments. The first on Kane's list, Helen Anderson, may have been a sex worker. She was being treated on the hospital's venereal ward for gonorrhoea, and Kane describes her sexual habits pejoratively as "promiscuous." Kane successfully diagnosed her pregnancy, and she gave birth to a baby prematurely. Isabella Smith was twenty-five and came into Kane's data set from the white obstetrical wards. She seemed to have a well-advanced pregnancy, but it had not been possible to do an internal examination because she had "epileptic paroxyms," which resulted in "her temporary removal to the women's lunatic asylum," where Kane acquired a urine sample from her, presumably under duress. Kane recorded her test as negative, which satisfied him "that she was an imposter." Then, "during a well simulated paroxysm of epilepsy, her dress gave way, and disclosed an abundant mass of hair padding ingeniously arranged over the abdomen." There is no hint as to her motive or why she might have needed to pretend. Another test subject, Maria Hero, was just fifteen and borrowed urine samples from her neighbour who wasn't pregnant to hide her condition from the doctors.

Little disguises the note of triumph that Kane sounds at being able to see through women's deceptions or, in cases where there is no attempt to deceive but a genuine confusion, to read against misleading symptoms. He understands his success to be measured in the admiration of his male colleagues, who send him samples in the post and marvel that he can invariably make a correct diagnosis. He shows no empathy for the women he researched and no concern about the emergencies which brought them into his case notes. Rather, there is a desire to gain an objective vantage point on the problem of pregnancy diagnosis, wresting it from female mendacity and subjectivity, rather in the forensic mode we encountered at the end of chapter 3. Like Elizabeth Holmes, Kane's own self-belief makes it hard fully to assess the capabilities of the system he claimed to master.

Of the nine edge cases that Kane narrates in detail, three were pregnant and clearly resistant to being so, like young Maria Hero. Others were not pregnant and knew they were not, like Isabella Smith, the "imposter" with the hair bump. But there are four women who clearly believed themselves to be pregnant, in whom "the evidences of pregnancy were well marked," but who weren't. One is an unnamed Black woman who thought herself to be six months pregnant. Her periods had stopped, her abdomen swollen, and her breasts enlarged. Both she and a nurse had felt foetal movement. But her urine test was negative, and Kane discharges her from the ward. The longest of Kane's case-note entries concerns thirty-seven-year-old Mary Welsh from the white obstetrical wards. Not only had her periods stopped (they were irregular anyway) and her abdomen become swollen, but milk had also come into her breasts; she too reported foetal movements. She was multiply examined internally and externally; doctors including Kane listened with a foetal stethoscope for a uterine "souffle" or foetal "pulsation." These different physical examinations proved inconclusive. Kane's observations of her urine convinced him that she was not pregnant. "Much against her own wishes and those of her fellow patients," he discharged her to the female working wards. Confirming Kane's diagnosis, Welsh was still undelivered of her false pregnancy at the time Kane was writing, perhaps as much as a year after she began to suffer.

Years later, as he voyaged through the Canadian Arctic Archipelago looking for John Franklin, Kane turned his considerable powers of observation and description from the urine specimen bottle to the snowy wastes. His journal is full of his detailed observations of landscape and people. He is particularly in awe of ice and icebergs and was attracted, as he was in his study of kyestein, to the impression of enlightenment that crystalline matter made on him. Kane's expedition never did find Franklin, although it came upon the remains of his winter camp. Experiments into kyestein similarly went nowhere and became one of history's dead ends. Whatever clarity kyestein gives Kane, it is firmly dismissed as nonsense by scientists and medics who came after him. In the early twentieth century, Selmar Aschheim, who with Bernhard Zondek developed the first biological pregnancy test, a forerunner of the frog test considered in chapter 1, explicitly divided off his own experiments with urine from the search for kyestein, declaring it illegitimate to see any continuity between old and new urine testing for pregnancy.[33] Neither Kane's work nor that of others who were also experimenting with kyestein fed into modern diagnostic practice. Experiments into kyestein were overtaken by other means and ways of discovering pregnancy.

The Eye's Evidence

Our internet uroscopers are not an isolated crowd. Urine testing of different kinds raises the question—often asked in trying-to-conceive internet forums—of the capability of the naked eye and the difficulty of interpreting what the eye sees. The test sticks—for both ovulation and pregnancy—treated with reagents are the subject of much macroscopic inspection as reported in internet forums. There are two kinds of test sticks: those that are meant to be read by the naked eye (which display a line) and those that are meant to be read by a battery-operated machine (as in a digital pregnancy test or fertility monitor). When I armed up with an ovulation kit of the first kind

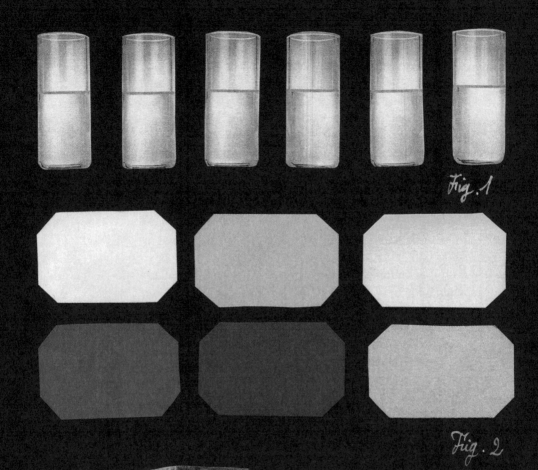

Fig. 1

Fig. 2

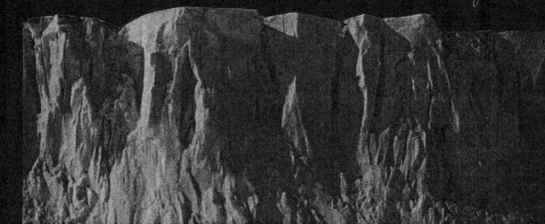

Table VI

Fig. 3

(piss and look), I found that, incompetent or infertile, even with much squinting, I could never get a clear result. Which was faulty: Me or the stick? If me, is it a fault in my reading or my ovulation? There I was, like William Montgomery failing to follow the uroscopers' method to success.

So I borrowed a digital ovulation monitor that my friend had invested in and used to get pregnant: disposable piss-on sticks that come with a machine reader to find "fertile" days. The machine took me, the subjective reader, out of the transaction by reading a urine test stick on my behalf. Like a dragon fed sacrificial victims to stave off its assault on the village, the machine demands these sticks from the end of menstruation for a couple of weeks. They are expensive, and you go through piles of them.

I got up before M. in the morning and brought the stick back; we lay in bed and watched the machine computing. "Roll up, roll up, place your bets—low, high, or peak?" I said, and then M. guessed, sometimes tentatively as if he were testing thin ice and sometimes impulsively as if a revelation had struck him. He shook his fist if he was wrong and punched the air if right. The first time the machine peaked, blinking an egg at the top of its screen, I felt pride as if I have achieved something, like ringing the bell at the top of the fairground high striker. But some months, there was nothing . . . a blinking nothing. Was I (anovulatory) or the machine (a bad reader, a rip-off) at fault?

So the next month, I didn't leave it to the machine, and like others on the forums, after the machine had its turn, I took the paper out of the stick, held it against the window, and gave my eye a go. Sometimes there was a line that the machine couldn't read but my eye could. So what is the machine for? The same is true of digital pregnancy tests, which are just the kind with a blue line inside an expensive plastic gadget with a lithium battery that uses LEDs and photosensors to detect the line, just like your eye could if it weren't obscured by gadgetry.[34] Technical computational aesthetics, the wonder of automated readers, get us every time. We are suckers for a great colour wheel or a comprehensive key to all the possible textures and grades of opacity, especially those that only experts can use or read. One morning, I catch myself concerned on behalf of the machine—that it might feel confused by my nontextbook results. Even more absurdly, I console myself that the machine has probably attended to worse, judging by the online reports of all the other outré cycles, as if my machine were part of a great Platonic machine, united with all the others blinking eggs in other women's bathrooms across the globe. It's a machine, I remind myself; it has no ghost.

M. likes fruit yoghurt, black cherry for preference. I cleaned the empty pots for tests. They weren't the best design for the purpose: the rim of the pot folded back on itself, holding, by capillary action, the urine within as if dipped in gold leaf. I really needed a medieval glass flask. But then the yoghurts got new packaging with a flat rim. M. is delighted: "Thank you, Activia, for the superior piss pots." I bought a new vitamin supplement that some modern mountebank persuaded me might help. The day after I started taking it, my wee was bright neon yellow, like Lucozade or the bottle of cheap limoncello at the back of our drinks cupboard left over from an Italian holiday. It was irradiated, resplendent, and clear. Not a cloud misted its sparkling translucency. "We're all monkey doctors now," I thought, peering in, entirely baffled.

Add-Ons

How much are we prepared to pay expert readers? Let's take our eyes away from the urine flask and look, instead, over the shoulder of a modern lab technician in a fertility clinic. We look now at images produced by an *embryoscope*: time-lapse imaging for embryo selection in IVF.[35] The embryoscope is both an incubator and an imaging system, so an embryo doesn't have to be removed from its protective environment to be evaluated. Thousands of images can be taken, rather than just the few snapped of embryos kept in conventional incubators—one every five to twenty minutes. Embryos can then be selected according to the speed between stages of their development. Run together, these images make mesmerising black-and-white films, extraordinary new sights of the first hours and days of a living fertilized egg and a potential foetus. Cells framed by the circular zona pellucid fizz as if affected by static. They divide. New cells seemingly pop into existence. Then the inner barriers come down, and the cells merge into a morula, a unified mass from which cells emerge and group, pockets forming between them, different parts differentiating themselves as the embryo becomes a blastocyst ready for transfer, if all goes well. This is by any reckoning amazing new technology, truly a glimpse into the "secrets of generation" for which those who came before us so fervently looked.

The idea is that this sequence of images can be analysed and a blastocyst can be designated as being at low, medium, or high risk of failing, based on how it relates to a standard or ideal in terms of cell division over time. If low-risk embryos can be identified and transferred into the uterus rather than their higher-risk siblings, then

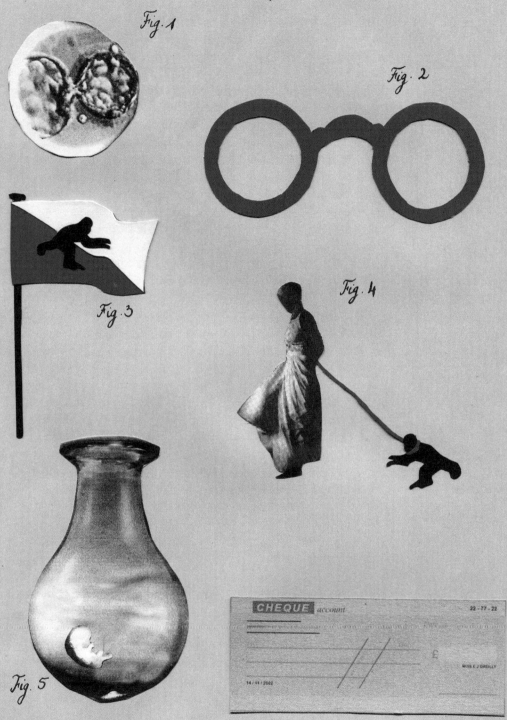

Table VII

Fig. 1

Fig. 2

Fig. 3

Fig. 4

Fig. 5

Fig. 6

the successful live birth rates in IVF might go up. This stands to reason: those embryos that look better will fare better. This is similar to the aesthetic logic that sustained and built trust in the practice of uroscopy. Both are imaging technologies; they work by taking something from within the body and exteriorising it, holding it out for view. Like uroscopy, the embryoscope is based on qualitative principles: embryos are selected according to how they compare to an ideal, whose cells divide evenly. What is less clear is that "ideal" embryos result in higher birth rates. Clinics argue, in their defence, that this is a learning technology which increasingly becomes quantitative as results are fed back into its algorithms. Selection may even become machine automated. Currently, though, this treatment relies on individual readers. I am a better reader, argues Thomas Brian's uroscoper narrator: my results are true, but I can't answer for my competition. The scientific aesthetic, the thing that pulls us in, is our own inability to interpret the marvellous and beautiful things we can see but not personally read.

The UK's regulatory body, the Human Fertilisation and Embryology Authority (HFEA), describes time-lapse imaging for embryo selection as an "add-on," one of several optional extras being sold to IVF patients.[36] In information for patients, the HFEA sets out a traffic-light system to grade these extras. Time-lapse imaging was initially given an amber light, although that has since been altered to black because, while it is unlikely to be harmful and graded red, available evidence shows it has "no effect on the treatment outcome."[37] At least this is how it is evaluated today; by the time you read this, it may have changed again. Who knows? Here is how the HFEA described this add-on when they classified it as amber:

> There have been various studies to try and see if time-lapse imaging can improve birth rates. Initial research has shown some promise, but it's still very early days. There's certainly not enough evidence to show that time-lapse imaging improves birth rates, which is something you may want to consider if it's being offered to you at an extra cost.[38]

Hopeful readers, coming to this from the firmer promises in the advertising of fertility clinics, have a bias that this confirms. There is a supposition ("still early days") that the embryoscope will eventually show results. Setting out a traffic-light system inadvertently implies that research or perhaps IVF patients travel in one direction to green. Readers have a reason to buy: this is amber, not red. Who wouldn't want to be a pioneer for science? And whatever the

outcome of your IVF round, you at least get a keepsake: a star-
tling, captivating video which might become a first image in a family album or a visual memorial of life temporally conjured up but
unsustained. So the wonder is that the early embryo now can not
only be seen developing (or not) but can be recorded and played
back. The last solemn warning in the HFEA statement is the key
reason for issuing advice to patients: money. There is no other jeopardy here: the embryoscope works on something already necessarily
extracted from the womb, and, what is more, the embryoscope is
itself protective, imaging a blastocyst that would otherwise have to
be repeatedly removed from incubation.

I think I would give an amber light to uroscopy for pregnancy
diagnosis, which also showed unproven promise. Macroscopic urine
analysis proved inconclusive because whatever its capabilities, it
relied on the expertise of individual reader-practitioners. The difference is that uroscopy was always presented as a finished and
ancient science rather than as something new and in development.
Those turning to historical uroscopers were sometimes believers
paying for a service and sometimes sceptics reluctantly gambling.
The eyewatering payments being handed over by IVF patients to
fertility clinics for add-ons work like that too, with patients more
or less aware of the unproven nature of the technique. But there is
also a difference in that the payments for IVF add-ons are financial
investments in research.[39] People are paying for the studies being
done on their own bodies. But until the results are in, should patients
pay, or should clinics be asked to fund investment? Belief, desire,
and hope are very readily monetised, and that is true now just as it
was in the past.

Only some infertility memoirists mention the money. Money is
almost more embarrassing than the sticky bodily ooze we don't like
to talk about. Money and children should not be discussed together.
As the sociologist Viviana Zelizer tells us when writing about Western historical shifts, when children were "expelled from the cash
nexus" and no longer thought of as future labour, they were increasingly sacralised, becoming in effect "priceless."[40] If your story ends
with a baby, it looks ungrateful to mention the cost of conception
success. If it doesn't, the money becomes a symbol of misplaced
hope or trust, a humiliation added on to the already considerable
humiliation of not conceiving in the first place. "Trying" proliferates
add-ons: vitamins, test kits, acupuncture, thermometers, books, and
apps are all added on to the big-ticket assisted reproductive treatments. Individual costs might be negligible, a small stretch that it
seems painless to make. Yet added together, these smaller costs make

cumulatively large debts and fortunes, depending on which side of the till you happen to stand.

I paid money just like anyone else, crediting the fertility industry with the power to improve my chances. There is always the thought that it might make the difference, that you are investing in the best chance, making the payment that will end all payments. Lying on the acupuncturist's couch once a week in my trying-to-conceive years, I consoled myself with the thought that, whether or not there was anything in the claim that acupuncture could aid fertility, I was having a mindful hour in a calming room filled with chinoiserie, listening to a kind practitioner's poetic babble about qi, and that couldn't be a wholly bad thing. Memoirist Miranda Ward gets it right when she sums it up: "this is a luxury, all of it," the luxury to waste, to spend, to invest afforded to privileged women.[41] Monied people need things to buy, and capital steps in to supply. There is no science that can show whether any of it works in individual cases, because there is no control you, no way to check outcomes against choices. Yet little dislodges the current cultural conviction that people in the past were more gullible than people today. Whilst we are discerning consumers of rational science, they are pitiful sitting targets for scam artists peddling faith cures.

The internet has fully exposed modern speculative and faith-based inclinations. Indeed, it has brought magical practitioners and divinators into people's homes and even, through their smartphones, into their pockets, moving them from boundary phenomena more centrally into more people's lives. Women in trying-to-conceive forums discuss their consultations with psychics, astrologers, and tarot practitioners as well as conventional medics. Their reviews log prices, response times, and quality of service, usually gauged in level of generality or specificity. Reviews veer between "it's just a bit of fun" to complaints about being cheated. Many people are paying for regular readings from different psychics, astrologers, and tarot practitioners; they share readings online, marking the incorrect ones red and correct ones green in another version of the traffic-light system. Some women have long lists of red readings covering a year or more. That's not to say that there isn't scepticism. Memoirist Jessica Hepburn describes a visit to a Covent Garden tarot-card practitioner where she tries not to speak, like the reticent customers of Brian's Pisse Prophet.[42] If the tarotist really could read the cards, she would know why she was being consulted: "it doesn't really work like that, my love," she tells Hepburn. Women are, at one and the same time, buying from and calling out online spam merchants, posting the manipulative pressure selling that jams up their email inboxes: "when my secretary told me your email came in, I felt an

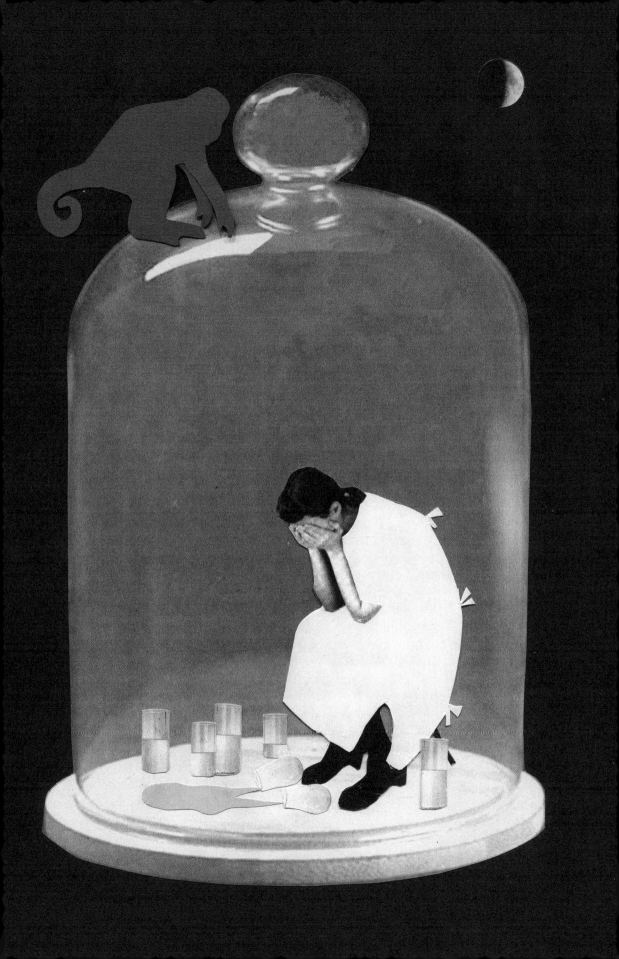

instant connection and a call from your spirit. I immediately stopped everything to personally do your reading."[43]

In his analysis of the *Los Angeles Times* astrology column in the 1950s, Theodor Adorno talks about the new detachment between astrologer and the print-reading audience: "They don't even see the sorcerers at work anymore nor are they allowed to listen to their abracadabra. They simply 'get the dope.'"[44] The internet gives users an even faster track to occult service providers. You can download ad-filled tarot and horoscope apps. New media and technologies counterintuitively enhance the aura of magical therapies and forecasts. I think of the allure of the machine blinking its egg, looking high-tech but no better (in fact, often worse) than my eye. When print replaced manuscript, the indulgences and icons that came off the press suffered no loss of authority, as one might expect.[45] Mass production, automation, and algorithms offer the prospect of a system sealed off from human interference. The readings, magical protection, promises, and fortunes that emerge from such systems must be paranormal, supernatural, divine, true. The light through the liquid crystal display technology that is your computer screen says it, so it must be true. Technological advances do not push faith into the past. We seem a long way away from the benighted confusions of people gazing into urine, yet our own intimacy with forms of bioinformation, mediated to us by light and glass, leaves us with similar "emotional and financial burdens."[46]

■

A friend of mine, let's call her Astra, once encouraged me to have my tarot cards read by her partner. He didn't exactly put on a silky turban, but together they talked up his North African heritage. Tarot, I read later, purports to have ancient and Egyptian roots but emerges from an Italian card game, not gathering its fortune-telling capabilities until the eighteenth century—in the Enlightenment, in fact.[47] Astra went first, asking if she would have another child soon. She had one already, just under a year old. He said that "soon" was too vague. "Two years?" she said. The answer was startlingly definitive: a yes. Don't these things work by fudging the answer, by meaning anything? And she did have another child, within a year of my trip. In fact, now that I think about the timings, she must have been, give or take a week or two, in her two-week wait.

Astra asked the questions that were pressing on me on my behalf, because I just felt too stupid. Silence came to me not as a premeditated test of the art but as a normal response to its claims. The first question was, "Would I have children?" The second was, "Would I have them with M.?" I was intrigued and amused by their pseudo-occult argot. I swilled wine round my glass and chuckled at them as if I didn't care. The answer to the first question was the Empress. "The pregnancy card!" Astra cheered. A yes, then? Shouldn't it show up the Nine of Wands or something less obvious and definitive? The second question returned the Fool. Ha, ha, ha. Too true, I thought, remembering the frustration which had sent me packing off on a trip on my own. But I'm told that the Fool is not just a big cosmic laugh but the card of new beginnings, of unexpected turn-ups, of slightly impractical but joyful change, neither a yes nor a no. The Empress and the Fool. That's us, for sure. But the glance into the future felt less fun than advertised. There was a weight to it somehow because of its uncanny perspicacity. No money changed hands, but trust had been solicited and, despite myself, given.

6 Jeux d'esprit: Testing the Limits

I had not been content with the results promised
by the modern professors of natural science.
With a confusion of ideas only to be accounted
for by my extreme youth, and my want of a
guide on such matters, I had retrod the steps
of knowledge along the paths of time, and
exchanged the discoveries of recent enquirers for
the dreams of forgotten alchymists.
—Mary Shelley, *Frankenstein; or, the Modern
Prometheus* (1831)[1]

Low-Tech Help

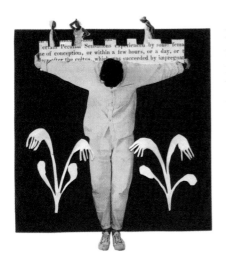

HE TREATMENT ROOM in an old church hall is divided from the waiting area by brown and orange curtains. I wait alongside two older men: one is coughing urgently, and the other can hardly walk. When my name is called, my blood is pulled from under papery blue-veined skin into a glass phial and labelled. I had gone to the doctor about something else and mentioned that we were taking a while to conceive. I left the room with the forms for two tests: mine was for a blood test, and M.'s was for a sperm test.

"Do I have to fill that?" M. says, turning the empty sample bottle for his semen test over in his hand. The bottle is accompanied with clear but intricate instructions in SHOUTING capitals:

> There are NO facilities at the hospital for producing the
> sample. Samples MUST be delivered within an hour.
> Samples MUST be delivered between 9 and 12. The sample
> MUST be produced after 3 DAYS of abstinence. NO testing
> will be done on weekends or bank holidays.

"Wank holidays," says M.

"Do you want to wait," I say, "to see if we get pregnant this month before bothering?"

"Nope," he says. "Never turn down an opportunity to have your virility confirmed."

I offer to help him by dropping him at the door, but he says he'd like to do it alone, as though he's circumnavigating the world solo, producing the sample, driving, parking, and running to the haematology department. Stop the clock!

My test is also time-sensitive and is to be done "seven days after you ovulate and on day twenty-one of your cycle," the doctor says.

I explain that I don't ovulate on day fourteen, so it wouldn't be seven days for me.

"But you'll do it on *your* day twenty-one," he says.

"Right . . . ," I say, unsure, and then, as if to point out the futility of my resistance to medical authority, I do ovulate around day fourteen after all.

A few weeks later, I am back in the doctor's surgery, this time with M. The doctor looks for my results first but can't find them.

"Well, never mind," he says. "If you have regular periods, we probably do know you're ovulating, anyway." Then he goes to look for M.'s test results. The only test result available for M. is a vaginal swab.

"No wonder we're having problems," says M.

"Well, they're pretty hard to interpret anyway," the doctor says. "This doesn't stop us moving forward."

The doctor dictates a referral to a hospital consultant into a tape recorder, using a soft tone like a late-night DJ: "Thank you for seeing this thirty-seven-year-old lady and her forty-one-year-old partner."

He turns off the machine and checks how long we've been trying. We give the agreed response of eighteen months, although it's not been that long.

"They've been trying for two years to conceive with no success so far," he dictates into the tape recorder. He explains that the consultant will see us sooner if we say we've been trying for longer, which is sensible "given your age."

Out in the car park, we collapse into giggles about the irresolution of our lost results for meaningless tests, like a miniature version of the whole trying-to-conceive experience. Objective information and real answers seem to be available, but, as you reach out for them, they dissolve.

"And what about the trying-time inflation!" I say.

"We're going to be someone's major success story. We're going to break medical history," says M.

That fantasy was as close as we came to infertility treatment, because somehow our referral also got lost, and a pregnancy put paid to the need to chase it up.

The Frankenstein Reflex

Here we are, then, at the cutting edge. This is the state of the art. I start with that rather low-tech encounter to remind us that we still have not met the future imagined by high-tech science fiction before I turn to consider science fiction that looks back to the past. This retrospective sci-fi looks over a dark and disturbing edge. The last chapter looked at some of the financial costs of trying to conceive at an experimental frontier and the reasons that we might pay them. This chapter looks at other costs: the human ones. I particularly look at some early nineteenth-century science fiction and the dance it did with science facts to discover the price that was paid in the reach for knowledge.

Other historians have also been interested in historical science fiction in relation to reproduction.[2] Science writer Philip Ball, for example, has considered the ethical and philosophical debates surrounding IVF but shows that those debates were already underway in historical stories about designing and making people.[3] He has searched through monster myths and accounts of people assuming or at least trying to assume godlike powers, finding the idea of "making life by art" to be very old.[4]

Whilst, like Ball, I consider IVF, mostly I am interested in somewhat different terrain: earlier inquiries about the different moving parts of conception, such as establishing timelines for the menstrual cycle and dating pregnancies—attempts to gather the kind of knowledge which "provided the medical groundwork" for the IVF project.[5] In chapter 1, I consider a breakthrough moment in this area with the separate research programmes of Kyusaku Ogino and Hermann Knaus in the twentieth century, but now I move back to a point where those breakthroughs were way off in the future. Breakthroughs depend on a prior culture of researching and imagining, and that prior culture is what concerns me here. In my first chapter, I ask that we hold in mind the women who contributed their bodies to that scientific research; in this chapter, women as test subjects are front and centre.

Perhaps the most famous of the making-people stories is Mary Shelley's novel *Frankenstein; or, the Modern Prometheus* (1818/1831). It is so famous that it is hard to write a book on the science of reproduction and not mention it. Philip Ball, for example, also discusses it and notes the "knee-jerk" ways that book is used to cast suspicion on modern assisted reproduction.[6] The unthinking use of the connection between *Frankenstein* and modern reproductive technologies causes pain to people who have used IVF to try for pregnancy and annoyed their doctors, and I do not want to aggravate those hurts here. I am not interested in warning against the dangers of modern therapies for infertility or in telling others what they should and shouldn't put their bodies through to come to parenthood. What interests me instead is the novel's position in time—written at the beginning of the nineteenth century but looking back to the Middle

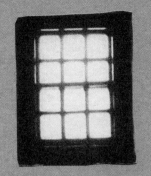
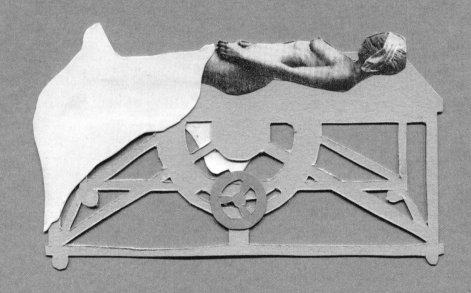
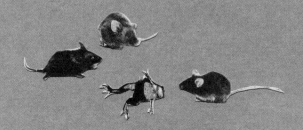

Ages as the source of secret knowledge about generation. This backwards glance is a different "knee-jerk," this one triggered by seeing the limits of modern scientific understandings of reproduction.

I want to return briefly to a quotation I considered when I first introduced this retrospective reflex. It is from Ariel Levy's memoir about growing up and coming to parenthood, as I did, after the IVF revolution:

> The shots and the pills, the sonograms and the ultrasounds, the ICSI and ovulation induction, the treatments at the very edge of modern technology, were miserable in a way that seemed, ironically, medieval. But they were not without a whiff of excitement. Because we were playing with a power much greater than even sexuality: nature herself.[7]

Levy is remembering how our generation's sex education syllabus was marked by the buzz around new reproductive technologies. We pitied the people who were subjected to scientific intervention, but the mood was one of excitement about what medical scientists were trying to do, which we mistook for what they could do. Before it mattered to any of us, we were consoled with the thought that if we ever needed them, we'd be held and helped by these advances. We envisaged this technological salvation bathed in the hygienic blue glow of the fantasy clinic but with a frisson borrowed from much older sorts of stories. New assisted reproductive therapies evoked for our generation a strange combination of horror and excitement both futuristic and anachronistic—as Levy says, medieval.

How can the newest most futuristic things we can imagine look or feel medieval? How is it that when we animate experimental monsters, we feel the pull of the past? In this chapter, I look back at the past and find it also looking back at the past to make the futures that we now inhabit. One of the uses of the Frankenstein reflex, I suggest, is that it enables both a rejection of the costs of science and experiment as well as an ownership of their advances. This book is centrally about the way that we disavow some immutable aspects of life—uncertainty, delay, disappointment, and, for this chapter, cruelty and violence—by imagining them to be more associated with the past than the present.

The Frankenstein reflex is part of that tendency, and locating it historically reminds us that people in the past also thought they were modern and, like us, spent time pretending that the things which they couldn't face were historical, even medieval. The phrase in my chapter title, "Jeux d'esprit," comes from a nineteenth-century science-fiction fantasy by a doctor and naturalist, Robert Lyall (1789–1831), which he described as a joke, a jeu d'esprit, although it lays out an elaborate plan for a cruel experiment involving the incarceration of women in a gothic "experimental conception hospital." As we'll discover, what Lyall's fiction refuses to see is the contemporary fact of slavery, which is patently interlaced in the problem that his imaginary experiment is designed to resolve. The Age of Enlightenment was also an age of slavery. These things are not opposites but coordinates.

The Frankenstein reflex is both contemporary and historical; it inspired both this book and also the historical material it explores. Lyall, writing in the early nineteenth century, saw his age as being modern but as facing research impasses which only the past, because of its lower ethical standards, could resolve. Holding the thought of Lyall's modernity in mind avoids an overly clarified approach to the history of medical ethics: on the one hand, thinking of the past uniquely as a place where men like Robert Lyall were taken up with the thrill of discovery and saw women and their bodies as research objects and little more; and, on the other hand, seeing the present as a time when medical science is altruistic and trained on empowering patients. We have already seen the confusion of research and treatment in chapter 5's discussion of the embryoscope, but there are other stories that challenge modern complacency.

When I began asking questions about how women in the past knew they were pregnant or how they thought about the am-I-aren't-I time, I first spoke with women who had had their children before home tests were available for purchase. Margaret, a friend of M., had her children in the late 1960s and early 1970s.

"Of course, there were no home tests then," I said to her, by way of a prompt.

"There *were*," she said. When she was breastfeeding her first child and her periods were disrupted, she had gone to the doctor wondering if she were pregnant again. He gave her what she described to me as a "disclosure tablet." I'd never heard of such a thing. Apparently, if you weren't pregnant, it would bring on your period. "But," she told me, "I didn't take it. For one thing it was huge, and I didn't fancy swallowing it. For another, I had read about the Thalidomide babies, and I wasn't sure I should."

I went away and started reading. What a snake pit of a disaster she avoided. Margaret was probably given a hormone pregnancy test called Primodos or something very like it. Primodos has since been shown to have caused birth defects in the children of some of the women who took it. Those women and their now-adult children are still, to this day, embroiled in seeking redress from the drug company (first Schering and now Bayer) and the government bodies that should have protected them. The story is complicated and devastating: silenced whistleblowers who had their careers blocked, stolen and suppressed documents, undercover investigators, cover-ups and denials, and the craven complicity of regulators.[8] In a weird moment, I discovered that my great-uncle, Cedric Carter, an expert in birth abnormalities at Great Ormond Street Hospital in the 1960s and 1970s, had written against his colleague, Isabel Gal, when she tried to raise the alarm and was making the comparison with Thalidomide that had instinctively occurred to Margaret.[9] The charitable reading here is that doctors like my great-uncle were defending the contraceptive pill, a revolutionary social good that was closely related to Primodos and was made of the same ingredients as that drug. Both were products of the same company. The problem, though, as Gal pointed out unheeded, is that it wasn't necessary to test for pregnancy like this; there were other ways. Primodos was marketed as a pregnancy test longer in the UK than it was elsewhere; money and corporate reputations were put over people's health.

But what about Margaret and her family doctor? I can't imagine that he wanted to harm her or her unborn child. A pill was cheap and a home test, something that Margaret could use herself to settle her am-I-aren't-I time. Medical culture was also immersed in trust: pills were modern, the future. Pharmaceuticals, most notably the pill and antibiotics, were changing medicine and improving and saving lives. There was a fantasy here though, too, fed by innovations in space exploration and the democratisation of air travel: the delivery of all sorts of things in pill form, in neat doses, on compartmentalised trays and in blister packs. Modernity was jet propelled, and, with it, all our needs and wants could be condensed into handy lozenges. A pill that could give you knowledge, a disclosure pill, could banish the unknown to the past.

The Primodos advertisements, aimed at family practitioners like Margaret's, featured the frogs discussed in chapter 1. Frog tests were expensive and slow, the ads pointed out. They looked historical and unmodern. Primodos, on the other hand, was progress: quick and more readily made available. The desire for a home test, as we have seen, is powerful: a dream of domesticating and mastering diagnosis. Lodged in the collaboration of people's desires to know and of others to help is an investment in the idea of our moment now being technologically advanced. A puzzle that I've not been able to resolve is that Primodos does not seem to have been a very large tablet of the kind that Margaret recalled.[10] Perhaps it loomed large in another way. Luckily, for whatever reason—her knowledge of Thalidomide and her better-safe-than-sorry instinct—it seemed to her to be a hard pill to swallow.

Inside the Experimental Conception Hospital

Imagine me as I stand before a great gate in a hundred-foot-tall perimeter wall (as high as a good-sized church steeple). When the gate opens, I am thrust through it by my abductors, whom I no longer bother to resist. Inside, when my eyes grow accustomed to the shadowy light, I find myself dwarfed by a dark Gothic-looking building. It seems old, medieval, but as I move closer, I see it is actually quite new. The gate shuts with ground-shaking finality. I am now trapped between the sky-high wall behind me and a forbidding entrance before me. The door is framed by a coat of arms displaying the words "Experimental Conception Hospital" above a motto, "Scientia Sit Potentia" (knowledge is power). A uniformed matron or a nun waits for me to make my way to the foot of the steps, which, seeing no alternative, I do, haltingly.

The date is 1830. I am young and friendless and have fallen on hard times. I own nothing but my clothes, and those are taken from me almost immediately after I am processed—brought to the dormitory space, washed in a communal bathroom, and given a uniform, a different one from the uniform worn by the staff members who have shepherded me through this process. A staff member fills out a form, but I manage to see only odd words and numbers, tables awaiting data, as it is filled out ("Unmarried," "Unknown," "#96") and then filed. Once dressed in my new clothes, I am taken to the great hall, which is full of other women who are sitting on benches at long tables and eating a midday meal. A few faces turn to look at me but with little curiosity. Some are older than I am, but many seem to be about my age. I am taken to a counter where a server gives me a tray of food, which I take, shivering, to a space amongst the other diners.

"New?" I am asked once the matrons have moved off.

I nod.

"You'll get used to it."

My new companion is trying to be kind, I can see, but this observation is the most frightening part of all.

■

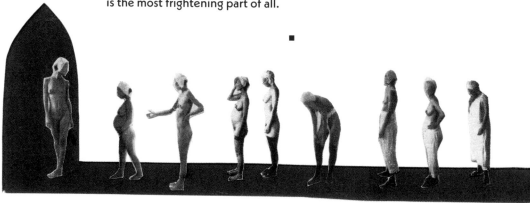

Chapter 6

This fictional institution isn't an invention of mine, although I've made up this firsthand account. The Experimental Conception Hospital was the brainchild of Robert Lyall, a Scottish medic, traveller, and botanist. He offers it as a humorous footnote—a "jeu d'esprit," he calls it—in his commentary on medical evidence on the duration of human pregnancy heard in a sensational peerage dispute over the fatherhood of a son born to Lord Gardner's adulterous wife, Maria, heard by the Committee for Privileges of the House of Lords in 1825 and 1826.[11] Lyall's "joke" is to imagine an experiment which would discover the true and precise length of human gestation by working out how to diagnose pregnancy and so how to determine from what point to date it. His solution is a purpose-built hospital in the medieval style which houses a hundred women. These are test subjects in a grand experiment who are "visited" with "physic and consolation" by vetted medical men. The statistics on their cycles, pregnancies, and childbirths are collected by matrons recruited from Catholic convents to ensure their probity and the accuracy of their record-keeping, although the matrons are also necessarily required to be hypocrites because they are overseeing an experiment which involves the repeated rape of a hundred women. This laboratory would need, Lyall reasoned, to be top-secret facility with a high perimeter wall, higher even than ordinary prison walls. He particularly worries about hot-air balloons (a new technology) because aeronauts might see in through windows or even carry off women from upper windows: "All aeronauts," he pronounces, "shall be forbidden from approaching the same edifice upon pain of death."

Lyall's hospital is a gothic fantasy building, the Frankenstein reflex in architectural form. It looks across at the dark and gloomy religious houses in contemporary novels like Matthew Lewis's (1775–1818) *The Monk* (1796), set around the Capuchin monastery in Madrid and a convent which houses a community of evil nuns of the kind that staff Lyall's hospital. Historical architectural settings and foreign Catholic villains give both Lewis and Lyall free rein to explore erotic desires about locking up and exploiting women: they pretend this is a vision of the past or of other cultures in other

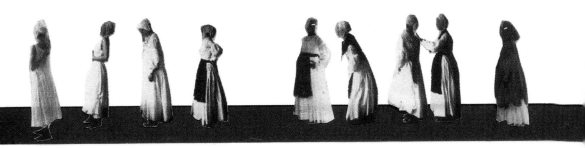

Jeux d'esprit

places somewhere unrelated to Britain. Lyall takes Gothic fantasy like Lewis's into the medical arena. Now sex might mean science, and its findings could be knowledge. For Lyall, only in the Middle Ages could a laboratory so abhorrent and so obviously at odds with modern practices exist. When he snaps back from his daydream to the reality of the present, he rules it out: "religion, morality, and decency equally forbid it," he says.

The minutes of the Committee for Privileges hearings are available to read in the UK Parliamentary Archives in beautiful manuscript booklets bound with hand-marbled paper.[12] In them, the Gardners' servants give a consistent account of domestic dysfunction: adultery and a secret birth. The medical evidence that the committee heard, however, was bewildering. Seventeen medical practitioners testified, and with every new witness called, the more confusing the issue of dating pregnancy became. No one could agree on the event to diagnose pregnancy from: a particular sexual encounter, the last period, quickening, or "certain peculiar sensations," which some witnesses understood to be the female orgasm and others thought of as a sensation felt hours or days after sex. The exact relationships between menstruation, intercourse, and conception were not known; every witness had a different theory and method of diagnosis. The medical witnesses' collective testimony was an anthology of strange tales from their case notes. The presiding judge commented later, when he was hearing another case that also revolved around a disputed pregnancy, that it would take much to surprise him after what he had heard in the Gardner case.[13]

Captain Alan Gardner, second Baron Gardner, had been at sea from early February 1802 until mid-July, yet the medical evidence didn't entirely rule him out as the father of a child born in early December (which would mean that the gestation was either five or ten months). The dates were fixed by the logbook of Gardner's ship and the compelling testimony of the crew. One witness told the committee that everyone was relieved that Mrs. Maria Gardner's visit to the ship before it sailed hadn't coincided with the execution of nine men for mutiny two days before. Lyall, in his commentary, was frustrated. How could it be that men of science had arrived at this supremely modern moment in an age of such extraordinary discovery and invention and yet knew so little about monitoring and understanding the female reproductive body, which was so familiar and near at hand and yet apparently beyond comprehension? His reference to the aeronauts shows him looking at the fact that people could now literally fly and yet this down-to-earth problem about pregnancy was still unresolved. Lyall complained that "we are nearly in the same state, on these points, as were the most ancient fathers of medicine," observing the same historical lag that Mary Shelley had fictionalised in *Frankenstein* less than a decade earlier.[14]

If you could build and secure such a place as the Experimental Conception Hospital, Lyall figures, then reproductive knowledge could be nailed down and used to serve the interests of the "Great British Parliament." The aim was to establish the right lineage for the transfer of property and title rather than anything more altruistic. He is amused by his idea and jokes that others would be, too, if it could ever come off, suggesting that he be given a £20,000 reward—a fortune in 1826—for sorting out this knotty aspect of medical jurisprudence. What selfless social duty and what dedication to all that's right! A contemporary review of Lyall's commentary in the medical journal *The Lancet* marvels at the sexual athleticism that the experiment would necessitate. "Few practitioners carry about them enough of 'physic and consolation' to dispense the Doctor's prescription," the reviewer observes, adopting Lyall's euphemistic "physic and consolation" to describe sex: "one would wonder, indeed, how an idea so wholly unprecedented, so far surpassing the conceptions of ordinary mortals, should have entered his [i.e., Lyall's] head; but he has travelled much, and doubtless has seen many wonderful things."[15] Critical though the review may be, it spares no moment for the experimental subjects who are holed up in Lyall's hideous erotic fantasy.

Lyall wasn't alone in writing science fiction about women in purpose-built research institutions. In one of the less commented on parts of his *Panopticon Writings*, Jeremy Bentham (1748–1832) invents a girls' school which has some striking similarities to Lyall's hospital. Bentham even uses the same phrase that Lyall uses, "jeu d'esprit," to license his frivolity and the words "experiment" and "experimental" in recognition of the "scientific" nature of panoptical social-engineering projects.[16] The Panopticon was a design idea for all sorts of institutions—prisons, factories, schools, hospitals, asylums, workhouses—which featured a blacked-out central surveillance tower which, with or without an actual superintendent inside, forced self-regulation on the inmates. Bentham enthuses that his panoptical design in girls' schools could ensure the pupils' virginity, outdoing old folkloric virginity tests, or enable an experiment in which "you keep up a sixteen or eighteen years separation between the male and female part of your young subjects; and at the end of that period see what the language of love would be."[17] Bentham's joke suggests that watching girls would be a way either to ensure their good sexual conduct or to discover the wholesome truth of human sexuality, shorn of the confected trappings of society and family. He imagines that these experiments would serve some social

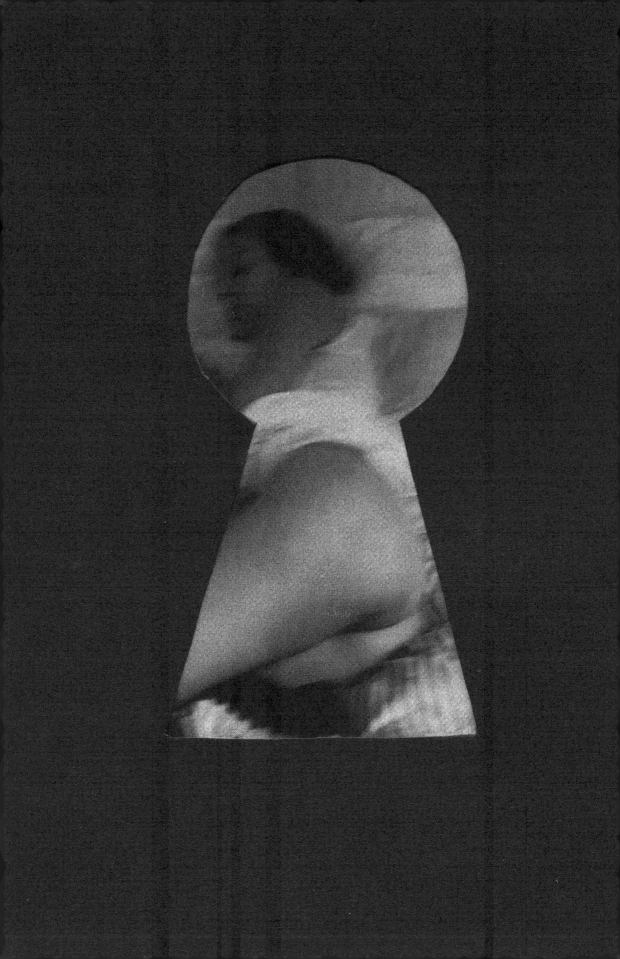

good, rather in the same way that Lyall pretends his experiment would be nothing more and nothing less than a patriotic service.

The problem with the idea that Bentham's and Lyall's science fantasies are hypothetical jokes, mere jeux d'esprit, is that women's reproduction and sexuality *were* being monitored and marshalled in all sorts of ways. Controlling reproduction was central to perpetuating European empires. Producing the next generation of powerful families, soldiers, and colonial administrators was a national duty. Women like Maria Gardner were clearly thorns in the side of this world order. But the Gardner case is not the story of only one family. It arose because Captain Gardner was away furthering British colonial interests in the Caribbean. Those interests remind us that whilst Bentham's and Lyall's plans for subjugating female sexuality and reproductivity were hypothetical, in truth something horrifyingly similar was widely practised. Many commentators on the history of slavery have written and are writing about the human breeding programmes that were pursued in Caribbean colonies. In an afterword to a poetry collection which explores the silencing of and violence experienced by Caribbean women, the poet M. NourbeSe Philip puts it like this: "In the New World, the female African body became the site of exploitation and profoundly anti-human demands—forced reproduction along with subsequent forceful abduction and sale of children."[18]

Fort St. George to London

Alan Gardner and Maria Adderley first met in the 1790s, not in the Caribbean but in another British colonial outpost: Fort St. George in Chennai (then Madras) on the east coast of India. Maria was the young stepdaughter of the governor, Lord Hobart (for whom the port city in Tasmania was named). In 1796, Alan Gardner was a young sea captain in charge of a warship, *The Heroine*, which was part of a force fighting the Dutch for control of Sri Lanka (then Ceylon). After a short courtship and marriage, Maria Gardner made the long sea journey with her new husband to England, eventually making home in a townhouse at 10 Portugal Street, London. Available evidence does not show how old she was; she couldn't have been older than nineteen and was possibly considerably younger.

In early February 1802, Gardner captained another ship, *The Resolution*, from Portsmouth to various destinations in the West Indies, leaving his wife behind in England. According to the later testimony of Mrs. Gardner's ladies' maid, Susanna Baker, whilst Gardner slept in his ship's cabin, rocking on the Caribbean Sea, his wife was in a "tumbled bed" in their house in Portugal Street with Henry Jadis, the nephew of the Earl of Strathmore. By the time Gardner returned in mid-July 1802, Maria was pregnant. Gardner was delighted and attentive, buying in linen from Abrahms of Houndsditch, the same shop that supplied the ship's stores. The longer the pregnancy went on, however, the more difficult Maria saw it would be to pass her baby off as Gardner's; she confided in Susanna that she didn't think the child could be "brought in on time." To try to precipitate the labour, she drove fast over cobbles in her carriage and, when that didn't work, told people that she wasn't pregnant after all but suffering from an illness which she had mixed up with pregnancy, a "dropsical" condition which manifested itself as spasms "occasioned by obstructions."

When she went into labour in early December, Captain Gardner was distracted by Maria's brother, who took him on a two-day excursion, and the baby was taken to a Mrs. Bailey, a wet nurse living in Swallow Street. Susanna Baker testified that the baby was "took out secretly" but did not remember, when cross-examined, how secretly, whether its "face was peeping through the flannel" or whether it was carried like a "child, a bundle of linen, or a parcel." Maria visited Swallow Street, sometimes accompanied by her brother and sometimes by a man disguised "in a large great coat and large handkerchief bound around his mouth." In July 1803, some eight months after baby Henry was born, a servant told Captain Gardner about the birth and his wife's infidelity, precipitating the couple's separation. After the Gardners' divorce in 1805, Maria married Henry Jadis, and he acknowledged baby Henry as his son. "Did he caress the Child and treat it as his own?" Susanna Baker was asked in the peerage committee hearing. "Yes he did," she said.[19]

Although Maria Gardner (by then, Maria Jadis) was alive in 1825 when the peerage dispute was heard in the House of Lords committee, she was never called to give her side of the story. Indeed, across three legal actions—a damages suit, a divorce, and a peerage dispute—her words were heard only secondhand by report from the household servants. We can only wonder at how she might have told her own story. Would she tell a pitiful tale of being ripped from her family and married very young to a naval captain who was frequently absent, maintaining cultures of violence in the Caribbean? The evidence we have suggests that she was a woman of considerable means and agency who was able to choreograph an elaborate ballet of medical professionals, including well-known London midwife John Clarke (1760–1815), and to manage a secret pregnancy and birth and the childcare that came in its aftermath. Captain Gardner's loyal manservant couldn't disguise his outrage about Maria's

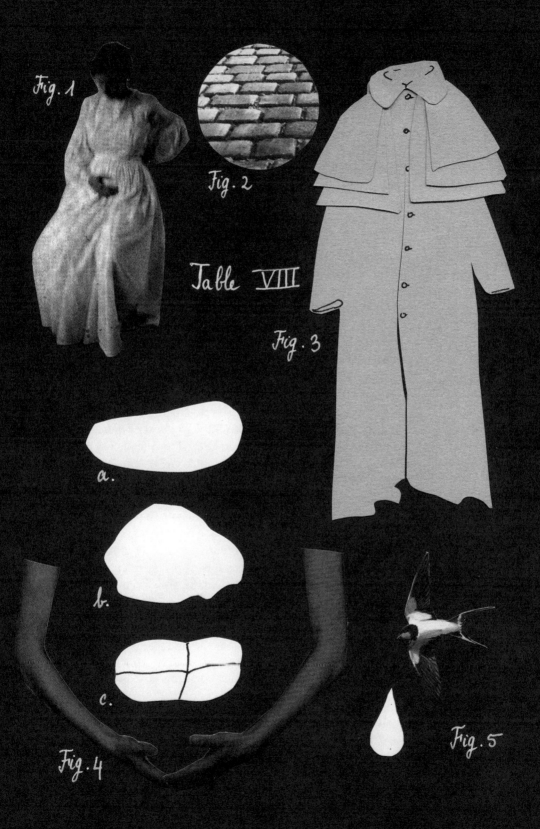

Fig. 1

Fig. 2

Fig. 3

Table VIII

a.

b.

c.

Fig. 4

Fig. 5

independent comings and goings from the couple's home as her ladies' maid walked a few paces behind carrying her lapdog. For several months into early motherhood, she maintained the fiction of herself as loyal to her husband and the larger structures of family and social respectability.

One of the things we can glean from Maria Gardner's story, albeit as it is told by others, is that the difficulty of diagnosing pregnancy was so normal, so anticipated, that it offered a ready-made cloak of fiction that could be taken down and put on by women like Mrs. Gardner whilst they anxiously worked out what to do. The am-I-aren't-I time gave women hiding nonmarital pregnancies, like Maria, a period in which they could make the world as they wanted it to be. Medical confusions around a pregnancy diagnosis and the length of gestation also held out opportunities for the legal team that later represented Henry Jadis, her son, in the peerage dispute. In the confusion of possibilities that emerged from the medical witnesses' testimony, there needed to be only one which proved that a successful pregnancy had extended to ten or more months. One example would trump all the servants' testimony, forcing the peerage committee to resort to the ordinary assumption built into medical jurisprudence in a world before paternity tests—that a man whose wife gave birth during their marriage was the child's father.

After all the paperwork was produced and all the speculation was generated, no one could definitively answer the questions which Maria Gardner's body raised. All the medical evidence was disregarded as confusing and contradictory. The one proven outlier that Henry Jadis's legal team sought could not be found. The case was settled in favour of Captain Gardner's son by his second wife, on the strength of the less technical evidence from the servants. In his commentary on the case, Robert Lyall is irritated by the fact that trying to work out legitimacy by using medical logic was a lost cause. Lyall is fixed on the fantasy of pinpointing everything and getting precise figures. He rolls his eyes about the lazy calculations that the medical witnesses make. In the end, he gives up his attachment to precision, throwing up his hands:

> Nature will not be limited by the opinions of man—she will not recognize human laws—she often delights in secrecy—she triumphs over the physiologist and the philosopher, by the incomprehensibility of her works, and by showing him his nothingness in the scale of her operations.[20]

Male scientists shrink to nothing when they are faced with the tricksy female reproductive body, written up here as the allegorical figure of nature herself. For Lyall, women *are* the limits of science.

In his 1837 textbook on pregnancy and gestation, the obstetrician William Fetherstone Montgomery (who we met in chapter 3) gives us a coda on the Gardner dispute, presented as an amusing anecdote (a jeu d'esprit, perhaps) that he heard from a colleague, a Dr. Reid. One of the female midwives who gave evidence at the Gardner peerage hearing (Montgomery doesn't name her, but based on his description, it must be Mary Ann Farrell) testified that she had gone beyond ten months with her final, seventh pregnancy. She knew, she said to the committee hearing the case, because in all her pregnancies she fainted at quickening and so couldn't mistake it. Since the hearing, however, she had consulted Dr. Reid as a patient, stating herself to be seven months pregnant with a new pregnancy: "the fainting had occurred as usual, the movements of the child were strong, and she had, in fact, all her established indications; on examination, she proved not to be pregnant at all."[21] Mary was a professional midwife, the mother of at least seven children, a woman of experience and knowledge, fighting her corner in a world overtaken by male midwives and sneering men like Montgomery and Reid, and yet she was humiliatingly outfoxed by her own am-I-aren't-I time. Montgomery's amusement, though, may well be a cover for his own anxiety, which as we saw earlier is never far from the surface in his writing on pregnancy diagnosis. Misdiagnosing pregnancy could dash a professional reputation. Montgomery's laughter is hollowed out by the intractability of the is-she-isn't-she time, which could afflict even very esteemed practitioners despite the strength of their knowledge and experience.

London to Kingston

There are other stories entwined with that of Captain Alan Gardner and Maria Gardner. Maria's adultery was given occasion by her husband's absences in the Caribbean. He was no stranger there. Members of the family of Gardner's mother were sugar planters and slave owners. His mother was born in Jamaica, and his grandfather had been born and buried there. At his death in 1774, Gardner's grandfather "owned" fifty-three slaves: twenty-eight men, seventeen women, and eight children.[22] Gardner had connections, then, that spanned the world from Kingston to London to Chennai, which meant that the Gardner scandal was the talk of the whole empire. Maria Gardner's adultery—her stepping away from her supposed responsibility for breeding the next generation of imperial servants— was shocking. When Gardner's brother, also a naval officer, paid a social call on Maria Nugent, the wife of the governor of Jamaica in

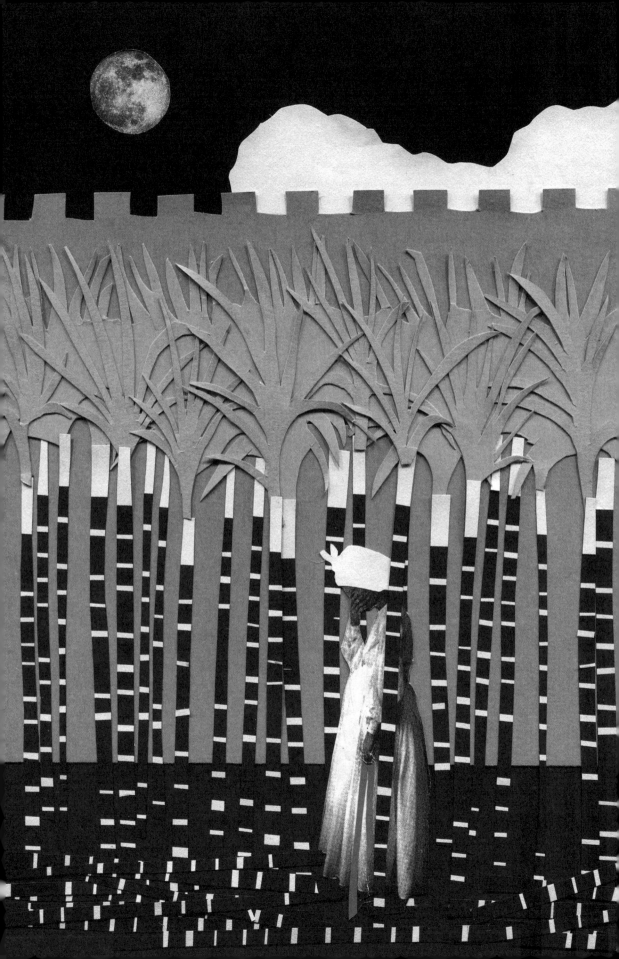

May 1805, a newspaper covering the Gardners' divorce case (then being trawled over in the London courts) lay open on the table between them. They sat together for hours as she discreetly tried to to close it, although later he surprised her by opening up "the whole history himself . . . discussing his brother's affairs fully," and she found that her "delicacy . . . was not at all necessary."[23]

Nugent's journal is full of these sensibilities and the complexities of etiquette involved in running a programme of society events like balls and dinners for resident and visiting dignitaries. Such niceties offer a shocking contrast to the fact of the slave plantations across Jamaica and the whole of the New World. The other hypocrisy is the anxiety threaded throughout Nugent's journal about the health of her children set alongside her participation in a system which had so little care for the health of African women and their children. Nugent manages these tensions by imagining herself in opposition to those bad actors who abused slaves—arguing that corrupt individuals rather than the whole institutional edifice were the problem. Nugent wasn't the only one who used that self-distancing argument. It is also on display in the journal of Matthew Lewis, who was the author of *The Monk* (1796), an English MP, and a Jamaican slave owner (referred to earlier in this chapter). On the death of his father in 1812, Lewis inherited two sugar estates which were much larger concerns than that of Gardner's grandfather, although by no means the largest in Jamaica. One year before Lewis came into his inheritance, his Hordley estate in the east of Jamaica and his Cornwall estate in the west together ran on the labour of 634 enslaved people.[24] Like Nugent, Lewis distances himself from a supposed bad side of slavery, fancying himself a "good" and even reluctant slave owner of "happy" slaves, contrasting his own character and conduct with the abusive owners and managers of other sugar estates.[25]

During the quarter century between the events hashed over in the Gardner divorce and 1825, when the Gardner peerage dispute came to the House of Lords and Robert Lyall was dreaming up the Experimental Conception Hospital, the English laws of slavery had changed. In 1807, the traffic of slaves was banned in the British empire, although British slavery continued until 1834. On the banning of the transport of enslaved people, slave owners had a greater vested interest in the health of their human "chattel" and in keeping them alive and fit for work by making improvements to their living conditions. This self-interest in the health of slaves also extended to slave fertility and maternity provisions. Although it was no longer legal to sell enslaved people newly arrived from Africa, there was still an internal market for their resale across the New World. Yet the easiest and cheapest way of acquiring new slaves was reproduction by human husbandry.[26] Many historians have written about the effects of this 1807 legal change. For example, Shauna J. Sweeney writes that it "pushed women's reproductive labor . . . to the center of transatlantic debates over the future of the British imperial economy."[27] Matthew Lewis's first visit to his Caribbean estates comes at the point at which the emphasis on reproduction—essentially, breeding programmes—had taken strong hold. Oversight of slave populations meant understanding reproduction in humans.

Lewis's journal is an important source for historians of slavery, particularly on the question of reproduction, but because of this emphasis, it is also dark and horrifying. Nakedly written from his point of view, any truth in this work of nonfiction is as a record of the self-justifications of slave owners. One of the first things Lewis notices as his gig carries him up the long drive to the estate house is a young woman holding out a child, offering it as if as a gift to him.[28] This scene strikes him so profoundly that he mentions it again later during reflections on the difficulty of breeding slaves. At this later mention, he multiplies the mothers; now he fancies that not just one but "every" mother on the estate is holding out her child to him. He recognises in these mothers' gesture their understanding of "their intrinsic value" to him as the source of the future workforce.[29]

Because of this overt sense of children as a potential "dividend," Lewis takes a vicarious interest in his slaves' partnerships and families. For example, he leans on his slave John Fuller to take a wife on the estate instead of or as well as the partner he has chosen on another part of the island, to whose offspring Lewis would have no legal right. Lewis threatens to auction John to the highest bidder amongst his slave women for yams or salt fish if he doesn't choose a mate from amongst them.[30] Lewis presents it as if it's a jeu d'esprit, which it is not. There was literally a market for men like John. Lewis is a farmer of people and finds that, unlike cockerels or bulls, male slaves can be half-jokily coerced into mating and increasing his "stock" with the threatening reminder that they could be goods in a market. Lewis writes a new code of conduct for his estates in which he bans whites at work on his estates from having sex with women married to his Black slaves. Lewis presents this as evidence of his magnanimity and his respect for his male slaves, whom he hopes to spare the humiliation of being cuckolded, with no care at all for the unmarried women that it consigned to systematic abuse.

Lewis takes even more of an interest in his female slaves' reproductive lives than in those of the men. We learn incidentally that Lewis has a "breeding book" in which he keeps lists of women. He is intricately appraised of who has miscarried and who has lost a child or children. One of his slaves tells Lewis that she has had fifteen children but only two are still living and then corrects herself: in fact, she says, she had "twelve whole children and three half ones," by which he understands her to mean miscarriages.[31] Lewis is prepared to own successes but never losses, blaming mothers for the deaths of their children.

He builds a new lying-in hospital whose conditions surpass the lying-in apartment that he had inherited. He also introduces a system of rewards in which women whose babies are "brought to the overseer alive and well on the fourteenth day" are given money and a commemorative silver medal on a scarlet girdle. The medal entitles the wearer to "marks of peculiar respect and attention": on showing it, they are to be served first at meals, given larger food portions, excused faults, or allowed favours. He sets aside a Mothers' Day, one of four annual "play days" that he gives the slaves off in addition to Christmas day.[32] In his speculations about slave breeding, Lewis is naked about the fact that good treatment of his slaves is in his interests and particularly stresses the privileges and comforts he affords pregnant women and mothers. Yet in his description of "every" woman holding out her baby to him, he writes a fiction that his female slaves share his interests. His petty rewards created a competitive reproductive hierarchy which tied his interests to theirs. The pressure on reproduction created a new and competing moral universe: any birth was understood to be a social good, regardless of the means through which it came about. Institutions have that power to launder abuse as apparent communal benefit. That's how Lyall's fantasy of the Experimental Conception Hospital works, too—by framing its unethical research curiosity as virtue and duty and the search for scientific knowledge as a moral and social good.

More than any of the silent women in this book, I wish I could hear the story of the enslaved woman who was named Psyche by Lewis's family. Lewis takes leering notice of Psyche: the number of children she has had and by which partners, her dancing, her facial expressions, and her beauty. Psyche was a Creole woman, the child of a Black slave and a white plantation worker or owner, and she worked in the house rather than in the production of sugar. She was probably born in the lying-in apartment on Lewis's Cornwall estate at the end of the eighteenth century. Could she be his half sister? We get a glimpse of one of her children, a little girl, fanning Lewis with an "orange bough" to keep the flies away while he eats his breakfast.

In one of the places in his journal where Lewis comments on Psyche's beauty, he adds disturbingly that "she really deserves her name." In Greek myth, Psyche, a great beauty, is carried by Zephyrus (the accessory to rape we met in chapter 4) to a sexual encounter with a lover she can't see. That lover is Cupid, and Psyche

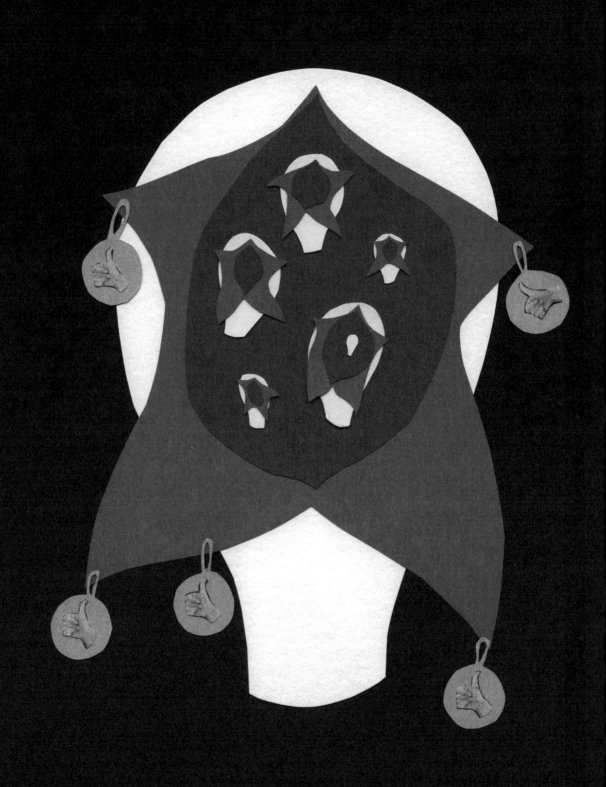

finds herself walled up, a prisoner in his grand otherwordly palace, "trembling and quivering, frightened most of what she knew nothing of."[33] First dreamed up in another slave culture, the Psyche and Cupid story was about sex, abduction, imprisonment, and the coercion of the female soul.

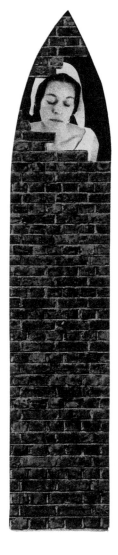

We do not get to hear the voice of Psyche and the other enslaved people that Lewis preyed upon, and as a result we see them rather as the victimised and objectified characters in his famous novel *The Monk* (1796), who are mostly seen through the eyes of the novel's antihero, the monk Ambrosio. Whilst the narrative apparently takes the moral high ground against Ambrosio's crimes, ending when he is thrown into hell by a demon, it also indulges in them:

> a single Lamp, . . . shed a faint light through the room, and permitted him to examine all the charms of the lovely Object before him. . . . He remained for some moments devouring those charms with his eyes, which soon were to be subjected to his ill-regulated passions."[34]

In a similar rhetorical move in his journal, Lewis pretends to hold the high moral ground, describing the institution of slavery as being undesirable but as now too big and structuring to be dismantled. He claims to be a passive, benign, and incidental beneficiary of the evil systems of slavery which he inherited.

One voice we can hear, though, is that of Psyche's near contemporary, Mary Prince (1788–1833), who leaves us her slave narrative, *The History of Mary Prince* (1831). "I have been a slave myself—I know what slaves feel," Mary says: "All slaves want to be free—to be free is very sweet."[35] Whilst Prince records cruelty and abuse, she also tells a story about resistance. Like Psyche, Mary was born into domestic slavery but in Bermuda rather than Jamaica. On being sold and resold, Mary was moved from Bermuda to Grand Turk Island in the Caicos archipelago, back to Bermuda, and then finally to Antigua before being brought to London in 1828, where she lived, walking the very streets where the events of the Gardner peerage case played out.

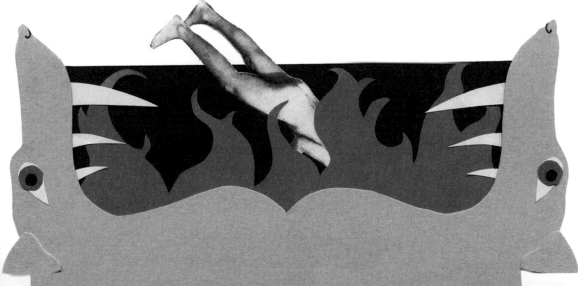

In London, Mary secured her freedom with the help of the Moravian Church and the Anti-Slavery Society. She did so through a petition to the "Great British Parliament," where the Gardner peerage dispute was settled. Her story is a catalogue of horrendous physical violence and also charts another kind of cruelty. In Antigua, she had met and married Daniel James, who was a free man, having bought his manumission from his owner. Whilst Mary managed to free herself in England, if she returned to Antigua to be with Daniel, she could legally be enslaved again. To return, she needed authority from her last owners, a Mr. and Mrs. Wood, who refused it out of spite. At the end of her narrative, Mary finds work as a domestic servant in England and declares herself to be "as comfortable as I can be while separated from my dear husband and away from my own country and all old friends and connections."[36] Notably, Mary never talks about children and what she felt about having her own or not. She refuses to dignify with comment the compulsory reproductive agendas she eventually escapes. Yet her life narrative is articulate about how the intervention and "management" of relationships, families, and reproduction extended even when women like Mary were supposedly free. Historians are clear that the fertility of former slaves and the ability to form families continued to be at issue even in the era of abolition; plantation owners still had an interest in the demographics of labour.[37] Prince's story exerted considerable influence over the public perception of slavery precisely because of its account of a family life disrupted.

We find evidence of enslaved resistance, even in Lewis's journal, including from Psyche herself. One mode of resistance was economic, and the other reproductive, and they were linked. Increasingly, as his journal goes on, Lewis grumps that on his own estate his "indulgences" are met with neither increased work productivity nor new babies. He complains, for example, that the enslaved people refuse to get out of bed early one day when cattle are trampling his cane, despite the holidays and other nugatory privileges he has given them. One of the ways in which Lewis thinks he manifests liberality and largesse to the slaves on his estate is by allowing them to run small commercial enterprises. We learn that Psyche and others, like John Fuller, are breeding cattle. In that, Lewis was not especially unusual or generous; indeed, he probably did not have much choice. Sweeney has described a thriving internal market for all sorts of things—firewood, foodstuffs, and other goods—which enslaved people, including and perhaps especially women, could legitimately take to market themselves and sell, giving their masters a cut.[38]

Some Black people in Jamaica were neither enslaved nor free but lived, disruptive and escaped, outside of the law. Sweeney paints a picture of the markets in urban centres, like Kingston and Spanish Town, as places where fugitive slaves could mix with legitimate enslaved traders, hiding in plain sight. In the hustle and bustle of people, it was impossible for the colonial authorities to tell who was who and what their legal status was. Psyche is involved in some of these commercial practices, maintaining her autonomy but also giving opportunity to runaway women to bring to market their cattle or whatever else they could grow, make, or raise. Lewis exposes his anxieties about this autonomy by winding them into his preoccupation with Psyche's sexuality. Psyche sells Lewis a steer (a calf raised for meat), which prompts him to wonder how she got it, although he says he's too discrete to enquire. His performative discretion implies that he covers an intimate secret, perhaps that Psyche is also selling sex. Lewis dwells on the threatening prospect of Psyche's economic independence, which he mixes up with her sexuality. Writing about slavery in the American South, Angela Davis reminds us that whilst repression works and "the wholesale rape of slave women must have had a profound impact on the slave community," it does so only partially: "it could not succeed in its intrinsic aim of stifling the impetus towards struggle."[39]

Enslaved bodies did their own thing. To Lewis's irritation, despite his system of rewards for mothers and mothers' days, birth rates were low. He had 330 slaves on his Cornwall estate at the point of writing but only twelve or thirteen babies were being born there each year. Historians agree that fertility rates were low and infant mortality high on all Jamaican plantations.[40] Not only were enslaved women subject to the ill health that was endured by all people in Jamaica, enslaved people and slavers alike (Lewis dies of yellow fever on his return from one of his Jamaican visits), but they were also subject to physical, sexual, emotional, and mental abuse.[41] Lewis fantasizes that slave women "can produce children at pleasure." When they do not, he decides, they resemble hens which won't lay on board ships because they don't like "their situation."[42] Lewis believes that wilfulness rather than anything more biological prevents the slave population being sustainable. Perhaps he suspected, as historians also do, that women were practising contraceptive or abortion techniques.[43] Regardless of the causes of these low fertility rates, they were read by Lewis as and stand as a testament to the essentially unbiddable nature of the Black female body.

When reproduction is aggressively overseen and monitored and women's care is deprioritised, pregnancy ambiguity begins to look like a positive benefit for women themselves.[44] The refusal, however conscious, to birth new slaves was a block on the power of slavers, and that was partly achieved by applying knowledge in the hazy time

Table IX

Fig. 1

Fig. 2

Fig. 3

Fig. 4

Fig. 5

Fig. 6

Fig. 7

before a pregnancy is common knowledge. These are the moments when botanical "menstrual regulators" or some other abortifacient measure may be useful, because they do not rely on a clear positive or negative pregnancy diagnosis. The possibilities of this fudge between knowing and unknowing are a burgeoning interest for feminist scholars who are working in cultures that criminalise terminations. Where the law extends its remit into the womb, there is clear motive for resisting knowledge technologies gathering data on women's cycles and conceptions.[45] The in-between can protect, and it is a consolation to me that someone in a difficult moment or place might have found useful or, indeed, still might find useful the ambiguity that I found so frustrating.

Outside the Experimental Conception Hospital

"When will it be?"

"As we leave matins after midnight. That's our only chance," comes the reply, whispered through the squint into my cell as number 70 pushes a linen bundle through. Then her footsteps hurry on.

Through the squint, I can see the candle in the tower guttering, and I am afraid and excited all at once. The procession from the chapel always moves in silence through the darkness. The sisters lead us, their heads bowed, back to our cells. I think about us there behind them and then . . . not there. We will need to be swift and silent, not flagging and shuffling as usual.

At first, today had been a day like every other: the great machine trundled from cell to cell to measure us and take samples just as it always does. I lay in bed waiting my turn, as usual. But as I came more into the waking world, I remembered that it wasn't going to be an ordinary day at all. This is the day I will get out, I whispered to myself, and not just into the yard but over the wall and into the fields or perhaps the streets or wherever takes my fancy. I try not to think about where I will really go. In truth, I have nowhere.

I hold out my arm to Sister Philomela and watch her fill out her tables: "Number," "Age," "Last menses," "Date of consolation and physic," "Quickening," "Labour," "Duration of gestation," "Number of weeks."[46] I laugh inside at how little she knows. The boxes are mostly blanks, but my face betrays nothing as I roll down the sleeve of my rough wool uniform and move away to sit in my chair. I imagine the whole experiment crashing down: the inspector shouting into Sister Philomela's cheerless hypocritical face.

As soon as the sun sets, I give the signal, holding my candle up to the window, obscuring it once, twice, three times, and keeping my body between the light and the squint shaft to avoid being seen by the invisible watcher in the tower. Then an answering star in the distance: once, twice, three times. I come away and continue as usual with the evening routine (I wash in the bucket, I kneel in prayer, I get into the cold bed), so as not to raise suspicions.

At matins, the three of us exchange covert glances, number 70 nods at me, nearly imperceptibly, and I nod back. Number 23 pinches my arm as she passes; I brush her finger in reply. As we move through the passage, pretending somnolence, 70 stops ahead, apparently to adjust her shoe, and, as she stands up, she slides the bolt on the chute swiftly and silently back, lifting the hatch. We climb through—first 70, then me, and 23 afterwards. Then 23 pulls the hatch shut.

We have minutes before we're missed, and we begin to climb the metal ladder that leads up to the roof. As we reach the top, we hear the knocking of the wind outside. Our cotton caps are thin. Icy but welcome air makes my scalp rigid as we climb out onto the roof, and the huge vista of the sky opens out above us. We are alone now, and the immensity of nothing swells around us who have grown accustomed to the close walls of our cells. The fear of nothing, of being found there unescaped, begins to set in. We brace ourselves for a wait.

And wait. Then, in time, over the wall, we see a great moon rising, a womb growing large or an enormous egg being laid slowly upwards: glowing white and venous even in the darkness beneath thick clouds. My heart rises in sympathetic anticipation. The balloon comes level with us, rises higher still, and drifts silently over our heads.

A ladder is thrown down, and there isn't time to disbelieve or hesitate. We climb it through the air, one by one, our fingers hurting from the cold and the rough rope, our eyes shut in fear. My hands are tough from sewing sacks, and the wheel we've exercised on in the yard over months taught me to put one foot and one hand in front of the other and just keep moving.

I am the first up, falling gratefully over the wickerwork side, and I am helped up by the aeronaut, her hair streaming from under her long cap. "Welcome to my laboratory," she says, but I'm too puffed to look at the world to which she gestures. The basket is tipping and rocking as the others pull themselves up over the edge. There are blankets here and brandy and a cloud travelling behind us in the wind stream.

There are some lights below, faint in the hospital's windows. The roof from which we flew off and the wall we thought we couldn't scale are falling away beneath us. Is that one of the sisters, shouting and shaking her fist impotently on the roof? It's too dark to see. The whole hospital is just a small speck, and then it's gone, along with its presiding gods: the law and the great British Parliament.

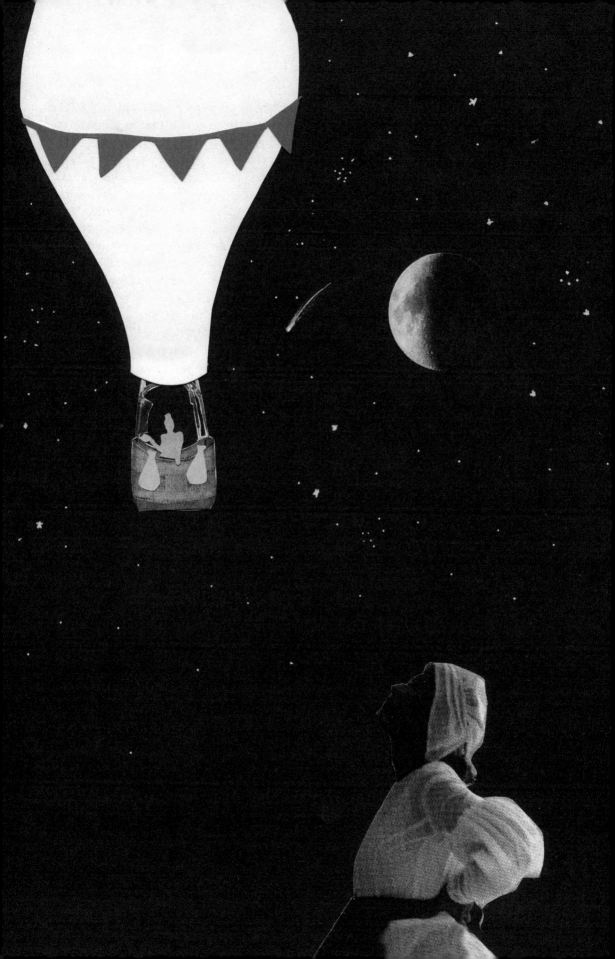

High-Tech Help

Let's shift now to a more evidently altruistic context, far away from the dehumanising Caribbean sugar plantations in the nineteenth century and Robert Lyall's mad plan for his hospital. In another time and another secretive experimental conception hospital, the first IVF babies, Louise Brown and Alastair Montgomery, were born. They were the two successes of a research study undertaken by Robert Edwards, Jean Purdy, and Patrick Steptoe which ran for nearly a decade (1969–1978) and involved at least 282 female volunteers hoping to be helped to motherhood.[47] Between them, the volunteers underwent 495 cycles of treatment from which 167 embryos were recorded and 112 embryo transfers were attempted, which resulted in eleven positive pregnancy tests, five pregnancies, and only two live births. The experiments were conducted in total secrecy for fear of press intrusion. There is no comparison between these experiments and those that Robert Lyall imagines. Not historical science fiction but modern science fact, they took place in a different world and were evidently backed by the laudable desire to improve the fertility opportunities for infertile couples. The assessments of scholars Martin H. Johnson and Kay Elder, on the "Oldham Notebooks" which document the research, are that Edwards, Purdy, and Steptoe worked with "deep ethical deliberation" and "extraordinary care and compassion" and that "they did at least strive to act ethically."[48]

Yet Johnson and Elder also raise some flags. Looking at those flags, we can reflect on the fact that the progress that was made at Oldham also incurred costs, which can sometimes be forgotten in our gratitude and wonder at what was enabled. And those costs should also be counted. At Oldham, volunteers seem not to have taken in the information about how experimental the work was. When they agreed to take part, some of them had no idea that the success rates were so low—indeed, were actually zero. Some patients were there to help the researchers perfect the skills of retrieving eggs and fertilising them in petri dishes. There was no prospect of their becoming pregnant. This group were effectively "purely experimental subjects." Medical ethics have changed between now and then, and current practice is mitigated by what has been learned. Yet medical trials must always weigh the harms done to and the sacrifices made by individuals in the present against the potential benefits to others in the future. And as every patient undergoing an invasive and gruelling treatment will know, every wish must be paid for in blood.

An odd effect of the entirely ethical desire to keep patients' private medical histories secret in the Oldham records is the substitution of numbers for names. Reading the transcripts of the Oldham notebooks, it is hard not to think about the nameless women in some of the records and sources I have used elsewhere in this book. When Robert Lyall urges his readers to resort to keeping careful records about their wives in their own "private practice," he also recommends anonymising the data: "we need not add that it will be unnecessary to tell the patients' names." A nameless army of women has contributed bodies, samples, and emotional lives to research into reproductive science. That army is still going to need recruits. A full picture of this technological scene should temper the tone of triumph that may otherwise characterise the celebrations surrounding Louise Brown's coming fiftieth birthday.

There is no doubt that the technologies that were developed in the Oldham study have changed the world and, since then, been improved. There is no doubt, too, that they have helped many people become biological parents who would otherwise not have been. Yet the promise that was held out of their democratisation has not been realised. What is more, the disparities in provision map the histories I have explored in this chapter. New science must always rely on old, whatever damage that earlier research or the culture that enabled that research caused. But its dividends are not universally shared, and there is a strong historical grip on the distribution patterns of medical knowledge and care. The majority of assisted reproductive procedures are available to a tiny minority concentrated in the global north. Nationally as well as internationally, too, there are demonstrable inequalities.[49] In the UK, for example, a recent report from the Human Fertilisation and Embryology Authority concluded that there are clear "disparities in access and outcomes of fertility treatment among ethnic minority groups," with the experience of Black parents being notably worst.[50] Such disparities are likely to be effects of history as much as contemporary prejudice and discrimination. Philosopher and historian of science Sarah S. Richardson, in her work on the "maternal imprint," draws our attention to the "efflorescence, in recent years, of scientific interest in the long-term effects of the intrauterine environment" and to how historical environmental stressors are inherited by generations at some distance from where those stressors are first felt.[51] This area of research has implications, for example, for the health outcomes of those people that descend from enslaved populations, such as British Afro-Caribbean people, who will be a significant part of the group of patients identified as worst off by the HFEA in their report. As Saidiya Hartman writes in a memoir about tracing her ancestry through slavery: "I, too, live in the time of slavery, by which I mean I am living in the future created by it."[52]

■

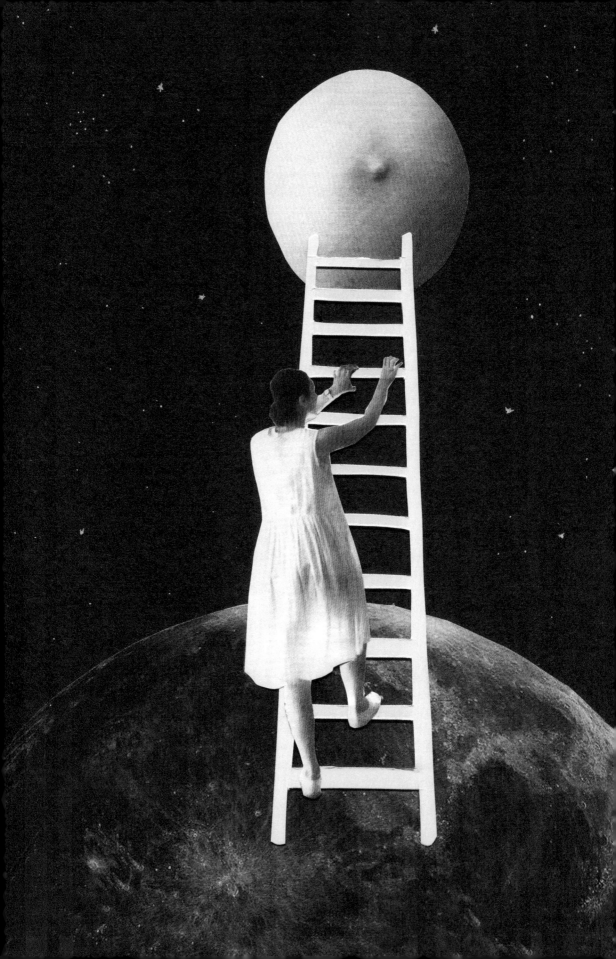

At one point, I became a test subject myself—a soldier in the army of the nameless—as part of a research project into recurrent miscarriage. If any historians of the future are reading this and want to know how I felt about it: it was no jeu d'esprit. But the staff I met there were kind and concerned to understand miscarriage for me and for others. They also weren't afraid to say that lots is still unknown. The cutting edge is where knowledge fails, and we are subject to the limitations people have always known. The copious tests they did on me seemed to turn up something for which I could be treated with daily self-administered anticoagulant injections. The bruises from these tracked and blossomed impressively across my tummy like Rorschach blots, but in the end, they lasted longer than the pregnancy the treatment was supposed to sustain. If the data I contributed helps in even some small way to the solve the research problems they were taking on, perhaps those experiences won't have been in vain.

"Unfortunately, there isn't a pill that I can give you that's going to make you have a baby," a doctor once said to me. She said it kindly but also wistfully, as if she herself half wished there were.

7 Wind-Eggs: Conceiving of Things

What makes you think there is anything creative about having babies? Would you call a plant-pot creative because seeds grow in it? It is a mechanical operation—and, like most mechanical operations, is most easily performed by the least intelligent.
—The words of a future historian, from John Wyndham, *Consider Her Ways* (1961)[1]

Imagining Pregnancy

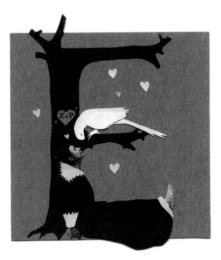

ARLY PREGNANCY symptoms appear like will-o'-the-wisps in a night marsh. "I can understand," I say to M., "imagining myself into nausea or feeling tired, but how can I imagine my breasts larger to the extent that you can see they are, too? What I would have to do," I say to him, after some thought, "is draw a semipermanent line around each breast and test by water displacement at different times of the month. That's the only way I know of to measure the changing volume of a still-attached body part."

"Come on, Archimedes," he says, by way of gently dismissing it. "Let's go out." Later he comes back to it: "But what would you be finding out there: that you were pregnant and repeatedly quickly miscarrying, or that you weren't but . . . ?" And then he seemingly can't think of what that other thing might be and trails off.

The first chapter of *What to Expect When You're Expecting*—for all that it urges women to trust their intuition, as I discuss in the introduction—also hints that a persistent but false impression of pregnancy might occur, concluding that it might have "psychological roots—possibly that you strongly do, or don't, want to have a baby."[2] Other self-help books on my home shelf refer to the "mind-body link." These coy allusions don't satisfy my curiosity or my mind or resolve its relation to my body.[3] What is that link? How does it work?

The novelist Angela Carter describes a series of what she terms "psychosomatic pregnancies" in her journals and letters to a friend in the late 1960s and early 1970s. These present to her as realistic pregnancy symptoms ("cessation of menstruation; vaginal discharge; sore breasts; & curious heaviness in the abdomen"), and some of those symptoms (her "larger bosom") are observable to others. "Dear Carole," she writes,

> Am in receipt of your "pregnancy" letter. It's okay. I was just doing my thing, with a good deal more conviction even than usual; I had a test, actually before I got around to posting my last letter; to the stunned surprise of those in my confidence . . . it was negative.[4]

In an earlier letter to the same friend, Carter describes another incident when she is shouted at by a doctor she consulted in the mistaken belief she was pregnant. What Carter describes as her "thing" bears some sort of resemblance to my "thing," to the "thing" encountered by the many other women whose existence is revealed because they report their symptoms on the internet, and perhaps also to the "thing" afflicting women today (for example, in rural Nigeria) who present to their doctors as if pregnant.[5] Yet those "things" cannot all be exactly the same because we live in different places and moments in time, with different resources and expectations, and in different bodies. There is a phenomenology to the encounter with spurious pregnancy symptoms—intersections between us, our personalities, our individual circumstances, and our historical and geographical cultures.

In a post entitled "My Imaginary Pregnancy," American blogger Marisa Costa self-diagnoses with "pseudocyesis"—a medical diagnostic term for a psychosomatic pregnancy. She goes straight to the question of history, lifting a quick account probably from the Wikipedia stub which lists as sufferers Mary Tudor and twelve women mentioned by Hippocrates (460–370 BCE). Over eighteen hundred years, just thirteen cases are cited, and only one of them is named. "Is it possible that I could really have such a rare condition that occurs in just one to six of every 22,000 births in the United States?" Costa asks, but she finally concludes: "Okay, so if it happened to Bloody Mary, it could happen to me, I guess."[6] At the same time, she admits that she has some sort of mild version, without a "distended belly or . . . labour pains . . . I'm not that crazy!"

So these are Costa's assumptions: she suffers from a condition that doesn't exist or is vanishingly rare in the modern developed world; there is a spectrum of severity within that condition from private surprise at not being pregnant to "crazy"; and the more severe form is a sign of serious mental ill health and still possible to suffer from in twenty-first-century America despite the cap created by testing and imaging technologies. Unlike Angela Carter or women in rural poverty in the Global South, where pseudocyesis was and is a recorded condition, Costa doesn't present to a medical professional. She is diagnosing herself using dozens of pregnancy test sticks at home every month. This means that she and others like her are not appearing in the statistics for the United States, although she nevertheless expects those stats to reflect the demographic profile of whatever condition she believes she suffers from. A "thing" will look rare if no one reports it. This chapter turns more fully to history to iron out the creases in assumptions like these.

My attachment to Carter's unspecific word "thing" points up my struggle with language. In this chapter, I plump variously for "psychosomatic" symptoms. I use the technical term *pseudocyesis* and investigate the concept of the imagination where it seems most appropriate. My aim is not to establish the truth of what happened to me or anyone else. It is not to name or diagnose but rather to investigate a particular intellectual puzzle presented by a body that acts as if pregnant whether in mild or strong ways, under the suspected influence of the mind. In my case, suffering from recurrent miscarriage further muddied the water: whether the intense impression of pregnancy was a pregnancy or a phantom once, always, or sometimes was unclear. Whatever the case, I wanted to know how the mind and body were thought to cooperate because I needed ways to think about thinking—how best to do it, what strategies to adopt, how to recognise habitual patterns, how to know what was healthy or normal, and how to protect myself from distress. Is there a psychologically healthy way not to conceive? Can I stay mentally well through the process?

How to Think

How to think whilst "trying" also matters because thought is regularly described as treacherous, affecting as much as being affected by fertility struggle. Often the advice written for women like me, living now, is to quell the mind. This is a message we get loudly from folk prescription: "stop worrying, and it will happen."[7] But it also filters into the self-help writing on my shelves. In advice on the two-week wait, fertility guru Zita West advises women not to obsess about symptoms, hinting at the potential power of autosuggestion at that vulnerable point. But can we stand the mind down when trying to conceive? Trying is a conscious effort, an intention; to try is to think. Is it possible to try or think too hard, to overthink? "I sometimes see women worrying over a year's worth of charts," West writes, disapprovingly.[8] Tacit here is an idea that to intellectualise "trying" is counterproductive and that the body can be overmonitored, a cause or manifestation of stress contraindicated for pregnancy. Research is being done on the question of whether stress inhibits reproduction; whether, say, tracking fertility or undergoing fertility treatment generates stress; and whether the problem is circular (that monitoring or treatment is not straightforwardly beneficial). What if trying, technologies, and treatments are undoing themselves? Some of that research is being funded by invested personal healthcare companies that are developing the monitors supporting women to chart their cycles.[9] Whilst funded science is not finding a direct causal link between infertility and the stress of trying, a possibly unshakeable public perception still holds that thinking too much or in the wrong ways—frequently demonised as worry and stress—comes back to bite and with physical effect.[10]

Stilling thought is easier said than done. The famous white bear experiments by Daniel Wegner and colleagues found that "people who try to suppress thoughts are in fact very bad at it." A conscious effort to think about something other than, in that case, a white bear is matched by an unconscious check for the unwanted thought, paradoxically making it more cognitively available than it would otherwise be.[11] Telling people not to think about something, especially something that excites them, is an "attempt to limit their experience of themselves" and risks making preoccupations into ungovernable obsessions: "trying not to think" can have "dire consequences." The attempt to control thought produces its opposite. You can't tell a person not to think, then, any more than you can tell a fox not to hunt. The advice to relax the mind also misses the fact that for lots of women, thinking, reading, and fertility monitoring are reassuring activities: these are things that can be done to try to take control and apply mind to matter and to biology. Intellectual endeavour represents a comforting human alternative to animal bewilderment.

Illustrated by pictures of women meditating and receiving a massage, West's advice is to get the mind "in tune" with the body and learn to "listen to ourselves."[12] Author Miranda Ward also uses audial imagery when she decides during her effort to conceive not to "worry so much about what the body, my body can *do*," resolving "to tune in" and declaring, "I want to listen."[13] But listening takes more interpretive effort than we sometimes imagine. Trying to tune into and listen to my own body produces strange echo effects, like listening to noises in the night. What is a loud noise far away (a door being pried open), and what is a quiet one nearby (the drumming of my own pulse)? The metaphors of tuning in and listening imagine that the mind is perceiving the body with the passivity of a radio audience. But the mind is within the body and has an agitated, active, even interfering curiosity. It doesn't have the advantage of objectivity. According to West, the two-week wait following embryo transfer is better spent "visualising the embryo implanting" than mentally checking for pregnancy symptoms.[14] This is a somewhat different proposition from passively hearing. Now I am generating an image to watch, like a conscious dream but one with wonderful power over physical matter. In this fantasy, the mind is so honed it can direct the unmoored embryo into the womb lining. I wish.

Even if conscious control is unavailable to me, I can see that my mind influences my reproductive biology. To return to the question of psychosomatic effects: my own experience was not especially spectacular. Privately, I would think for a while I was pregnant but then turned out not to be, and then a few months later, the same thing would happen again. When people relate stories of false pregnancy that they have heard through family and community grapevines and from the living historical record, they usually do so in hushed tones, like those adopted for telling a ghost story. What happened to me, though, was mundane and mild, not ghoulish at all. I did, however, recognise the surprise described by Angela Carter and Marisa Costa on receiving negative pregnancy diagnoses in the face of a reasonably strong conviction supported by physical indications. I did not, like Costa, identify with Mary Tudor in her dramatic and anomalous circumstances, but I did wonder where I might be without the limits secured by effective diagnostic technologies. Strong symptoms, with no clear organic cause and with no pregnancy, unsettled me. I had physically arrived in a historical argument about how female reproductive biology fell under the spell of the mind . . . or was it the other way around? The final humiliation, it seemed, was to be given forced glimpses into the active

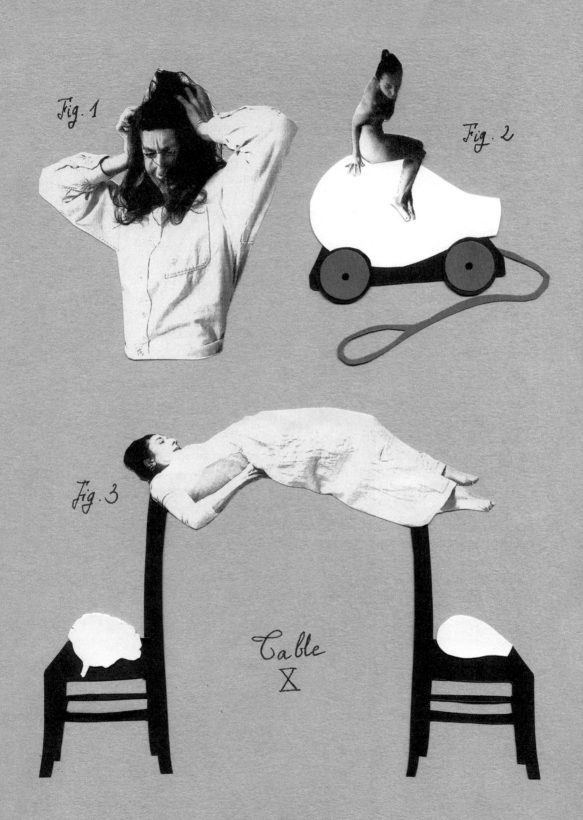

Fig. 1

Fig. 2

Fig. 3

Table
X

collusions of psyche and soma instead of a pregnancy and a baby like other people.

What do such enigmatic effects say about mental health? We measure madness or sanity in the distance between perception and illusion—between dreams and waking life. If symptoms are manifesting inappropriately, we assume some sort of psychological disorder: hysteria, perhaps. Everybody knows that the word *hysteria* derives from the Greek word for womb (ὑστερά; *husterá*) (literally, the word means "suffering in the womb") and that the etymology betrays the special association which was perceived to exist between the female reproductive system and the mind.[15] In the very broadest terms, historians of hysteria have tended to see a historical shift from physiological explanations (a wandering womb, neurological dysfunction, or other organic causes) to psychological ones in the psychoanalytic turn with Freud and others at the end of the nineteenth century. Every age, though, is characterised by debate on the exact nature of communication between mind and body, so it isn't as simple as this sketch history suggests. The sense of the special association between mind and womb has hung on through these various twists and turns, even through the discovery of male hysteria, and been given longevity in part by unthinking antifeminism.

During a spell in Friern Barnet asylum in the 1980s, by which time "hysteria was long out of fashion," historian and memoirist Barbara Taylor was asked by a duty psychologist if she had children. When she said no, he replied, "childless women tend to have poor mental health . . . nature didn't intend women to remain childless."[16] 'The female reproductive cycle," Taylor writes, "was viewed as inherently pathogenic."[17] What Taylor describes here is a misogyny which made lazy connections between the female (un)reproductive body and a diseased mind, connections which cannot possibly improve the care of women in mental health crises like Taylor. A huge feminist literature has faced up to hysteria's long and twisty history.[18] Memoirist and novelist Siri Hustvedt, in an account of her possibly hysterical shaking disorder, reminds us that hysteria's "history is far more complicated than misogyny."[19]

Because this isn't a book about hysteria or conversion disorders (to use the more modern neutral term) and because that topic could suck up all my words, I need to focus on the somewhat different but interestingly intersected history of spurious pregnancy. The most recent edition of the *Diagnostic and Statistical Manual of Mental Disorders* produced by the American Psychiatric Association (*DSM-V*) lists pseudocyesis as an "Other Specified Somatic Symptom and

Related Disorder," which means that now, at our historical juncture, pseudocyesis is considered to share something but not everything with other conversion disorders.[20] A clear difference from those other disorders is that the sufferer presents to a midwife or obstetrician as if pregnant rather than to a neurologist with, say, limb paralysis or a language impairment like aphasia. So the distinction is mapped by the configuration of healthcare disciplines. Another distinction is the effect of the diagnostic event itself, which, with some historical consistency, is said to dispel the problem quickly, whereas conversion disorder symptoms are often chronic and more complex to treat. Here is the natural birth activist and midwife, Ina May Gaskin, writing about a case in the early 1970s:

> I encountered my first case during my second year of midwifery practice. My friend had plenty of the presumptive symptoms of pregnancy, but when I palpated her uterus, I found nothing in it. When I showed her a reference to a false pregnancy in a medical book, she readily accepted my diagnosis, and her "pregnancy" symptoms quickly subsided.[21]

And here is Thomas Hawkes Tanner, a mid-nineteenth-century obstetrical writer, who we've met before:

> It is due, however, to my patient to add, that she did not maintain her delusion very long; since she listened to a simple statement of the facts, and was apparently convinced of her mistake by the end of twenty-four hours.[22]

This is perhaps why psychosomatic pregnancy exists (statistically if not exactly in fact) only where diagnosis is mediated by a doctor in a clinic rather than by a pregnancy test kit at home. Pseudocyesis is usually easily treated through diagnosis itself and is often less severe than pathologies which mimic neurological damage.

On the other hand, there are some similarities between psychosomatic pregnancies and other conversion disorders, and they can be understood through tools developed for the wider category. Historian and medic Philip R. Slavney has compared hysteria to grief. Both are physical phenomena triggered by "bad news"; that is, they take in cultural information. In the case of conversion disorders, that information taken in may be more diffuse and more difficult to isolate and identify than in the case of grief, but nonetheless some sort of emotional catalyst or trauma is looked for. Information in the case of a psychosomatic pregnancy is plainer, more like grief than hysteria. Social and cultural expectations about childbearing meet either a personal desire for a child or, as in Angela Carter's case, anxiety or ambivalence about pregnancy and motherhood. Sex is not quite "bad news," like a message about a death which sparks a grief, but is nonetheless also information taken in. This is how it works in Carter's case:

> I went off the pill because all these feminists I know say
> you ought to from time to time; & none of them ever get
> pregnant, damn it. Either Kō dislodged the diaphragm,
> which is perfectly possible, or it was before I got the thing.[23]

She is moving between two different forms of contraception and so creates or at least recognises a chink, no matter how small, through which pregnancy might have squeezed. Expectation, also a known active ingredient in placebo and nocebo conversion, is generated by the information taken in whilst trying for or trying to avoid pregnancy. So social, familial, personal, and cultural pressure is followed by the more specific local *expectation* generated by having sex.[24] *What to Expect When You're Expecting* could do with another chapter. After all, what is expectation?

Because of the adjacency between pseudocyesis and other conversion disorders, we can also accept some help from feminist cultural historians working on hysteria. We might even consider that the special case of psychosomatic pregnancy may give something back to the feminist project of reckoning with the gendered history of psychogenic conversion. Feminist philosopher Elizabeth A. Wilson, whilst acknowledging the extensive feminist work on the political and cultural oppression at the root of female hysteria, draws attention to the lack of feminist interest in the bodily mechanisms that effect it: we are, she writes, "well equipped to answer why hysterics convert, but . . . collectively mute in response to the question of how."[25] Rather than repudiating biology and anatomy, Wilson focuses on the neurological body, an integrated rather than a dualist system, a model of mind which is not contained by brain and head but extends to other parts and organs of the body through the peripheral nervous system "Formulated this way, hysterical diversion is not forced on the throat, legs, or eyes from the outside, it is already part of the natural repertoire of biological matter."[26] Turning to the historically central place of the womb in hysteria, she suggests we redeploy the old Platonic idea of its errancy but that we recognise errancy to be a habit of all and other parts of the body, regardless of sex. "Perhaps all biology wanders," she says, giving us a way to think not just about pathological hysteria—paralyses, language, or sensory impairment—but rather about a generalised proclivity to conversion, which is also available, although less pronounced, in good health.

Wilson suggests we return to historical models to correct our sense of the mind and body as separate and opposed. She particularly finds the early work of Sigmund Freud on the animal nervous system—studies which predate his work on the psychological nature of hysteria—instructive. In the rest of this chapter, I focus on psychosomatic pregnancy and its difference from hysteria, using a different historical tack from Wilson by selecting an earlier, premodern example: William Harvey's work on generation from the mid-seventeenth century. Like Freud, Harvey was speculating about how the mind operated in relation to gendered and sexual health, and he also develops his hypotheses from animal studies. He is asking the questions that Wilson is asking: What is the biology of "imagined" symptoms? And what psychology can we impute to body parts beyond the brain, including those apparently beyond the reach of the conscious will?

In chapter 4, I talk about sixteenth-century ideas which saw the body and the environment as interwoven. The environment was not a body box. Rather, the four environmental elements made up the body, bringing climatic influence into and through it. In this chapter, I explore a similarly intricate idea of the enmeshment of mind and body which Harvey finds in his chief scientific influence, Aristotle, and in his cultural milieu. One way in which this entanglement was understood is in the very bodily idea of the Aristotelian tripartite soul. The soul's three parts—the vegetative, sensitive, and rational souls—corresponded to different somatic and psychological faculties. The vegetative soul is the part that humans and animals share with plants, and it governs processes like growth, reproduction, digestion which are outside conscious control. The sensitive soul is shared by humans and animals, and it oversees, for example, locomotion and sensory perception. The rational soul is a peculiarly human faculty that people grow into but also potentially out of with age. This is the organising scaffolding for William Harvey's sense of how mind, soul, and body closely relate in the process of conception.

Roundly dismissed in its own time and also more recently by historians of science and medicine, I rethink Harvey's ideas on generation and the potential for parts of the body well beyond the head—the breast, uterus, and abdomen—to register as pregnant. I also ask what Harvey can give back to the wider question of conversion disorders. An imitation pregnancy offers a new vista on the "mind-body link" because the thing which it imitates is not illness but a healthy physiological process. Whilst nausea and breast tenderness are supposedly negative symptoms, they do not augur disease, and in pregnancy they can even be welcomed. It is strange that we talk about pregnancy diagnosis. *The International Classification of Diseases* lists pregnancy as a life stage, along with the other hormonal transitions like puberty and menopause, which are also symptomatic but rarely gather the label "diagnosis." One of the things the exchange between Harvey and Wilson might do is to enlarge our understandings of what is healthy. Wilson is pushing us to see that our bodies—all our bodies and not just sick ones—have a psychological and encultured function. Harvey is also keen to describe conversion effects which are available even in good health. Part of his description of good health includes maternal desires and behaviours even in the absence of a foetus or a child, which he describes compassionately and respectfully as a sign of fertile biology. We don't have to quell the mind or tune it into the body; the two are fundamentally and irrevocably intertwined whatever or however we consciously think.

Elizabeth's Parrot

During an autopsy on his wife's pet parrot, William Harvey was surprised to find that it was female rather than male, as he had first thought. Elizabeth's bird suffered "convulsive motions" before it "did at length deposite his much lamented spirit in his Mistresses bosom, where he had so often sported."[27] The autopsy confirmed the cause of death as a retained egg stuck in the bird's cloaca. Harvey had assumed the animal was male because it was plainly in love with Elizabeth, as indeed she was with him. If the parrot found her absent, "he would search her out, and when he had found her, he would court her with a cheerfull congratulation," he flew to her when she called, walking up and down her shoulder, responding to her requests for him to sing and talk to her, even in the darkness of night. There is perhaps even an erotic edge to these nighttime assignations and, more broadly, in the way Harvey characterises their bond:

> Many times when he was sportive and wanton, he would sit in her lap, where he loved to have her scratch his head, and stroke his back, and then testifie his contentment, by kinde mutterings, and shaking of his wings.[28]

Harvey sounds charmed by the parrot's tameness, impressed by how "well instructed" Elizabeth had got it, but also jealously relieved to have outlived and dissected it. He is describing a love triangle with the parrot as a sexual rival. Some aspects of the bird's behaviours seem inappropriately intimate. The bird, Harvey says, has "now grown so familiar, that he was permitted to walk at liberty through the whole house," and its sitting in Elizabeth's lap is part of its "customary familiarity and obsequiousness."

One of William's biographers tells us that "William and Elizabeth had no children; all that we know of her from Harvey's own words was that she kept a parrot."[29] What a suggestive semicolon. What is the connection between being childless and keeping a parrot? The oblique implication comes from Harvey himself, where the account of the parrot is implicitly about Harvey and Elizabeth's own reproductive fortunes. The parrot anecdote appears in Harvey's study *Exercitationes de generatione animalium (Exercitations on the Generation of Animals)*, the work that Harvey went on to write after his more celebrated account of the heart and circulation of the blood. Birds' eggs, so usefully exteriorised and laid in the lap of scientific observation, offered clues as to what was going on in the hidden processes of mammalian reproduction. Elsewhere Harvey had described his investigations of animal biology as a proxy study of humans: "homo enim the text, the other the comment" (for man is the text and the other—i.e., the animal—is the commentary).[30] His investigations of eggs and birds were a case in point.

Harvey is drawing different points out of the anecdote about the parrot. The most apparent is his concern with pathological lovesickness and illnesses that look like lovesickness—such as those he terms "hysteria" and "green sickness"—in young unmarried girls.[31] In his view, this is the cause of the parrot's premature death: it fatally retains the egg because it cannot consummate its impossible cross-species and same-sex love for Elizabeth. We are clearly at a different moment in the long and twisty history of hysteria that I mentioned earlier, where the principal symptom of hysteria was thought to be the stopping or "retention" of menstruation, and lovesickness was typically the cause. If some women "be too long detained from [marriage], they are assaulted with dangerous symptoms." Harvey warns that in some cases they may "grow frantick for love; and this extravagancy is so outragious in some, that they seem bewitched, planetstrucke, or possessed."[32] Expressing love in marriage and having sex, according to Harvey, can keep women who desire it healthy, and blocking that desire makes them ill. Birds can sometimes get sick like this "when they covet the society of the cock," Harvey says. We

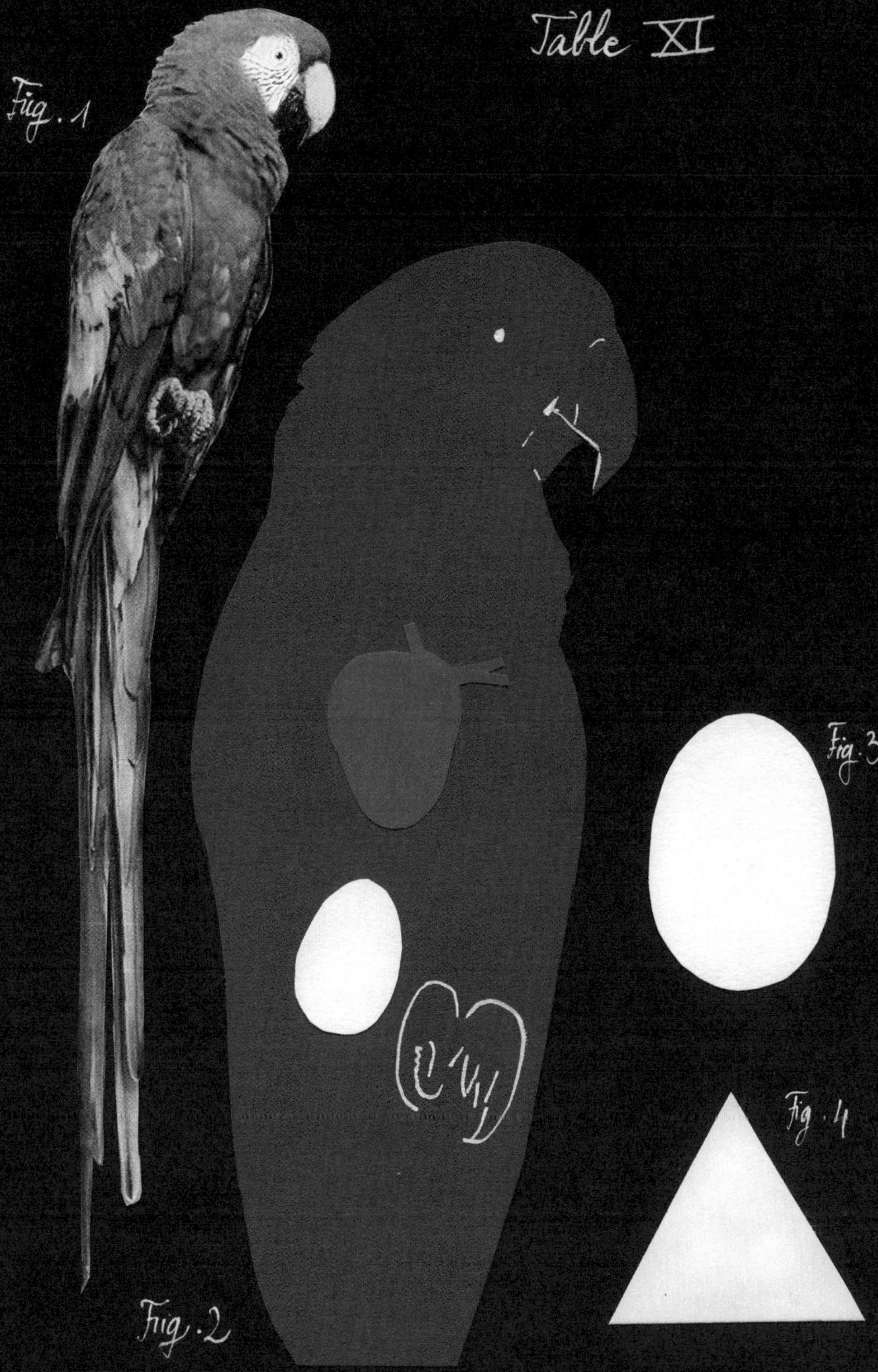

Chapter 7

Table XI

Fig. 1

Fig. 2

Fig. 3

Fig. 4

may detect here some of the thinking that assaulted Barbara Taylor in the Friern Barnet Asylum in the 1980s, but with important differences. Most particularly, Harvey is recommending that women's desires and sexuality are best not blocked rather than suggesting that reproduction should be compulsory. As we will see, Harvey is not of the view that childlessness is a cause or sign of illness.

However, there is also another argument going on around the story of Elizabeth and the parrot which is less explicit, this time about Elizabeth rather than the parrot. By piecing together clues across Harvey's writing, I think we can see Harvey puzzling out psychosomatic pregnancy as it happened in his own marriage. Harvey repeatedly returns to the problem of spurious pregnancy, giving several case histories. This one, he tells us, is close to him personally: "I know a young Woman," Harvey writes,

> who was the Daughter of a Physitian, who was of my neer acquaintance, which being Big, felt all the Symptomes incident to Women in that condition; and continuing healthy and sprightly, after the fourteenth week she perceived the motions of a Foetus in her Womb; and having finished her time for going with Child, conceiving the hour of her delivery to be nigh at hand, she had her Bed furnished, her Cradle ready, and all the implements appertaining to the purpose laid out for use. But all these preparations came to nothing, and Lucina was cross to her wishes; for her customary paines quite left her, and her Belly as it rose by degrees, so it sunk againe, and shee never sicke for the matter, but she remained barren ever after.[33]

I suspect that this empty cradle was in the Harveys' own home and that he is talking about something that happened to Elizabeth without using her name. I am reminded of Robert Lyall's call to his professional medical readers to scientifically observe their own wives, omitting their names. Elizabeth was the daughter of Launcelot Browne (d. 1605), court physician first to Queen Elizabeth (for whom she was presumably named) and then to King James. The English translator's choice of "neer acquaintance" sounds more casual than Harvey's Latin, where either the physician or his daughter (it isn't clear) is described with a superlative as "mihi familiarissimi" (most intimate with or most familiar to me).[34]

My reading of Harvey's work on conception is different from that of many other historians. The difference is based on what it means to work—as Harvey did—without microscopic imaging technologies. Microscopes were just available by Harvey's day, but Harvey

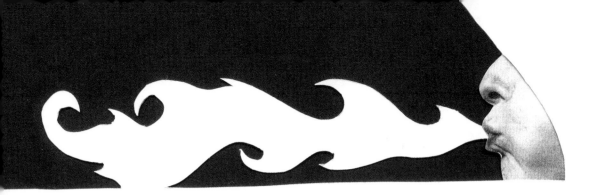

wasn't an early adopter. Some historians of science have felt disappointed that Harvey, a proto-modern in his work on the circulation of the blood, wasn't in the magnification vanguard, and, for them, it blights his work on generation because there were things he could not see. On the other hand, I have an experience of trying to use my intellect—my perceptions, reason, and imagination—to understand my body. I don't even have the advantage on Harvey with his extensive dissection practice. I cannot vivisect myself and see what is happening either micro- or macroscopically. Ordinary living bodies cannot be sliced and mounted on glass slides. I would say that Harvey and I share a blindness, but the truth is that he could see much further.

Harvey's parrot story is interrupted by a digression about the influence of the wind in pregnancy and fertility, invoking the tradition that I discuss in chapter 4. In that digression, Harvey understands wind to be both potentially fertilising and potentially vacant. He cites Virgil's *Georgics* on the erotic dramas of the natural world in spring and Aristotle on the idea that some hen birds—partridges, in this case—can conceive when they are sitting downwind from a cock, when they hear his courtship song and feel desire, or when he flies overhead covering them with breath.[35] The birdsong is the prompt for the digression; he is thinking about how Elizabeth's parrot's singing misled him to think it was a cock parrot. The other thing which ties the digression to his personal anecdote is Elizabeth's body. Harvey keeps using the same Latin word for Elizabeth's lap—*gremium*—a word which could also mean womb; it had a general application to the warm and incubating parts of the female body. This is the place the parrot likes to be petted and where he eventually gives

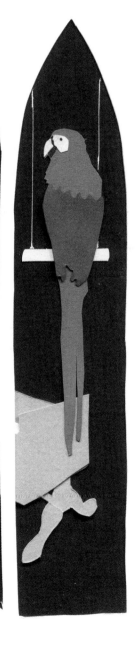

up the ghost. Elsewhere Harvey uses it in a discussion of artificial egg incubation, giving an example of a woman who kept eggs in her cleavage, skin to shell.[36] *Gremium* is a word suggested to him by Virgil's description of the fertile descent of Aether as rain into the womb (*gremium*) of his consort, Earth. By using it to refer to Elizabeth, Harvey includes her in springtime fertility, with all the erotic potential it was given in classical poetry like Virgil's, even though she didn't have any children. So Harvey's windy digression is about how his childless wife and marriage are also a part of the natural world and under the influence of healthy seasonal cycles.

When he talks about conception in this windy tangent, Harvey is drawing on an idea that runs through all his work on generation: there are some "conceptions" that do not result in a foetus or an eventual baby. Springtime fertility was universal; it covered everything, not only animals and plants but humans and not only those who had children but also those who did not. So how else might fertility be experienced if not by the conception and birth of children? What did spring mean for the childless? In the discussion of the three Armada portraits of Queen Elizabeth in chapter 4, I consider how avian and wind imagery together—eggs, feathers, and rounded-out things—articulate a kind of fertility which is not about chicks and children. In those portraits, fertility resided in English expectations of the New World, ripe for colonial exploitation. Harvey, however, had a very different idea of how conceptions which do not result in offspring might be fertile, and that was in a very biological form of the imagination.

Harvey was a physician in the court of Charles I who dissected deer fresh from the royal hunts. He describes working alongside the hunting party, cutting open animals still quivering from the chase. He gives the king an exclusive view inside his dissections, and he argues with the huntsmen about when the rest of the herd will calve that year. His fellow physicians are also part of these dissections as they trot along behind. The theory he is intent on proving to his sceptical audience is that there is a gap between two macroscopically visible things: the spermatic fluid left over from intercourse and an early embryo. Despite extensive searches in the "crannies" of hens and mammals, he could see nothing:

> since I plainly see that nothing at all doth remain in the
> Uterus after coition, whereunto I might ascribe the principle
> of generation; no more then remaines in the braine after
> sensation, and experience, whereunto the principle of Art
> may be reduced; but finding the constitution to be alike
> in both, I have invented this Fable. Let the Learned and

ingenious stock of men consider of it; let the supercilious reject it: and for the scoffing ticklish generation, let them laugh their swinge [i.e., at full liberty].[37]

And laugh they did. It is this apparent absence of male seed that those around him cannot credit. How did the sperm influence the ovum if it was not appreciably there? Harvey's answer—and this is the bit that historians of science (the supercilious?) don't like because it is wrong—was that the spermatic influence was immaterial, working like thought in the brain rather than through physical contact. His proof came with the assistance of the king, who helped him "separate about a dozen Does from the society of the Buck, and lock them up in the Course neer Hampton Court." These are a group that have been mated and isolated to establish that they have not mated again beyond the observation of this royal research team. Some of these does are dissected to show that there was "no seed at all residing in their Uterus." The other does go on to fawn at their "appointed time" despite the gap, "by the virtue of their former Coition (as by Contagion)."[38]

To understand this gap, Harvey reached for different analogies, finding contagion (as here), smell, and magnetism useful to think about how a force could be exerted or transferred without physical contact being made. However, the analogy that he prefers is of the way ideas form in the brain. The womb, he decides, is like a brain, both in the way that it can look and feel in its fertile season (so soft that "did not your own eyes give evidence to that touch, you would not believe your fingers were upon it") and in the way that it operates by taking in information or external influences (sights, sperm) and processing them as conceptions.[39] "Nature," he says,

hath contrived the Womb, which is a no lesse admirable Organ then the Braine, and hath framed it of a like constitution to execute the office of Conception, hath designed it also to a like function, or at least to one which beareth an Analogy with it.[40]

He prefers this brain analogy because an idea—unlike a magnet, an odour, or an infection—had more to say about resemblance, which made it useful for trying to understand the transfer of physical traits from father to child. I should say here that Harvey understood the female "seed" to play a full and equal part in the creation of a child, but his perception of the noncontinuity between male sperm and the embryo made the question of how children looked like their

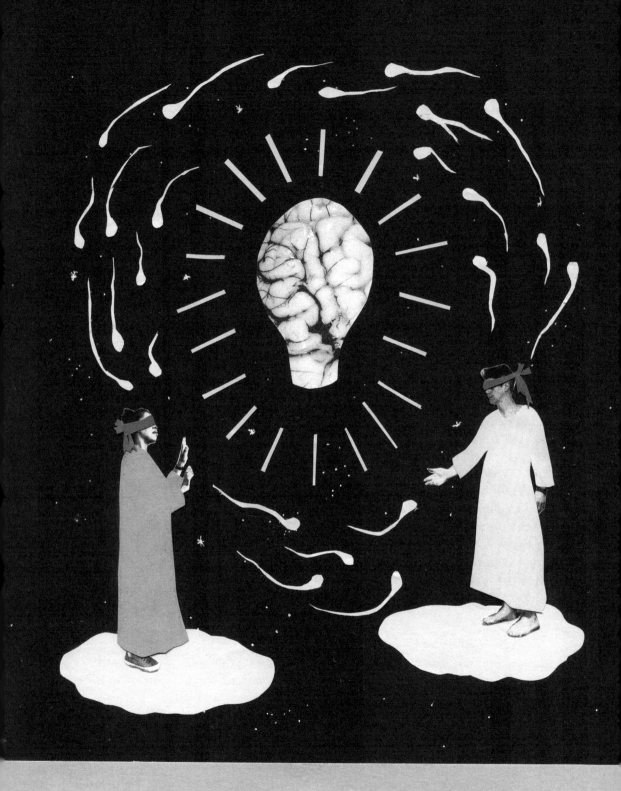

fathers more puzzling and pressing. The idea of the seasonality of the uterus is ingenious: because the endometrial wall changed in thickness and texture across the menstrual cycle, it was more brain-like and so more susceptible to conceptions at some junctures and in some "seasons" more than at others. He also notes that the word *conception* has two meanings used for talking about both ideas and reproduction. And in that etymological coincidence resided a truth.

I think, though, that the other reason for Harvey's mistake—his sense that the influence of sperm was remote or virtual—is that he makes a distinction between conception and generation. Harvey's extraordinary idea of the uterus as brain-like is motivated by a discussion not only of how sperm contributes to the generation of a foetus but also of how it contributes to a "conception" which may or may not result in a foetus:

> For though the female sometimes (conceiving after coition) doth not produce a Foetus: yet we know that those Symptomes did ensue, which gave a cleare testimony of a conception set on foot, (though it came to nothing).[41]

In the absence of a foetus, the appearance of pregnancy symptoms looked like a psychological phenomenon but a kind of psychology that was beneath or outside of consciousness. The uterus, after all, was part of the vegetative soul (what we might term the *autonomic nervous system*), the portion of the tripartite soul which was shared with animals and plants. Women cannot instruct and manoeuvre the uterus as they can their arms and legs. Harvey, writing before the psychoanalytic revolution, does not anticipate the unconscious here but instead arrives at what was available to him: the idea that parts of the body that are not the brain, like the uterus, are themselves intelligent and can think. This notion was not peculiar to Harvey, who lived in a world which understood human psychology, regardless of sex, to be body-wide rather than brain-bound in this way. Harvey operates with understandings of mind and body as mutually corroborative and culturally embedded, well before he specialises to focus on the female reproductive system and the nature of generation.

Scholars have variously referred to this sense of the integration of mind and body as "psychophysiology," or the "intelligent body."[42] Moreover, in humoral medicine, as we see in chapter 4, these integrated psychosomatic individuals were also thought to be inextricably entangled with their wider world. This entanglement is sometimes referred to by historians and philosophers of cognition as the "extended mind" or "distributed cognition."[43] Far from dismissing these models as historical oddities, these extended and integrated ways of understanding humans in their world are increasingly proving useful now to account for evidence of the intersubjectivity and phenomenological way in which humans are constituted, as body and mind combined, which is also mutually shaped by and shaping of nearby material objects and tools, the climates we inhabit, the specificities of our times and cultures, and the demands of our families and communities. And Harvey's incorporation of the uterus into this systemic view may be similarly useful for us, particularly for rethinking mind-body relations in the trying-to-conceive experience.

Harvey sees foetus-less conceptions in his animal studies, too. Bitches, he says, are sometimes mated but don't have puppies, yet they behave or present symptoms at the appropriate time as if they do, becoming "sluggish," producing colostrum when they are due, and afterwards proving "obnoxious to the distempers incident to those that have really puppied."[44] Birds offer another comparator. Their generation "is mainly differenced by their Nest," Harvey notes, who sees the egg as an external uterus and the nest an equivalent to the mammalian body.[45] Nesting behaviours can be observed even in cases where birds "lay no eggs at all, or subventaneous ones onely."[46] "Subventaneous" eggs are wind eggs, eggs which don't hatch, so named because they were the unfruitful products of the wind, evoking once again the poetic and scientific tradition about the part the wind played in nonreproductive as much as generative conception.

Everywhere that he talks about foetus-less conceptions, Harvey is careful to mention that conceptions like this happen only after mating—"if they admit coition at the wonted time." The historian Thomas Lacqueur is dismissive, quipping that, if Harvey's account were true, "women should be able to conceive by just thinking about it."[47] Harvey might reply that, properly stipulated, with all the correct terms and conditions, his theory goes more like this: women may well be able to "conceive" (remembering that conception might result in a foetus but equally might not) first by having sexual intercourse and then afterwards by doing something very like thinking about it, except in the uterus rather than the brain, in such a way that the woman herself would not be aware of those thoughts passing.

Harvey's theory about the brain-uterus has been roundly rejected, but I think unfairly. Historians have dismissed it for various reasons. James Lennox, for example, is concerned that the analogy assigns purpose and sentience to the uterus, anthropomorphising it.[48] Lennox is suspicious of "animism" and the projection of feelings or intentions onto things. Yet the uterus is not inanimate. Harvey is writing not about rocks or plants but about animals and often the human animal, where psychosomatic explanations are entirely appropriate. Making a different objection, the historian Georges Rousseau, picking up the same comparison between dogs and humans as I did earlier, complains that Harvey "explicitly drew a parallel between bitches in heat and hysterical women" and that he described the womb as "insatiable, ferocious, animal-like" and women as "slaves to their biology."[49]

Yet because for Harvey *all* conceptions are immaterially produced, conceptions without foetuses are perceived to be neither hysterical nor a sign of ill health. We have already seen, in the story about the parrot, that Harvey marks a difference between hysteria (a pathological lovesickness in young women who are barred from sexual and reproductive lives) and conception which follows only from sex. Whilst the parrot was so sick that it died, in the story of the physician's daughter, Harvey twice stresses her good health; not only did the woman seem "healthy and sprightly" as her symptoms came up, but she also did not seem unwell as they died down. Whilst the parrot is not able to express its desire sexually, a sexual life lived produces expectations—in both dogs and humans—which are not always realised in puppies and babies.

When Harvey talks about the independence of the uterus, he does so, for example, like this:

> The cavity of the Womb being laied open
> immediately after the killing of the Deere, I
> have often discovered a slow waving motion,
> (such a one as is seen in the bottom of
> a creeping Snailes belly) as if the Womb
> were Animal in Animali, one living creature
> in another; and had a peculiar independent
> motion of its own.[50]

Here Harvey observes contraction waves with some wonder and describes them with precision in comparison to gastropod locomotion. He sees them in the mammalian uterus and also in animal testicles and intestines. The apparent independence of certain organs was not peculiar to women, although in his work on generation Harvey necessarily focuses on and singles out the uterus.

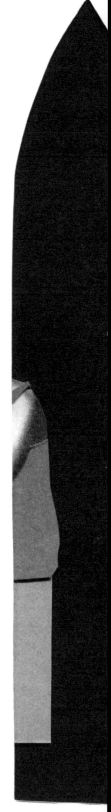

Indeed, in his study of the heart and circulation of the blood, he has a similar awe of the heart, another organ of the autonomic rather than the voluntary nervous system. The heart, according to Harvey is "a kind of internal creature . . . like the prince in a kingdom," although inevitably it is also different from the uterus.[51] Organs like the heart and uterus were always ready to overrule the brain, because they were centres of intelligent power and yet outside of the conscious will. All animals, and humans were no exception, were subject (slaves, if you want to be negative about it) to their biology and its intelligence.

Harvey is not responsible for the abuses suffered by hysterics in nineteenth- and twentieth-century asylums; he writes about something completely different when he draws his brain-uterus analogy. My own reading of Harvey does not find him to be misogynist or dehumanising, as some others have done. Scientists do compare us to animals. "I've finished my mouse-work," I once overheard a man on the tube say to his companion, "and I've just got my human studies to do." They do this not to dehumanise us but to develop *comparanda*. Dogs, birds, frogs, flies: these creatures have things to tell us about human biology and psychology. Harvey used animals as analogies in his biological studies, but they were also sites of wonder that exceeded their biology. He marvelled at webs, nests, and songs as examples of animal artistry, and in his observations of Elizabeth with her parrot, Harvey also recognised the animal capacity for love. It should not be beneath us to draw human lessons from the dog.

We might differentiate Harvey's tone from the tone of those physicians who are dotted through the rest of this book who see women as liars and fools and themselves as the detective-heroes who will catch them out. In contrast, Harvey stands ready to credit what women say about their symptoms, finding a theory into which those truths can fit. I am touched by the wonder Harvey articulates at the tenderness of hen birds towards wind eggs ("the Birds affection towards the dull, liveless egge, is exceeding wonderful, which is altogether incapable of making any return of friendship or respect") and hatchlings from eggs that they have incubated but not laid:

> Who can refrain smiling, to see a Henne follow young
> Ducklins, and having hatched up that suppositious brood
> (apprehending them to be her own) pursue them when they
> are now swimming in the pond.[52]

In these descriptions, he makes physiological narratives about fosterage, adoption, and biological parentage, naturalising those

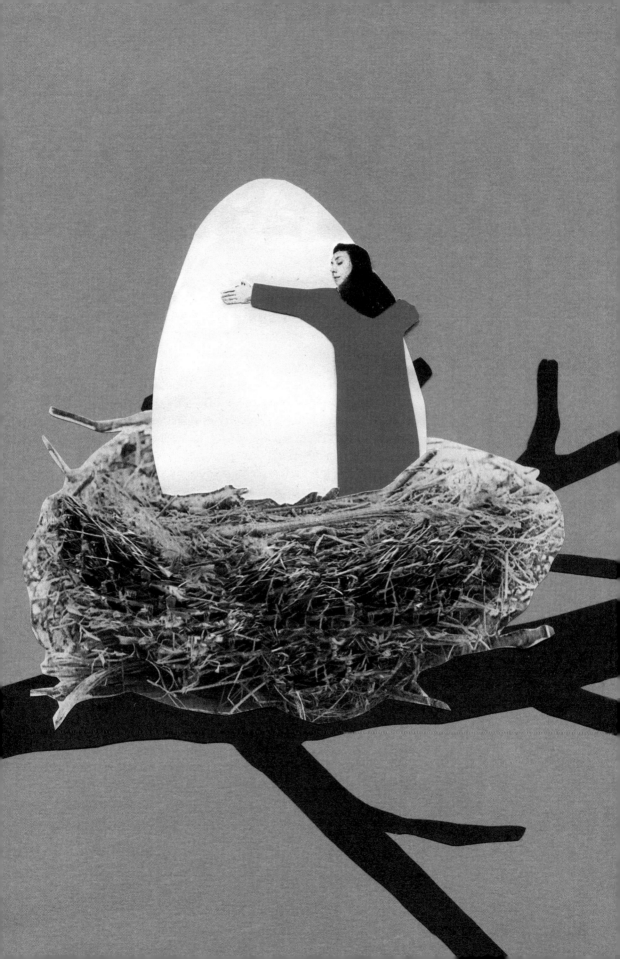

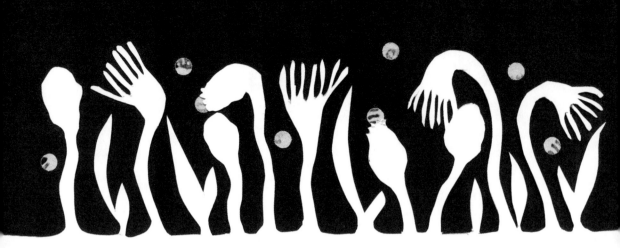

arrangements. Harvey writes with respect and admiration about maternal behaviours in both nonhuman animals and women, even, and perhaps particularly, in the case where there are mixed or nonreproductive results: wind eggs and addled eggs, or no "egges to sit upon, or chickens to discipline" at all.

Returning to the tableaux of the pet parrot in Elizabeth's "lap," which may also figure an incubating "womb" or a "bosom," we might read Elizabeth's love for the bird as motherly and further evidence of her participation in, rather than exclusion from the fertile warmth of spring. There are lots of ways to parent, and pets offer a vital possible outlet for our capacities to love. Harvey's own relationship to the parrot is hard to ascertain. Does he also see it as a substitute child? What is clear is that Harvey describes himself as fertile in relation to his ideas and intellectual labour. His brain-uterus analogy may also be useful for his sense of self.[53] Elizabeth and her parrot—as lovers? as mother and child?—take part in seasonal and natural dramas, and Harvey's observation of their mutual affection gives him a new perspective on his marriage and family. It is in the context of that practice of behavioural observation and the insights it brings him that Harvey can also see himself as a scientist and writer as well as a husband and as part of a reproductive and fertile world. Although he had no literal children, Harvey wanted to father and found out a way to do it. Ideas were babies, his conceptions.

■

I sent off for a sensitive basal body thermometer and awaited its delivery eagerly, hungry with curiosity about it. The thermometer would, hopefully, record a biphasal temperature shift on ovulation. Every life problem has a stationary solution, and I got ready with a template chart and some coloured pens. The temperature must be taken at the instant one wakes from a sleep that must have lasted at least three hours and at the same time every day. Does thinking or raising the head from the pillow affect your temperature and fluff the results? I think of the Pisse-Prophet's claims that his results would be completely reliable if the sample had only been produced correctly by his client. Human fallibility is always a good cover for inconclusive results. The thermometer beeps every four seconds to show it is working. I try to muffle it so as not to wake up M., holding it with the metal prongle under my tongue and the other end in a fistful of duvet. As winter gives way to spring, the thermometer's cheeps join the dawn chorus.

"You've woken up the birds now," M. complains sleepily.

And it's as if I have: they're all stirring. A female blackbird sits on top of the wheelie bin when I go to make the tea in the morning, its beak filled with bright green moss and head cocked. She doesn't want me to see her go into the hedge where nest construction is underway. Everything in its season. Do I have a season?

That night I dream that I am a plastic toy bird and I can see myself from above. My mechanical cheeping attracts a flock of finches who are so mesmerised that they fail to build their nests and instead fly in circles and sing ditzy songs.

Conclusion:
Seeing the Unbecoming

One does not think of the foetus as it is—a goldfish, a tadpole, a clot of red phlegm, a gobbet of scarcely stiff jelly, but as minute and perfectly formed from the first month, homunculus, like the new-born kangaroo in the pouch.
—Angela Carter, unpublished journal (1965)[1]

Unbecoming Books

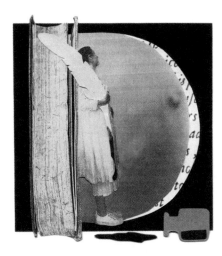

ESPITE ITS BEING a commonplace, I can't help comparing the difficulty of conceiving this book to its subject. As we've seen, William Harvey uses the same association between his ideas and uterine conception; the analogy was and is a commonplace. He took that association, though, and developed a clear sense of *how* these two different sorts of conception might be comparable. Because Harvey is a useful guide on the intellectual and imaginative work of conception, I suggest we travel with him a little further to the final pages of this book. His insight concerns how incoming information is internally processed and, crucially, imaged in the rational soul and also in the vegetative soul to which we have no conscious access. Both are intelligent and, crucially, image making. The difficulty I encountered with conceiving this book is a reason that it also comes illustrated. Perhaps you have been wondering why or how this book came to acquire its images or how these images came to acquire their book? What have imaging and looking got to do with it?

The brain that Harvey found to be most similar in function to the conceiving uterus was that of the artist:

> The brain of the artist, or the artist himself by virtue of his brain, doth form things which are not present with him, but such as he only hath formerly seen.[2]

The womb was an artistic organ operating in the apparently empty space that Harvey saw between sex and conception: "there is no Sensible thing," he reiterated, "to be found in the Uterus, after coition," "no more then remains in the braine after sensation, and experience, whereunto the principle of Art may be reduced."[3] When I first met Anna, the illustrator of this book, I had been working and reading for some time and had made attempts to articulate what I wanted to say. I was reaching for but could not quite touch my subject. How should I articulate the common but culturally invisible experience of not being pregnant, despite reasonable expectations, for month on month? Part of the difficulty is not being able to see quite what is happening whilst trying to conceive and being reliant on ideation and imagination in the absence of a clear sight. That experience is even harder to see if it isn't happening or if it is sort of happening but not coming out as expected. How do you research and write a history of pregnancy nonevents, the struggle to know a diffuse and moving object?

Whilst, as so many have pointed out, it was a mistake for Harvey to think that nothing existed just because he could not see it, he nonetheless correctly sections off a phase of time, a gap, which is still effectively closed off from view. Harvey's gap, where a very early pregnancy might or might not be developing, is the black box into which many of us are curious to see. It corresponds to the "two-week" postovulation, postimplanation wait, not in duration exactly but in its obscurity, in the difficulty of knowing future outcomes, in the impossibility of sight and knowledge. The collaboration with Anna has made it possible to picture that blacked-out space and time because, as Harvey says, the artist "doth form things which are not present," envisaging things beyond ordinary sight.

Artists have often stepped in to produce surrogates for the scientific study of the moving process of conception and the development of the embryo and foetus. Harvey's identification of the artistic brain as the best figure for the conceiving womb must partly have been informed by his consultation of illustrated anatomy books like those of his Paduan teacher Hieronymus Fabricius (1533–1619), whose embryological work, *De formato foetu* (On the Formed Foetus, 1600), had thirty-four engravings of human and animal foetuses by an unnamed artist and whose study of the chicken and egg, *De formatione ovi et pulli* (On the Formation of the Egg and Chicken, 1606), was illustrated with seven plates showing the uterus of the hen, the composition of hens' eggs, and eggs and embryos at different stages of development, some of the first of their kind. "By employing both illustrations and written description," Fabricius writes in the preface to *De formato foetu*, "I shall enable anyone hereafter to understand

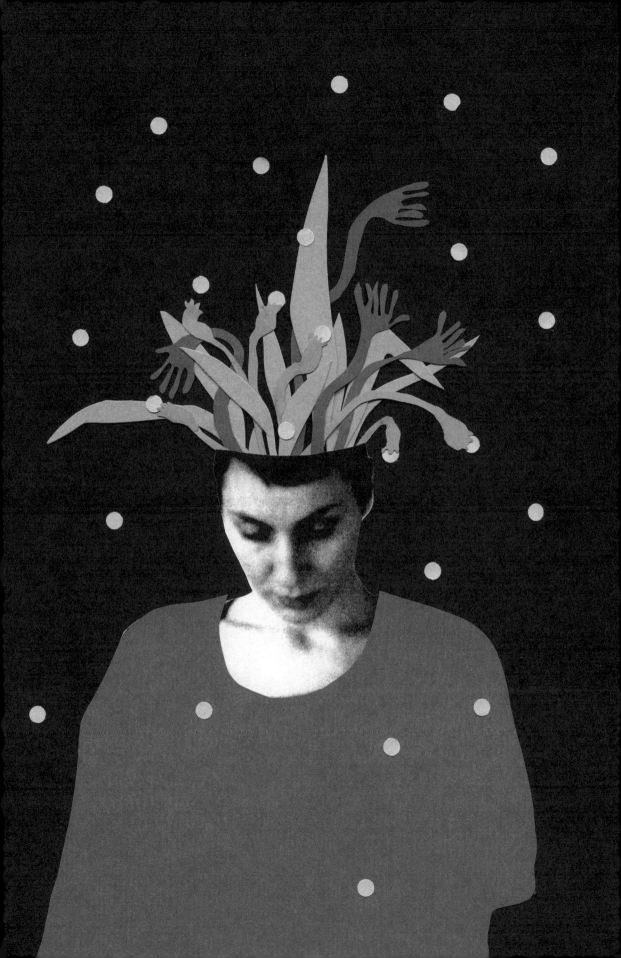

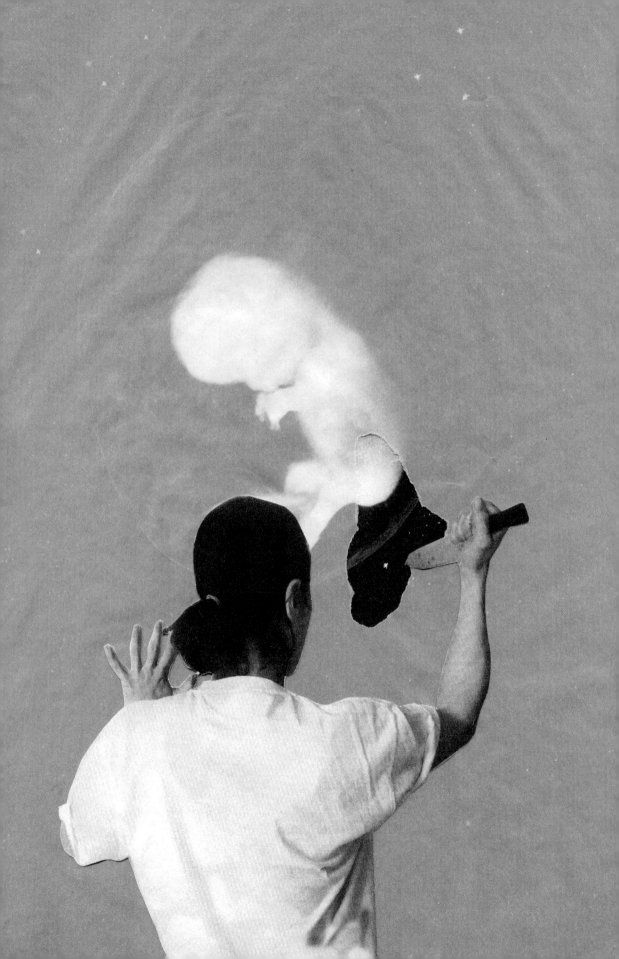

and behold for himself the first beginnings of life in every animal."[4] Artists make historically ephemeral sights perpetually present: conceiving and bringing knowledge of prior things into existence.

Harvey rarely agrees with Fabricius, although he names him as a formative guide. Acknowledging that "Fabricius hath indeed recounted many miraculous things, concerning . . . Birth," he pushes his own sense that "wee meet with more things worthy our wonder concerning . . . Conception."[5] Harvey has the sense, then, that Fabricius's embryological research was tending forwards in time from the embryo to birth, whilst his own was pushing backwards, trying to fathom the phase before that and before that and before that:

> A Man, was first a Boy (because from a Boy he grew up to be a Man;) before he was a Boy, he was an Infant; and before an Infant, an Embryo.
> Now we must search farther, what hee was in his Mothers Womb, before he was this Embryo, or Foetus; whether three bubbles? or some rude and indigested lump? or a conception, or coagulation of mixed seed? or whether any thing else?[6]

These are the research questions in the preface to Harvey's work on generation. In this range of starting hypotheses, he got closer to accurately describing very young embryonic life than he did in his eventual conclusion: that there was nothing and that spermatic influence moved aerially. In reaching for descriptions of what he imagined he might see if he kept working backwards, Harvey is trying to understand how formed or formless, how combined or separate, were the parts of whatever preexisted the things that had so far been seen and drawn. These speculations about what was not yet fully established and shaped drew Harvey more to Fabricius's work on the formation of the egg and chicken than to his study of the formed foetus. Fabricius and Harvey are both landmark figures in histories of epigenesis—the idea (which has turned out to be right) that embryos develop from undifferentiated matter. If you weren't an epigenesist like Harvey, you were a preformationist, holding the alternative view that the embryo begins complete and just enlarges over time. The quotation illustrates the strong epigenetic line that drives Harvey's research. Fabricius's studies of chickens and eggs in series spoke more to this interest in the process of formation, to epigenesis, than did his work on the formed foetus.

In the production of study tools for embryological scientists, artistic practice has had to grapple with how to depict epigenesis, emergence, and metamorphosis over a duration. Cultural historian of science Janina Wellmann has described Fabricius's work on the developmental stages of the embryo in the chicken's egg as inaugurating the "tradition of chronological visualization in embryology, a tradition in which the picture refers to the time of the observer" by presenting eggs in series.[7] The series as a representational form came to define embryological illustration. Wellmann has charted the way that scientific media in embryological study turned to longstanding artistic methods of depicting movement in series (in instructional works on dance and combat, for example) to capture change over time. These imaging habits she refers to as "epigenetic iconography"—that is, as attempts to capture the process of becoming rather than the finished form. These imaging techniques anticipated the "moving pictures . . . later deployed by cinematic technology."[8] Indeed, the embryoscope discussed in chapter 5 is the logical extension of "epigenetic iconography," enabling the sight of a developing blastocyst by speeding up freeze-frame images from a slower process. Image specialists—artists, if you like—are needed to produce and select stills and to run them at an appreciable speed.

Anna's work in this book is also about making surrogates for study but for students of experience rather than of embryological science. Anna's and my tasks were different from those faced by anatomists or embryologists and their artist collaborators: we hoped to picture and articulate some of the lived experience of trying to conceive. In an essay about pregnancy, art, and the female imagination, the feminist art historian Rosemary Betterton brings to our attention "an aesthetic of embodied becoming," in which category she also considers the idea of the series. For example Susan Hiller's documentation of her pregnancy in the work *10 Months* (1977–1979), a grid of ten black and white photographs of her pregnant abdomen, shares something with Fabricius's illustrations of staged embryogenesis.[9] Anna and I are interested in finding a way to represent something different about epigenesis. Perhaps we should call it "unbecoming": not gestation and development exactly but the experience of those processes not happening or not happening in exactly the way that

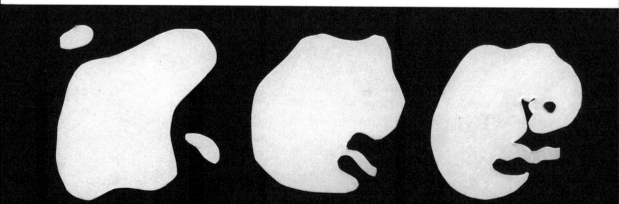

one might either hope or expect. Unbecoming points up the lie in
the series: Fabricius's chicken embryos charted a series of unbecoming individuals rather than the life of one, from laying to hatching.

Under the Microscope

If he had put samples from his dissections under a microscope,
Harvey might have seen defined cellular forms, like the bubbles he
imagined before he set out on his observational studies. Bioethicist
Jane Maienschein insists that we should all get to know the character and stages of embryological life by seeing them magnified:
"accepting enlightenment," she argues, "is our social responsibility."[10] Before the microscope, she reminds us, the embryo was necessarily "hypothetical." Harvey's bubbles have turned out to be good
descriptions of blastocyst development, but they are imagined rather
than observed structures. The hypothetical embryo of the prefor-
mationists was a different prospect: a little man, a homunculus or
animalcule, fully formed and steadily enlarging from day one. An
evident precursor is the tiny perfect Christ homunculus carried to
the Virgin Mary's womb in images of the annunciation that I discuss at the beginning of this book. The view afforded by microscope
technologies, however, settled the argument, teaching us that the
embryo does indeed go "through stages of development, each of
which is biologically very different" from the next, which discounts
preformation.[11] The persistence of preformationist views in modern
American abortion politics, Maienschein argues, is a relic of the
historical hypothetical embryo which ought to have been banished
by scientific observation.[12]

Maienschein is making a case about the importance of providing
good and unpoliticised access to healthcare for pregnant women to
seek terminations. She is convinced that true sight has the power to
dispel the historical hypothetical embryo for good. It makes no sense,
she argues, to give "a cluster of unformed cells" human rights.[13] If we

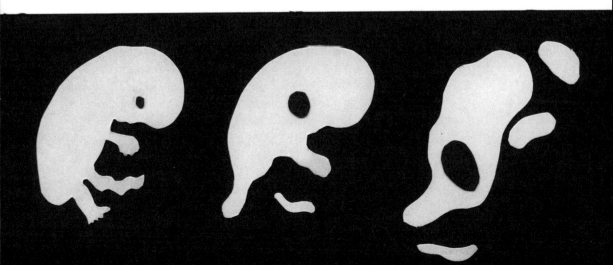

could see what we were looking at, there would be no political opposition to early abortion. I share Maienschein's position on women's rights to access good reproductive healthcare and the importance of not assigning personhood to the very young embryo. My doubt here is that modernity is ever going to be clear eyed. Maienschein's book is all about how epigenesis, which is actually the older Aristotelian idea, has historically always competed with preformationism. If we take the Middle Ages as an early marker, the Christ homunculus was a perfect preformed exception to the natural epigenetic rule.[14] There are few grounds for identifying preformation more than epigenesis with the past. Maienschein's sense that preformationism *ought* to be a thing of the past does not and will not make it so. There is no dispelling folk authority; it is intrinsic to modernity, however ancient it looks. Modernity is mixed—a mash-up of the "hypothetical" and the scientifically observed, of folk traditions and technical authority.

And how clear is our view, in fact? Maienschein also notes the gap that I have been stressing throughout this book—the post-implantation news blackout when "the embryo disappears from direct view: now it is inside the gestating mother" and is dependent on her; this is the gap that Harvey also saw.[15] Epigenesis is a moving target and is also so close to— indeed, so fully within us—that it is hidden from view. I love this account by New Zealand blogger Little Red Hen of seeing her embryo transferred to her uterus:

> The next thing I knew, the embryo was on its way over to my side of the room. I watched the monitor next to the bed as the doctor dropped it into me, and it floated gracefully down in the blackness—a glowing white dot that finally nestled into the bottom and disappeared from view.[16]

The embryo in this description seems to have its own agency, making its own way across the room and floating down into "me," nestling like a wild animal beyond sight. Magnification mediates this sight, although it isn't mentioned. Yet this is the best vista we have: those high-tech monitors in the clinic have a horizon in the uterus beyond which we cannot see. In *Conceiving Histories*, I have been trying to marry up an understanding of epigenesis hidden inside the womb with an account of what that process looks or feels like from the perspective of the person whose womb is doing the hiding. What is going on out of sight? Can it be felt and sensed, if not seen?

But furthermore, sight of the embryo before or of the foetus after that gap is mostly mediated; all images must be interpreted. Like a great deal of scientific knowledge, laypeople like me must

Conclusion

rely on the authority of experts and knowledge produced by sights we have not personally seen. I have no rights to go into a clinic or lab, take a human blastocyst out of its incubator, and slip it under a magnifying lens. Direct sight of a magnified living embryo is rare. The best we have are recorded image sequences from the embryo-scope which, as is shown in chapter 5, mediate in interesting but not wholly straightforward ways. And anyway, counterintuitively, early microscopy often seemed to support hypotheses on embryogenesis that have since been discredited.[17] The eye is already an unreliable mediator, even before it is enhanced by the glass lens; people saw what they expected. To really see, you must know what you're look-ing for and at. Decontextualised, Little Red Hen's "dropped . . . glowing white dot" does not speak for itself. Historian Nick Hop-wood has made this point in his work on the wax models of embryos cast by Adolf Ziegler and Friedrich Ziegler for universities and other institutions.[18] These were three-dimensional, colour representations of much-magnified embryos, again produced in series. They could be held, turned, and compared and were extensively used to train scientists to understand what they might observe when they put their eye to the microscope. A direct sight is not enough; it needs the educational apparatus supplied by models, images, and textual instructional glosses.

Moreover, Maienschein's "hypothetical" embryo is not the only alternative to the microscopically inspected embryo. Her focus on the gestating embryo and the ways it can and should be seen loses sight of miscarriage. In miscarriage, there is an unmediated but also unmagnified sight of the embryo or foetus which is very far from hypothetical. Hopwood tells us that the Ziegler brothers had to rede-scribe as embryos the "clots" and "lumps" that they sourced from midwives or women directly. They then applied the microscope to those lumps, seeing distinct forms in them before they could begin modelling.[19] In chapter 1, I talk about the paucity of our language and visual resources for fertility awareness and changes across the menstrual cycle; we have also lost those languages for reckoning with miscarriage. The lack of sociocultural tools is an effect of our difficul-ties with facing the topic, which means that women are struggling to find the terminology about texture, quantity, and other specifics of blood loss that are important for triaging their care. Maienschein's conviction is surely correct that embryos and foetuses are not peo-ple with independent rights; she means this as a reassuring thought about early-stage termination.[20] Yet the common encounter in mis-carriage with one's offspring in arrested formation equally shakes up our sense of what it means to be human. How do we face the half-formed thoughts of the intelligent womb? Such sights are grim but also enlightening; they represent knowledge, although knowledge that uncomfortably sits on the borders of death. Such scenes are certainly of a very different sort from the technical images generated by magnification and presented in stately greyscale series. Yet perhaps if we use art to rehypothesise these difficult sights and if we consciously use rather than reject the hypothetical embryo, we may be able to face, however indirectly, epigenesis interrupted and rebuild the languages we need.

Maienschein's arguments about seeing remind me of those put to us by Fabricius in his preface to *De formato foetu*. Both writers are winningly in awe of the sights they have personally seen of embryological life and urge their readers to look at the same wonders. Both also take the view that ignorance of what embryos look like is not OK: "it should not be acceptable . . . to know nothing about a topic of public concern," writes Maienschein, whilst Fabricius argues that it is "unfitting [Fabricius's Latin *indignum est* could also be translated as "shameful"] that such great wonders of Nature should be concealed."[21] Look, though, at how Fabricius reads the story about the emperor Nero's gynaecological anatomical experiments, which I look at in chapter 1:

> Could one tell or invent a tale more magnificent, more mysterious, or more wonderful than this? They say that the Emperor Nero himself (fascinated perhaps by the wonder of this theme) wished to look into the corpse of his dead mother and gaze upon that first domicile of man, from which he himself had issued.[22]

Here Nero is evoked as only a positive precursor, as someone straightforwardly and understandably curious to see inside the female cadaver and especially the uterus. Nero is feted as a man who looked. Seeing is uncomplicatedly wonderful for Fabricius. Fabricius imagines a counterposition against which he defends his work, but it seems to be that the embryo might be too mundane or practical and not as valuable as the usual gifts that people gave aristocratic patrons like his dedicatee. He has no qualms, no squeamishness, no nervousness about whether his subject might cause offence in other ways. He does concede that his subject may be "difficult" but uses an old proverb to reassure readers that "everything beautiful is difficult."[23] For Fabricius, Nero is unquestioningly right to want to see inside his mother; the murder and Nero's monstrous desires are not the point. But Maienshein's mode of looking at the preimplantation embryo in the fertility clinic does not rely on dissection. I don't accuse her or Fabricius of being an apologist for crimes like Nero's. Yet she shares with Fabricius this sense that looking is an unequivocal social good and that when we look, we will see and know with all clarity.

■

I asked for some tissue from one of my failed pregnancies to be viewed under the microscope in a laboratory. When I asked for it, the consultant gynaecologist who treated me said something like, "You can have this if you want, but you won't find out anything." Do not look; there will be nothing to see. I did find out something, though. This is the letter that came back: "I now have the genetic results of your recent miscarriage and the result does show an abnormal male consistent with trisomy 15." Trisomy 15 means that part of the fifteenth chromosome appears three times rather than twice in the embryo's cells. People are sometimes but rarely born with trisomy 15. Most affected embryos are miscarried. So it is very uncommon that people live with the condition. My trisomy 15 embryo was unviable. That is the way it is. Loss is sometimes what happens. Seeing can aid acceptance.

But trisomy 15 has a history and a visual context. Pejoratively, people born with trisomy 15 were historically described as having "happy puppet syndrome."[24] They were labelled like this because of their supposed facial similarity to the subject of a strange portrait by the sixteenth-century painter Giovanni Francesco Caroto (1480–1555). The painting was of a redhaired child showing his or her drawing of a stick man (historical figure 9). Sixteenth-century children drew stick men too! Let's assume, because of my "male consistent with trisomy 15," that Caroto's child is a boy. He is looking at me and holding my gaze but asking me to look at his picture rather than at him. His smile tells me that he is pleased with it: "Look," he seems to say. As if to underscore the point, his figure drawing is accompanied by a sketch of an eye. Look with your eyes, he specifies. And when we look, we see the artist in formation within the child, and his drawn figure is also half-formed and rudimentary. I feel connected to, comforted by, and intrigued by this picture. It represents a part of me that I had to let go, arrested in formation—a picture of the beauty of a developmental process that interrupts me and which I, in turn, interrupt.

So here I am trying to be rational—having pushed for microscopic analysis and for scientific knowledge, out science-ing my

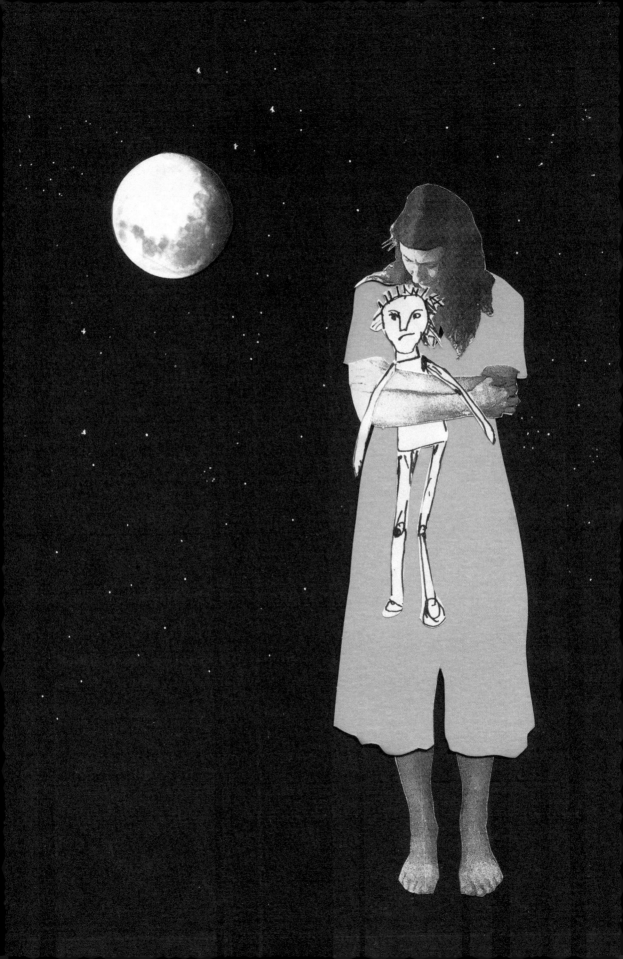

medical consultant and accepting enlightenment. I am holding the consultant's letter, trying to dispel the thought that this never-child stepped into me from the Renaissance past, out of the frame of this captivating portrait, with the thought that the term "happy puppet" is now rejected from the trisomy diagnosis. Sorrow makes connections where none exist. Only the letter, with its technical language and this tissue cytogenetics report, is real. The five-hundred-year-old Caroto portrait is history. But then I learn that the new term, the unpejorative term, is Angelman syndrome. The condition is named for Harry Angelman (1915–1996), who first described it in three children in 1965, which was a feat because of its rarity, and who drew the connection to Caroto's smiling child.[25] Angelman doesn't mean "angel man," even though the Caroto child looks so beatific and even though he resembles those who are born with the condition; Angelman just happens to be Harry Angelman's name. Angelman is a coincidence. In Caroto's day, though, coincidences were revelations. And whether mundane coincidence or revelation, I cannot erase this half-person half-angel from my dreams—dreams into which the Enlightenment does not reach and where this child sits with a packet of crayons doing his child's drawings.

The question here is: who or what starts "it"? Here I am, living my own life, misconceiving, turning to medicine and science to help where it can. At the same time, a history of curious outcomes constantly drags the past into my present, demanding my attention. Mixed forms of understanding happen to us all.

Monsters Un-Inc.

A powerful historical idea about how the imagination intersected with conception and pregnancy concerned the maternal impression: sight or the imagination itself could carry an image, like a print block, down to the womb and into the impressionable stuff of the forming foetus.[26] From this perspective, pregnant women had to be careful about what they looked at or thought about for fear of causing disability, or transferring the features of someone or something other than the child's natural father. In this exoticising view, if a white pregnant woman with a white partner looked at a Black person or an image of one, her baby would be Black. If she looked at an image of a monster, her child would resemble it, or if she looked at an icon of John the Baptist, the baby would be covered in a thick pelt of hair. The language that surrounded

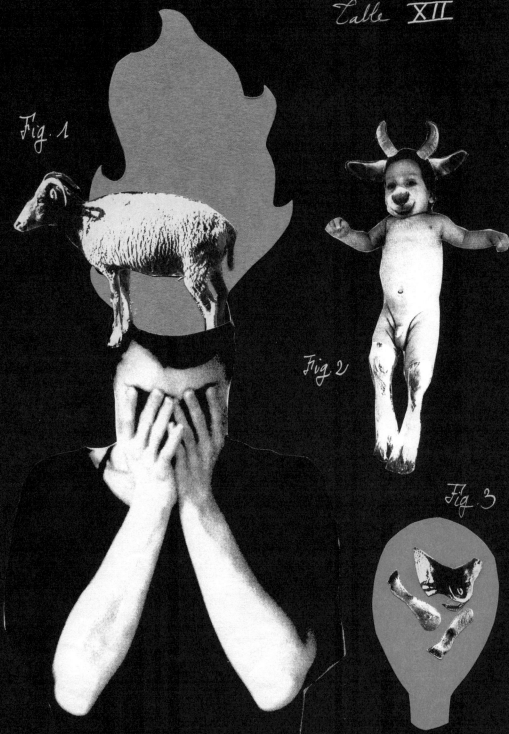

Table XII

Fig. 1

Fig. 2

Fig. 3

this notion was of monstrosity, bizarre animal-human births, and other extraordinary natural reproductive phenomena. The fullest description of the maternal impression is found in Ambroise Pare's (1510–1590) *On Monsters and Marvels*, which, paradoxically, also fully illustrated the scenes on which the pregnant woman was not advised to look.

This was a thesis that William Harvey directly rejected and, instead, he contributed his own, which I have been presenting to you, about how the uterus—"a no lesse admirable Organ than the Braine"—can think about and copy "information in" without material influence.[27] He thinks of the womb's creative process as analogous to the way that artists make art, birds make nests, and spiders make webs: sometimes the original is absent but can nonetheless be reproduced by instinct or skill. Harvey's thesis is less suspicious of thought and the imagination generally and of women more specifically than those contemporaries who signed up to the idea of the maternal impression. Unlike those contemporaries, Harvey is not primarily concerned with the securely formed and eventually birthed foetus and its unexpected forms—with "monsters and marvels"—but rather with the prior question of conception itself and embryogenesis as a process. He is interested in the time before reproductive outcomes are known, in living with the possibilities but also the doubt of the epigenetic process, and with becoming but also, radically, unbecoming. What is more, he owns up to the role of the imagination and fiction in the making of new knowledge. He sees a gap, and in that knowledge void he creates a "fable" that can effectively explain it. But, he reminds us: "all those Opinions (which we now cry up) were at first meere figments, and imaginations, untill they wrought a solid credit in us, by sensible experiment."[28] He knew that his "conception" was thus conjectural and fictional and that it may or may not come to be credited—that ideas take shape and are proved (or not) over time.

This book had a different body to investigate than the one which confronted Harvey: not the flesh and blood of women or animals or the foetus exactly, but fragments and figments from the historical archive. That task also presented the challenge of duration over time, like epigenesis: of seeing and capturing the metamorphic nature of history. What I have found is that my research objects did not present themselves neatly lined up chronologically, one giving way to another that showed slightly more advancement, like embryos in eggs between laying and hatching. I did not find a history of development and progress but rather a more anarchic hybridity to the way that conception experience is lived in any period. History is more unbecoming than becoming. Ignorance does not straightforwardly give way to knowledge, and neither does faith to reason nor myth to science. One consistent change over time, however, is the increasing inability to acknowledge the coexistence of those apparently contradictory forms. The things we choose to renounce—unknowing, faith, folklore—must be pushed out of modernity, backwards into history, even though in practice, they sit all around us amongst everything we categorise as modern, although in what exact combination it is difficult to assess. Whether they are "bubbles? or some rude and indigested lump? or a conception, or coagulation of mixed seed? or whether any thing else?" we cannot tell.[29]

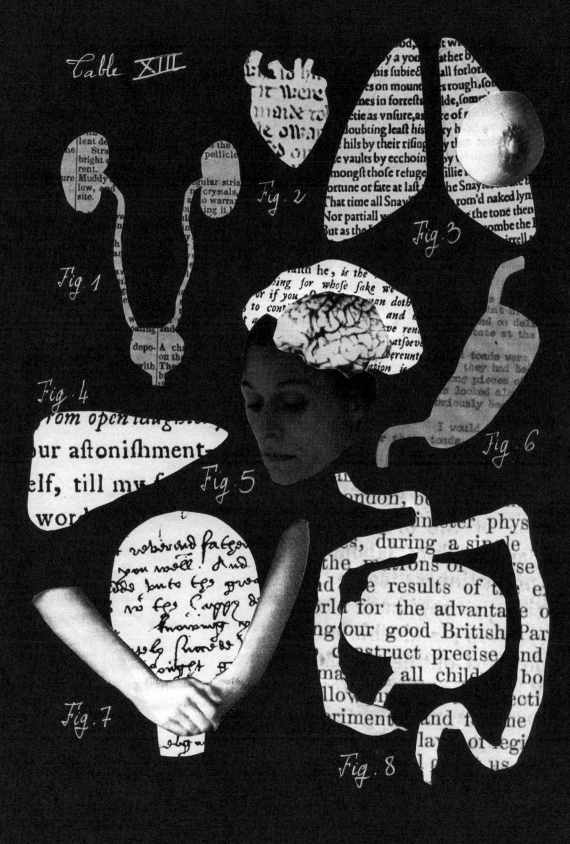

Historical Figures

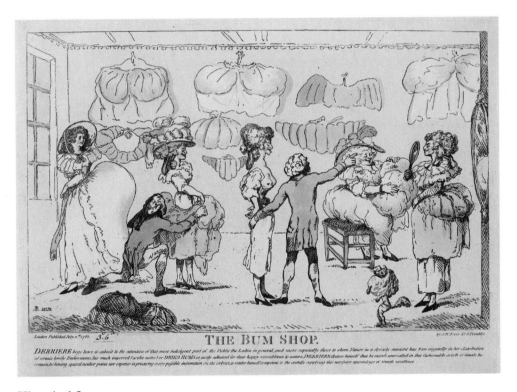

THE BUM SHOP.

Historical figure 1
The Bum Shop, 1785, etching, published by S. W. Fores,
British Museum Prints and Drawings,
London, registration number 1932,0226.12.
© The Trustees of the British Museum.

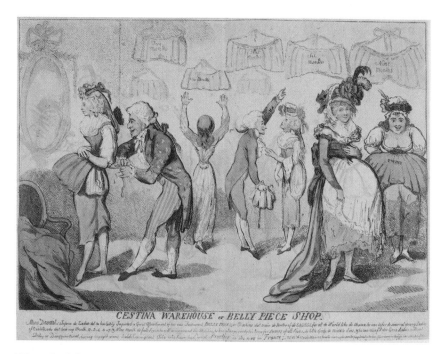

Historical figure 2
Isaac Cruikshank?, *The Cestina Warehouse or Belly Piece Shop*, 1793, etching, published by S. W. Fores, British Museum Prints and Drawings, London, registration number 1935,0522.8.28. © The Trustees of the British Museum.

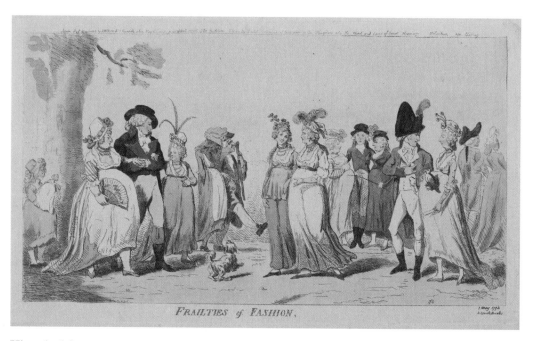

Historical figure 3
Isaac Cruikshank, *Frailties of Fashion*, 1793, etching, published by S. W. Fores, British Museum Prints and Drawings, London, registration number 1868,0808.6292. © The Trustees of the British Museum.

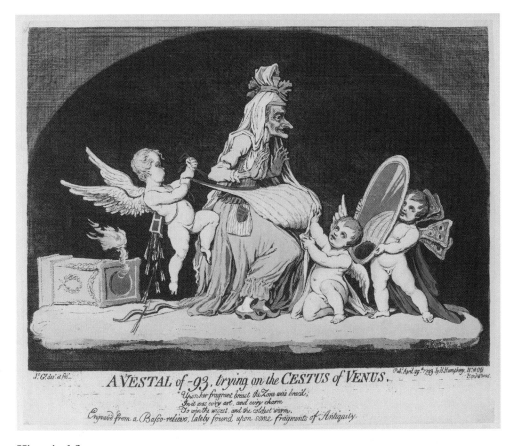

Historical figure 4
James Gillray, *A Vestal of '93 Trying on the Cestus of Venus*, 1793, etching,
published by Hannah Humphrey, National Portrait Gallery, London,
registration number NPG D13015. © National Portrait Gallery, London.

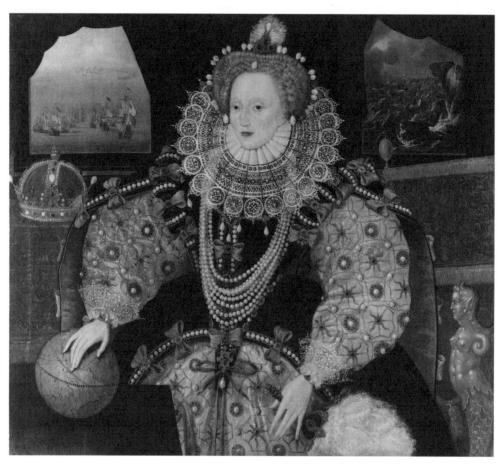

Historical figure 5
Armada Portrait of Elizabeth I, ca. 1588, Queen's House,
National Maritime Museum, London, ID number ZBA7719.

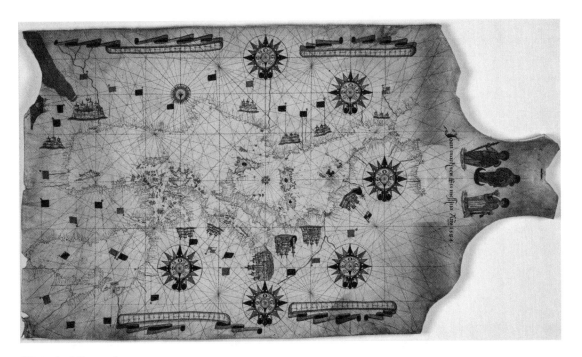

Historical figure 6
Joan Martines, Royal Cartographer to Philip II of Spain, *Portolan Map of the Mediterranean*, 1584, hand-drawn and coloured on vellum, Trinity College Library, Cambridge, MS. R.4.50. © The Master and Fellows of Trinity College, Cambridge.

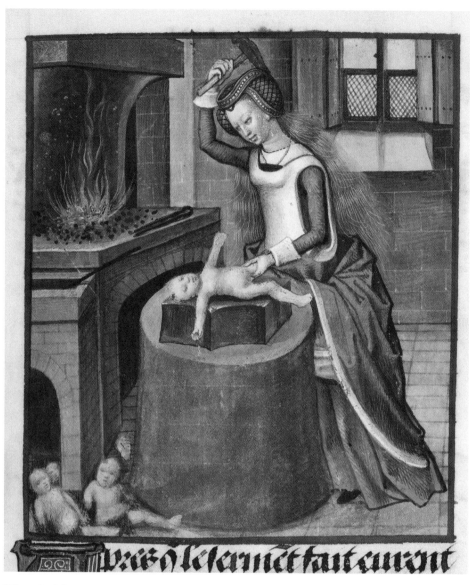

Historical figure 7
Nature in Her Forge, ca. 1490–1500, paint on parchment, 39.5 × 29 cm,
British Library, London, MS. Harley 4425, f. 140.
© The British Library Board.

Historical Figures

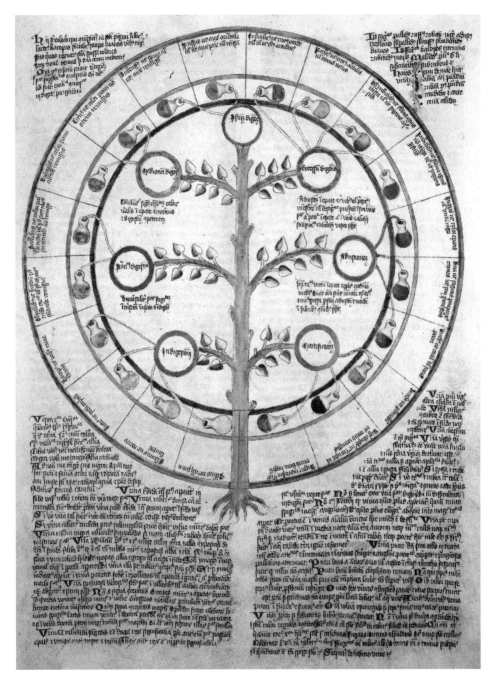

Historical figure 8
Urine image, from *Wellcome Apocalypse*, ca. 1420. Wellcome Collection, London, Wellcome MS. 49, fol. 42r, https://wellcomecollection.org/works /du9ua6nd. Public domain mark.

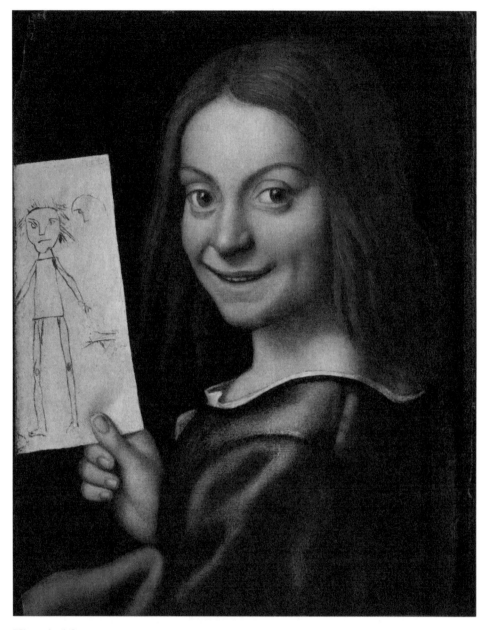

Historical figure 9
Giovanni Francesco Caroto, *Ritratto di giovane con disegno infantile*
(*Portrait of a Child with Drawing*), 1515–1520, oil on wood, 37 x 29 cm,
Museo di Castelvecchio, Verona, inv. 5519–1B130. Photography credit:
Archivio Fotografico dei Musei Civici, Verona (Gardaphoto, Salò).

Acknowledgements

Anna and I have incurred many debts in the making of this book and are unable fully to articulate our gratitude. We are particularly thankful for the support we received when we faced rejection, delay, and uncertainty. I received funding for library and archives research from Birkbeck's Wellcome Trust Institutional Strategic Support Fund in 2016 and 2017.

Thanks to our families who have lived with this project for so long: Mark Perrott, Jaime Valtierra, Lewis Perrott, Alma Valtierra Burel, and Otto Valtierra Burel.

Thank you to Katie Helke, Justin Kehoe, Suraiya Jetha, Deborah Cantor-Adams, Rosemary Winfield, their colleagues, and the peer readers at the MIT Press. Thanks to Jess Farr-Cox for the index.

We are also grateful for the support of Leah Astbury, Anthony Bale, Lisa Baraitser, Richard Barnett, Robin Basu Roy, Heike Bauer, Cordelia Beattie, Suzannah Biernoff, Mike Bintley, Joanna Bourke, Elma Brenner, Julia Bueno, Carolyn Burdett, Rémy Burel, Sarah-Lou Burel, David Burel, Emma Cheatle, Hanya Chlala, Catherine Clarke, Zaza Curran-Griffiths, David Davis, Mary Davis, Dennis Duncan, Wendy Earle, Carmen Fracchia, Montse Gallego, Agathe Geiger, Eliane Glaser, Jeremy Goldberg, Grace Halden, Anna Hartnell, Karen Hearn, Jessica Hepburn, Julie Hipperson, Nick Hopwood, Fiona Johnstone, Sophie Jones, Susie Latta, Mary Beth Long, Tracey Loughran, Julia Martins, Emily Mayhew, Cathy McClive, Nicola McDonald, Clare Monagle, Tabitha Moses, Jesse Olszynko-Gryn, Kim Phillips, Jane Reavley, Felicity Riddy, Catherine Rider, Peter Riley, Jutta Rolf, Laura Salisbury, Benedicte Siewe, Stephanie Trigg, Marion Turner, Gabby Vautier-Farr, Margot Waggoner, Fintan Walsh, Rosie Wanek, Marina Warner, Diane Watt, Rebecca Whiteley, and Jo Winning.

Particular thanks to Luisa Calé, Mark Perrott, and Sue Wiseman, who read and commented on multiple drafts across many years.

I/we have learned a lot from academic conference audiences at the Universities of Brighton, Cambridge, Essex, Exeter, Leeds, Oxford, Southampton, Strathclyde, Sussex, and York; de Montfort and Swansea Universities; The Centre for the Study of Medicine and the Body in the Renaissance, Pisa; gallery visitors and staff at the Peltz and Hundred Years Galleries in London, and festival goers and participants at the Being Human Festival, Birkbeck Arts Week, and Fertility Fest. I am also grateful for the help of archivists and other staff at the British Library and Wellcome Collection Library in London.

Thank you, too, to my former colleagues and students at Birkbeck, University of London, who created such an exceptionally rich and generative research environment in which to conduct this research.

Notes

Introduction: Annunciations

1. Angela Carter, Unpublished journal, 1961–1962, British Library, London, Additional MS. 88899/1/87, f. 9r.
2. There is a huge literature on menstrual regulation. See, for example, Jennifer Evans, *Aphrodisiacs, Fertility and Medicine in Early Modern England* (Woodbridge, UK: Boydell Press, 2014), 171; Angus McLaren, *Reproductive Rituals: The Perception of Fertility in England from the Sixteenth Century to the Nineteenth Century* (London: Methuen, 1984), 102–103.
3. A rich body of work is emerging on historical infertility and miscarriage. For a discussion of why those histories have taken time to be written, see Christina Benninghaus, "Silences: Coping with Infertility in Nineteenth-Century Germany," in *The Palgrave Handbook of Infertility in History*, eds. Gayle Davis and Tracey Loughran (London: Palgrave, 2017), 100.
4. Shannon Withycombe, *Lost: Miscarriage in Nineteenth-Century America* (New Brunswick, NJ: Rutgers University Press, 2018), is a particularly interesting example from a growing historiography.
5. Donna J. Drucker, *Fertility Technology* (Cambridge, MA: MIT Press, 2023), 166.
6. Lauren Kassell, Michael Hawkins, Robert Ralley, John Young, Joanne Edge, Janet Yvonne Martin-Portugues, and Natalie Kaoukji, eds., *The Casebooks of Simon Forman and Richard Napier, 1596–1634: A Digital Edition*, The Casebooks Project, University of Cambridge, accessed January 27, 2021, https://casebooks.lib.cam.ac.uk.
7. Miranda Ward, *Adrift: Fieldnotes from Almost-Motherhood* (London: Weidenfeld & Nicolson, 2021), 113.
8. Ariel Levy, *The Rules Do Not Apply* (London: Fleet, 2017), 86.
9. This is particularly the case in the 1831 edition of the novel, where medieval science is given a greater hold over Frankenstein's experiments. Mary Wollstonecraft Shelley, *Frankenstein; or, the Modern Prometheus* (London: Colburn and Bentley, 1831), 38.
10. Shelley, *Frankenstein*, 26.
11. Pregnancy ambiguity is a prominent topic in reproductive history with an expanding literature. See, for example, Suzanne O. Bell and Mary Fissell, "A Little Bit Pregnant? Productive Ambiguity and Fertility Research," *Population and Development Review* 47, no. 2 (2021): 505–526; Cathy McClive, "The Hidden Truths of the Belly: The Uncertainties of Pregnancy in Early Modern Europe," *Social History of Medicine* 15 (2002): 209–22.
12. I am grateful to Lisa Surridge and Mary Elizabeth Leighton for this observation, through personal communication.
13. J. Allan Mitchell, *Becoming Human: The Matter of the Medieval Child*

(Minneapolis: University of Minnesota Press, 2014), 8.

14. Lara Freidenfelds, *The Myth of the Perfect Pregnancy: A History of Miscarriage in America* (Oxford: Oxford University Press, 2019).

15. The quotation comes from S. B. Shigley, "Great Expectations: Infertility, Disability, and Possibility," in *The Palgrave Handbook of Infertility in History*, eds. Gayle Davis and Tracey Loughran (London: Palgrave, 2017), 45. See also Davis and Loughran, "Introduction," 5.

16. Miriam Stoppard, *Conception, Pregnancy and Birth: The Childbirth Bible for Today's Parents*, rev. ed. (London: Dorling Kindersley, 2008), 32–33.

17. M. C. Seymour, ed., *On the Properties of Things: John Trevisa's Translation of Bartholomaeus Anglicus, De Proprietatibus Rerum: A Critical Text*, 3 vols. (Oxford: Clarendon Press, 1975–1988), vol. 1, book 6, chap. 3, p. 296.

18. Heidi Murkoff, Arlene Eisenberg, and Sandee Hathaway, *What to Expect When You're Expecting*, 3rd ed. (London: Pocket Books, 2002, first published 1984), 2.

19. Stoppard, *Conception, Pregnancy and Birth*, 60.

20. *Oxford English Dictionary*, s.v. "intuition (n.)," esp. entry 4, accessed July 2023, https://doi.org/10.1093/OED/1096866985.

21. Robert Lyall, *The Medical Evidence Relative to the Duration of Human Pregnancy* (London: Burgess and Hill, 1826), ix.

22. Thom Gunn, *Selected Poems, 1950–1975* (London: Faber & Faber, 1979), 6–7.

Chapter 1

1. Edward Topsell, *The Historie of Serpents* (London: William Jaggard, 1608), 183, ESTC S122051.

2. Mary Douglas, *Purity and Danger: An Analysis of Concept of Pollution and Taboo* (London: Routledge, 2002, first published 1966), 217.

3. Jacob Grimm and Wilhelm Grimm, "The Juniper Tree," in *The Complete Folk and Fairy Tales of the Brothers Grimm*, trans. Margaret Hunt (Ballingslöv, Sweden: Wisehouse Classics, 2016), 122.

4. It reads "man se kregen keen und kregen keen." Jacob Grimm and Wilhelm Grimm, "Von dem Machandelbaum," *Kinder und Hausmärchen* (Göttingen, Germany: Dieterich, 1857), no. 47, 232.

5. Grimm and Grimm, *The Complete Folk and Fairy Tales*, 13.

6. Grimm and Grimm, *The Complete Folk and Fairy Tales*, 14.

7. Grimm and Grimm, *The Complete Folk and Fairy Tales*, 132.

8. Mary Karr, *Cherry: A Memoir* (London: Picador, 2017), 125.

9. Mary Wollstonecraft, *A Vindication of Woman*, in *A Vindication of the Rights of Man; A Vindication of the Rights of Woman; An Historical and Moral View of the French Revolution*, ed. Janet Todd (Oxford: Oxford University Press, 1993), 204–205.

10. Wollstonecraft's school is discussed in Susan Skedd, "Women Teachers and the Expansion of Girls' Schooling in England, c. 1760–1820," in *Gender in Eighteenth-Century England: Roles, Representations and Responsibilities*, eds. Hannah Barker and Elaine Chalus (London: Routledge, 1997), 111.

11. See, e.g., Monica H. Green, "Secrets of Women," in *Women and Gender in Medieval Europe: An Encyclopaedia*, ed. Margaret Schaus (London: Routledge, 2006), 734.

12. Many historians have written about this fascinating text. See, e.g., Mary Fissell, "Hairy Women and Naked Truths: Gender and the Politics of Knowledge in *Aristotle's Masterpiece*," *William and Mary Quarterly* 60 (2003): 43–74.

13. See, e.g., Monica H. Green, *Making Women's Medicine Masculine* (Oxford: Oxford University Press, 2008), 244.

14. I owe this observation to Rebecca Whiteley, through personal communication.

15. Emilie Pine, *Notes to Self* (Dublin: Tramp Press, 2018), 42.

16. Elizabeth Grosz, *Volatile Bodies: Toward a Corporeal Feminism* (Bloomington: Indiana University Press, 1995), 203.

17. Alfredo Pérez, "General Overview of Natural Family Planning," *Genus* 54 (1998): 77.

18. On the differences, see, e.g., Toni Weschler, *Taking Charge of Your Fertility: The Definitive Guide to Natural Birth Control, Pregnancy Achievement, and Reproductive Health* (London: Harper Collins, 2006, first published 1995), 4–5.

19. E.g., M. Guida, G. A. Tommaselli, S. Palomba, M. Pellicano, G. Moccia, C. Di Carlo, and C. Nappi, "Efficacy of Methods for Determining Ovulation in a Natural Family Planning Program," *Fertility and Sterility* 72, no. 5 (1999): 900–904.

20. Keith Thomas, "The Meaning of Literacy in Early Modern England," in *The Written Word: Literacy in Transition*, ed. Gerd Baumann (Oxford: Clarendon Press, 1986), 109.

21. There are parts here from Pliny, Suetonius, Tacitus, Boethius, Jacobus de Voragine, and Jean de Meun. See Alastair Minnis, "Aspects of the Medieval French and English Traditions of the *De Consolatione Philosophiae*," in *Boethius: His Life, Thought and Influence*, ed. Margaret Gibson (Oxford: Oxford University Press, 1981).

22. Jacobus de Voragine, *Golden Legend: Readings on the Saints*, trans. William Granger Ryan (Princeton, NJ: Princeton University Press, 2012), 346–348. The story is discussed in Katherine Park, *The Secrets of Women: Gender, Generation, and the Origins of Human Dissection* (Chicago: Zone Books, 2006), 151–157.

23. See, e.g., *Roman de la rose*, ca. 1525, manuscript, Morgan Library and Museum, New York, MS. M.948, fol. 63r, a digital surrogate is available at *Roman de la Rose* Digital Library, Sheridan Libraries, Johns Hopkins University, https://dlmm.library.jhu.edu/viewer/#rose/Morgan948/063r/image.

24. Lazzaro Spallanzani's experiments, putting frogs in trousers to collect sperm, are not discussed here because they are covered thoroughly elsewhere. See, e.g., Clara Pinto-Correia, *The Ovary of Eve: Egg and Sperm and Preformation* (Chicago: University of Chicago Press, 1997), 183–210.

25. Lorna Sage, *Bad Blood* (London: Fourth Estate, 2000), 236.

26. Ann Oakley, *The Captured Womb: A History of the Medical Care of Pregnant Women* (Oxford: Basil Blackwell, 1990, first published 1984), 98.

27. The history of pregnancy testing is also told elsewhere. On the British context, see Jesse Olszynko-Gryn, *A Woman's Right to Know: Pregnancy Testing in Twentieth-Century Britain* (Cambridge, MA: MIT Press, 2023), which has a detailed account of the use of *Xenopus*. Page numbers not available. I am grateful to Jesse for letting me read the prepublication manuscript.

28. Family Planning Association Archive, "Pregnancy Diagnosis Laboratory." Wellcome Collection, London, SA/FPA/A3, 11–13.

29. Jesse Olszynko-Gryn, "The Demand for Pregnancy Testing: The Aschheim-Zondek Reaction, Diagnostic Versatility, and Laboratory Services in 1930s Britain," *Studies in History and Philosophy of Science* 47, part B (2014): 233–247.

30. J. B. Gurdon and N. Hopwood, "The Introduction of *Xenopus laevis* into Developmental Biology: Of Empire, Pregnancy Testing and Ribosomal Genes," *International Journal of Developmental Biology* 44 (2000): 45; H. Zwarenstein, "The Frog Pregnancy Test: The First of Its Kind in the World," *Bulletin of the Adler Museum of the History of Medicine* 11 (1985): 9–10.

31. This dispute is covered in Olszynko-Gryn, *A Woman's Right to Know*.

32. William Beinart and Lotte Hughes, *Environment and Empire* (Oxford: Oxford University Press, 2007), esp.

chap. 4. For discussion of the phrase "commodity frontier," see 2.

33. Beinart and Hughes, *Environment and Empire*, 64.

34. Beinart and Hughes, *Environment and Empire*, 66–67. On diamonds and gold, see Martin Meredith, *Diamonds, Gold, and War: The British, the Boers and the Making of South Africa* (New York: Simon and Schuster, 2007), 30.

35. Gurdon and Hopwood, "The Introduction of *Xenopus laevis*," 43–44.

36. Olszynko-Gryn, *A Woman's Right to Know*.

37. Edward Elkan, "Sketches from My Life," 1983, unpublished memoir, Wellcome Collection, London, MS. 9151.

38. Elkan, "Sketches from My Life," 56.

39. "Heritage Statement by Beacon Planning," November 2015, Application number PP/15/07206, Royal Borough of Kensington and Chelsea, London, accessed July 5, 2021, https://www.rbkc.gov.uk.

40. Internal FPA note by Beric Wright to chairman of finance committee, "Correspondence and Papers," in Pregnancy Diagnosis Laboratory. Family Planning Association Archive, Wellcome Collection, London, SA/FPA/A3, 11.

41. Lance van Sittert and G. John Measey, "Historical Perspectives on Global Exports and Research of African Clawed Frogs (*Xenopus laevis*)," *Transactions of the Royal Society of South Africa* 71 (2016): 157–166.

42. A. W. Wells, *South Africa: A Planned Tour of the Country To-Day* (London: J. M. Dent, 1949, first published 1939), 28.

43. Joy Cobern, *Fish Hoek, Looking Back* (Fish Hoek, South Africa: Fish Hoek Printing and Publishing, 2003), chap. 1, https://gosouth.co.za/wp-content/uploads/2016/05/FISH-HOEK-Looking-Back-Pdf.pdf.

44. Letter from FPA to Thomas Cook, May 31, 1950, in "Correspondence and Papers," in Pregnancy Diagnosis Laboratory. Family Planning Association Archive, Wellcome Collection, London, SA/FPA/A3, 11.

45. Letter from Thomas Cook to FPA, February 11, 1949, in "Correspondence and Papers," in Pregnancy Diagnosis Laboratory. Family Planning Association Archive, Wellcome Collection, London, SA/FPA/A3, 11.

46. Shipping journalist Michael Grey, speaking in "The MV Stirling Castle," *On Your Behalf*, BBC World Service, December 9, 1998, https://www.bbc.co.uk/sounds/play/p033jx6n. See also Harriet McKay, "'It's Fun in South Africa': Interior Design for the Union Castle Shipping Line, 1948–1977," in *The Politics of Design: Privilege and Prejudice in Aotearoa New Zealand, Australia and South Africa*, eds. Federico Freschi, Farieda Nazier, and Jane Venis, 231–253 (Dunedin, New Zealand: Otago Polytechnic Press, 2022). A Union-Castle brochure from 1930 can be seen at Union-Castle Mail Steamship Company, "South Africa, East and West Africa," 1930, brochure, Cayzer Family Archive, https://cayzer.com/business/shipping/union-castle-s-s-company/union-castle-line-motorships-brochure.

47. Rodney Gascoigne, "Life at Sea with Union Castle," 2003, Wayback Machine, https://web.archive.org/web/20060212220823/http://rgascoyne.canadianwebs.com/LifeAtSea.htm.

48. Beinart and Hughes, *Environment and Empire*, 63.

49. Edward R. Elkan, "The *Xenopus* Pregnancy Test," *British Medical Journal* 2 (1938): 1253.

50. Ché Weldon, Atherton L. De Villiers, and Louis H. Du Preez, "Quantification of the Trade in *Xenopus laevis* from South Africa, with Implications for Biodiversity Conservation," *African Journal of Herpetology* 56 (2007): 77.

51. Letter from Thomas Cook to FPA, July 15, 1954, in "Correspondence and Papers," in Pregnancy Diagnosis Laboratory. Family Planning Association Archive, Wellcome Collection, London, SA/FPA/A3, 11.

52. Weldon, De Villiers, and Du Preez, "Quantification of the Trade in *Xenopus laevis*," 80.

53. Van Sittert and Measey, "Historical Perspectives," 157.

54. See, e.g., The Convention on Biological Diversity (1992) and The Nagoya Protocol (2011).

55. Klavs Skovsholm, "The Right to Vote in South-Africa—A Hundred Years of Experience," *Law and Politics in Africa, Asia and Latin America* 32 (1999): 239–240.

56. Janet Remmington, "Solomon Plaatje's Decade of Creative Mobility, 1912–1922: The Politics of Travel and Writing in and beyond South Africa," *Journal of Southern African Studies* 39 (2013): 427.

57. McKay, "'It's Fun in South Africa,'" 237.

58. "Union Castle Line (Race Segregation)," House of Commons Debate, December 6, 1948, Hansard, vol. 459, cols. 30–31, https://api .parliament.uk/historic-hansard /commons/1948/dec/06/union-castle -line-race-segregation.

59. G. R. Berridge, *The Politics of the South Africa Run: European Shipping and Pretoria* (Oxford: Oxford University Press, 1987).

60. Max Price, "Health Care as an Instrument of Apartheid Policy in South Africa," *Health Policy and Planning* 3 (1982): 161.

61. Aziza Seedat, *Crippling a Nation: Health in Apartheid South Africa* (London: International Defence and Aid Fund for South Africa, 1984), 12.

62. Seedat, *Crippling a Nation*, 12–13.

63. Amnesty International, *Struggle for Maternal Health: Barriers to Antenatal Care in South Africa* (London: Amnesty International, 2014), https://www .amnesty.org/en/documents/afr53 /006/2014/en; Njeri Wabiri, Matthew Chersich, Olive Shisana, Duane Blaauw, Helen Rees, and Ntabozuko Dwane, "Growing Inequities in Maternal Health in South Africa: A Comparison of Serial National Household Surveys," *BMC Pregnancy and Childbirth* 16 (2016): 8, https://doi .org/10.1186/s12884-016-1048-z.

64. Chelsea Morroni and Jennifer Moodley, "The Role of Urine Pregnancy Testing in Facilitating Access to Antenatal Care and Abortion Services in South Africa: A Cross-Sectional Study," *BMC Pregnancy and Childbirth* 6 (2006): 1–3, https://doi.org/10.1186/1471-2393-6-26.

65. Angela Carter, "The Baby," ca. 1961, unpublished story, British Library, London, MS. Additional 88899/1/42.

66. Letter from FPA to general secretary of the BMA, Dr. S. J. Hadfield, December 1, 1949, in "Correspondence and Papers," in Pregnancy Diagnosis Laboratory. Family Planning Association Archive, Wellcome Collection, London, SA/FPA/A3, 11.

67. N. J. Van Abbee, Letter to *Pharmaceutical Journal*, July 23, 1949, Family Planning Association Archive, Wellcome Collection, London, SA/ FPA/A3, 11.

68. Olszynko-Gryn, *A Woman's Right to Know*.

69. "Radar for the Stork," *Reveille*, August 27, 1949, clipping available in Family Planning Association Archive, Wellcome Collection, London, SA/FPA/A3, 11.

70. Jesse Olszynko-Gryn, "The Feminist Appropriation of Pregnancy Testing in 1970s Britain," *Women's History Review* 28 (2019): 871.

Chapter 2

1. Isobel English, *Every Eye* (London: Persephone, 2000, first published 1956), 32.

2. Naomi Mitchison, *You May Well Ask: A Memoir 1920–1940* (London: Flamingo, 1986, first published 1979), 52.

3. See, e.g., Adrienne Rich, *Of Woman Born: Motherhood as Experience and Institution* (New York: Norton, 1995, first published 1976), chap. 2.

4. See, e.g., "Ring," 1300–1400, bronze, engraved with "O mater dei memento" (O mother of God, remember me), Victoria and Albert Museum, London,

V&A accession number 995-1871, https://collections.vam.ac.uk/item/O377756/ring.

5. Mitchison, *You May Well Ask*, 52.

6. Mitchison, *You May Well Ask*, 45.

7. Cited in Barbara Charlesworth Gelpi, *Shelley's Goddess: Maternity, Language, Subjectivity* (Oxford: Oxford University Press, 1992), 46.

8. "Fashion: A Guide to Chic for Maternity Clothes," *Vogue*, June 7, 1930, 82–83, 102, 106, 126.

9. Thomas Hawkes Tanner, *On the Signs and Diseases of Pregnancy* (London: Henry Renshaw, 1860), 26.

10. Leslie Tuttle, *Conceiving the Old Regime: Pronatalism and the Politics of Reproduction in Early Modern France* (Oxford: Oxford University Press, 2010), 5.

11. *The Pad, a New Ballad, Sung by Mr Dighton* (London: 42 Long Lane, ca. 1795).

12. Lisa Freeman Cody, *Birthing the Nation: Sex, Science, and the Conception of Eighteenth-Century Britons* (Oxford: Oxford University Press, 2005), 17.

13. See, for example, Gelpi, *Shelley's Goddess*, 46–47.

14. Mireya Navarro, "Here Comes the Mother-to-Be," *New York Times*, March 13, 2005, 1.

15. Maggie Nelson, *The Argonauts* (London: Melville House, 2015), 100–101.

16. Robert Woodbridge, *The Pad, a Farce, in One Act* (London: J. Parsons, 1793), ESTC T043545. See also Gelpi, *Shelley's Goddess*, 59–60.

17. "Review of *The Pad: A Farce, in One Act*, by Robert Woodbridge," in *The Monthly Review: or Literary Journal Enlarged* 11 (1793): 348–349, https://hdl.handle.net/2027/hvd.hxjg9t.

18. Woodbridge, *The Pad*, 20.

19. Elizabeth Inchbald, *Every One Has His Fault* (Dublin, 1793), ESTC T20768.

20. Woodbridge, *The Pad*, 3.

21. Woodbridge, *The Pad*, 9.

22. Woodbridge, *The Pad*, 23–24.

23. Woodbridge, *The Pad*, 35.

24. Woodbridge, *The Pad*, 34.

25. Woodbridge, *The Pad*, 7.

26. Woodbridge, *The Pad*, 36.

27. Woodbridge, *The Pad*, 37.

28. Benjamin Zephaniah, "I'm 64 and My Infertility Still Brings Me to Tears," inews.co.uk, August 5, 2022, https://web.archive.org/web/20220812031319/https://inews.co.uk/opinion/benjamin-zephaniah-64-infertility-tears-1772217. See also Robin A. Hadley, *How Is a Man Supposed to Be a Man: Male Childlessness—A Life Course Disrupted* (Oxford: Berghahn, 2021).

29. Woodbridge, *The Pad*, 7.

30. Gelpi, *Shelley's Goddess*, 60.

31. Homer, *The Iliad of Homer*, trans. Alexander Pope, 2 vols. (Edinburgh: A. Donaldson, 1769, first published 1715), 2:150.

32. Chris Brooke, "Why College Girls Are Missing Out on Motherhood," *Daily Mail*, October 1, 2004, 17. See also Eir Nolsoe, "What Is the Ideal Age to Have Children," YouGov, June 21, 2021, accessed November 12, 2022, https://yougov.co.uk/topics/lifestyle/articles-reports/2021/06/21/what-ideal-age-have-children.

33. Cari Rosen, *The Secret Diary of a New Mum Aged 43¼* (London: Vermillion, 2011), 5.

34. E.g., Joyce Harper, *Your Fertile Years: What You Need to Know to Make Informed Choices* (London: Sheldon Press, 2021), 51–71.

35. Kate Spicer, "Leaving It Too Late," *Sunday Times*, October 2, 2011.

36. See, e.g., Arwa Mahdawi, "It Is Time to Reassess Our Obsession with Women's Fertility and the Number 35," *The Guardian*, April 10, 2021; Nicholas Raine-Fenning, "Hard Evidence: Does Fertility Really Drop Off a Cliff at 35?," *The Conversation*, July 15, 2014.

37. Harper, *Your Fertile Years*, 54; Ulla Larsen and Sharon Yan, "The Age Pattern of Fecundability: An Analysis of French Canadian and Hutterite Birth Histories," *Social Biology* 47 (2000): 34–50.

38. There is a huge literature on the age at marriage and first birth. A classic study

of England, e.g., is E. A. Wrigley and Roger Schofield, *The Population History of England, 1541–1871: A Reconstruction* (London: Edward Arnold, 1981).

39. Ursula A. Cowgill, "Marriage and Its Progeny in the City of York, 1538–1751," *Kroeber Anthropological Society Papers* 42 (1970): 75; E. A. Wrigley, *Population and History* (New York: McGraw-Hill, 1969), 116–127; Wrigley and Schofield, *Population History*, 255–266.

40. Office for National Statistics, "Standardised Mean Age of Mother by Birth Order, 1938–2020 England and Wales," Information on Births by Parents' Characteristic Statistics, UK Statistics Authority, January 13, 2022, https://www.ons.gov.uk/file?uri=/peoplepopulationandcommunity/birthsdeathsandmarriages/livebirths/datasets/birthsbyparentscharacteristics/2020/finalparentscharacteristics2020 workbook.xlsx. It is very hard to do historical comparisons, because of the difficulty of comparing like with like in vastly differing data sets.

41. There are caveats here: the historical figures exclude the illegitimacy rates and aren't corrected for the numbers of never married. These bring these numbers lower.

42. Rosen, *Secret Diary*, 6.

43. Grace Halden, Mel Johnson, Shalaka Kamerkar, Nancy Milligan, Genevieve Roberts, and Rebecca Ward, "Independent Family Planning: Choosing Solo Parenthood through Gamete or Embryo Donation," Wellcome Trust, March 2023, https://www.drgracehalden.com/_files/ugd/8699d5_e8afa75dcc4c42919081e495f5dd4aea.pdf.

44. Rosamund Urwin, "Having a Baby Takes a Bit of Forward Planning," *London Evening Standard*, January 31, 2011, 17.

45. BBC News, "Where Have All the Men Gone?," April 6, 2004, http://news.bbc.co.uk/1/hi/magazine/3601493.stm; Danny Dorling and Ludi Simpson, "Where Have All the Young Men Gone?," BBC Radio 4, April 2004 and January 2, 2005, http://www.radstats.org.uk/news/censusradio4.htm.

46. Nora Ephron, *Heartburn* (London: Virago, 1996, first published 1983), 75.

47. Jack Kerouac, *On the Road* (New York: Viking, 1955), 111.

48. Kerouac, *On the Road*, 74.

49. Carolyn Cassady, *Off the Road: My Years with Cassady, Kerouac, and Ginsberg* (New York: Morrow, 1990), 30.

50. Cassady, *Off the Road*, 50.

51. Nelson, *Argonauts*, 16–17, 22.

52. Mary Wollstonecraft, *A Vindication of the Rights of Woman*, in *A Vindication of the Rights of Man; A Vindication of the Rights of Woman; An Historical and Moral View of the French Revolution*, ed. Janet Todd (Oxford: Oxford University Press, 1993), 109.

53. Betty Friedan, *The Feminine Mystique* (London: Thread, 2021, first published 1963), 95–96.

54. Friedan, *The Feminine Mystique*, 43.

55. *The Pad, a New Ballad, Sung by Mr Dighton.*

Chapter 3

1. Hilary Mantel, "Royal Bodies," *London Review of Books* 35, no. 4 (2013).

2. Sheila Heti, *Motherhood: A Novel* (London: Penguin, 2018), 32.

3. Rachel Chrastil, *How to Be Childless: A History and Philosophy of Life without Children* (Oxford: Oxford University Press, 2020), 2 and, for discussion about suspicion, 48.

4. P. J. P. Goldberg, ed., *Women in England c. 1275–1525* (Oxford: Oxford University Press, 1995), 133.

5. Tina Reid-Peršin, "The People of Lamberhurst Are Horrified," *Tina Reid-Peršin* (blog), September 24, 2012, https://tinamreid.wordpress.com/category/photos-ill-never-take-2/page/4/.

6. I base this account of the tale on the Middle English version available at

Anne Laskaya and Eve Salisbury, eds., *The Middle English Breton Lays* (Kalamazoo, MI: Medieval Institute Publications, 1995). There is also an earlier Anglo-Norman version by Marie de France in which she claims she is translating a still earlier oral Breton tale.

7. Karen Harvey, *The Impostress Rabbit Breeder* (Oxford: Oxford University Press, 2020); Susan Juster, "Mystical Pregnancy and Holy Bleeding: Visionary Experience in Early Modern Britain and America," *William and Mary Quarterly* 57, no. 2 (2000): 249–288; Kate Williams, *Becoming Queen: The Tragic Death of Princess Charlotte and the Unexpected Rise of Britain's Greatest Monarch* (New York: Ballantine, 2008), chap. 40.

8. Judith M. Richards, *Mary Tudor* (London: Routledge, 2008), 174.

9. Henry Machyn, *The Diary of Henry Machyn, Citizen and Merchant-Taylor of London, 1550–1563*, ed. John Gough Nichols (London: Camden Society, 1848).

10. *Calendar of Patent Rolls. Philip and Mary 1555–1557*, vol. 3 (London: Her Majesty's Stationery Office, 1938).

11. John Foxe, *Acts and Monuments*, all four editions (1563, 1570, 1576, 1583) available at John Foxe's The Acts and Monuments Online, Humanities Research Institute, Sheffield University; *Acts and Monuments,* 11:1621 (1583 ed.), https://www.dhi.ac.uk/foxe/index.php?realm=text&gototype=&edition=1583&pageid=162.

12. "200. Giovanni Michiel, Venetian Ambassador in England, to the Doge and Senate," August 27, 1555, in *Calendar of State Papers Relating To English Affairs in the Archives of Venice, Volume 6: 1555–1558*, ed. Rawdon Brown (London: Her Majesty's Stationery Office, 1877), 173.

13. Thomas Wright and James Orchard Halliwell, eds., *Reliquiæ antiquæ: Scraps from Ancient Manuscripts*, 2 vols. (London: John Russell Smith, 1845), 2:16–17.

14. Foxe, *Acts and Monuments*, 5:1205 (1563 ed.).

15. Foxe, *Acts and Monuments*, 12:2122 (1583 ed.).

16. "124. Giovanni Michiel, Venetian Ambassador to England, to the Doge and Senate," June 6, 1555, in *Calendar of State Papers Relating To English Affairs in the Archives of Venice, Volume 6: 1555–1558*, ed. Rawdon Brown (London: Her Majesty's Stationery Office, 1877), 100.

17. Anna Whitelock, *Mary Tudor: Princess, Bastard, Queen* (London: Random House, 2009), 327.

18. "Queen Mary—Volume 5: June 1555," in *Calendar of State Papers Domestic: Edward VI, Mary and Elizabeth, 1547–80*, ed. Robert Lemon (London: Her Majesty's Stationery Office, 1856), 67.

19. Karen Hearn, curator, *Portraying Pregnancy: From Holbein to Social Media*, Foundling Hospital, London (January–August 2020).

20. J. A. Froude, *History of England from the Fall of Wolsey to the Death of Elizabeth*, 12 vols. (London: Longmans, 1858–1870), 6:490.

21. Ann Ward Radcliffe, *The Mysteries of Udolpho*, ed. Bonamy Dobrée (Oxford: Oxford University Press, 1980, first published 1794), 232.

22. A. F. Pollard, *The History of England from the Accession of Edward VI to the Death of Elizabeth* (London: Longmans, 1910).

23. Walter Carruthers Sellar and Robert Julian Yeatman, *1066 and All That: A Memorable History of England* (London: Methuen, 1930), 57.

24. There are many recent biographies of Mary, and all touch on her false pregnancies. See, e.g., Richards, *Mary Tudor*, 173–178. See also Linda Porter, *Mary Tudor: The First Queen* (London: Little, Brown, 2007); Judith M. Richards, "Reassessing Mary Tudor: Some Concluding Points," in *Mary Tudor: Old and New Perspectives*, eds. Susan Doran and Thomas Freeman, 206–224 (London: Macmillan, 2011); Whitelock, *Mary Tudor*, 257.

25. For example, Laura Gowing, *Common Bodies: Women, Touch and Power in Seventeenth-Century England* (New Haven, CT: Yale University Press, 2003), 119.

26. George David Bivin and M. Pauline Klinger, *Pseudocyesis* (Bloomington, IN: Principia, 1937).

27. Jessica Hepburn, *The Pursuit of Motherhood* (London: Troubador, 2014), 47.

28. Maggie O'Farrell, *I Am, I Am, I Am: Seventeen Brushes with Death* (London: Headline, 2017), 263–264.

29. Jane Sharp, *The Midwives Book or the Whole Art of Midwifery Discovered* (London, 1671), 102, ESTC R203554.

30. Sharp, *The Midwives Book*, 85.

31. Sharp, *The Midwives Book*, 110.

32. Sharp, *The Midwives Book*, 111.

33. My translation of Sweiten's Latin in W. F. Montgomery, *An Exposition of the Signs and Symptoms of Pregnancy* (Philadelphia, PA: Blanchard and Lea, 1857), 55–56.

34. Montgomery, *Signs and Symptoms*, 60 (1857 ed.).

35. Montgomery, *Signs and Symptoms*, 28 (1857 ed.).

36. Montgomery, *Signs and Symptoms*, 30 (1857 ed.).

37. The history from short entry to full book is given in the preface to the 1837 edition: W. F. Montgomery, *An Exposition of the Signs and Symptoms of Pregnancy* (London: Sherwood, Gilbert & Piper, 1837), v.

38. Montgomery, *Signs and Symptoms*, 468 (1857 ed.).

39. Montgomery, *Signs and Symptoms*, 72–74 (1857 ed.).

40. Thomas Hawkes Tanner, *On the Signs and Diseases of Pregnancy* (London: Henry Renshaw, 1860), 74.

41. Montgomery, *Signs and Symptoms*, 75 (1857 ed.).

42. Montgomery, *Signs and Symptoms*, 79 (1857 ed.).

43. Whitelock, *Mary Tudor*, 330.

44. Montgomery, *Signs and Symptoms*, 86 (1857 ed.).

45. Montgomery, *Signs and Symptoms*, 74 (1857 ed.).

46. Barbara Duden, *Disembodying Women: Perspectives on Pregnancy and the Unborn* (Cambridge, MA: Harvard University Press, 1993), 55.

47. Duden, *Disembodying Women*, 76–78.

48. Randi Hutter Epstein, *Get Me Out: A History of Childbirth from the Garden of Eden to the Sperm Bank* (New York: Norton, 2010), 200.

49. See the intersectional take on this problem in Rayna Rapp, "Real-Time Fetus: The Role of the Sonogram in the Age of Monitored Reproduction," in *Cyborgs and Citadels: Anthropological Interventions into Techno-Humanism*, eds. G. Downey, J. Dumit, and S. Traweek (Seattle: University of Washington Press, 1997).

Chapter 4

1. Jane Sharp, *The Midwives Book or the Whole Art of Midwifery Discovered* (London: Simon Miller, 1671), 101, ESTC R203554.

2. John Hill, *Lucina sine concubitu. A Letter Humbly Address'd to the Royal Society* (London: Cooper, 1750), 32 ESTC T124780.

3. Trevor G. Cooper et al., "World Health Organization Reference Values for Human Semen Characteristics," *Human Reproduction Update* 16, no. 3 (May/June 2010): 231–245, published November 24, 2009, https://doi.10.1093/humupd/dmp048.

4. Miriam Stoppard, *Conception, Pregnancy and Birth: The Childbirth Bible for Today's Parents*, rev. ed. (London: Dorling Kindersley, 2008), 41.

5. Zita West, *Plan to Get Pregnant: Ten Steps to Maximum Pregnancy* (London: Dorling Kindersley, 2008), 58–59.

6. "116. Giovanni Michel, Venetian Ambassador to England, to the Doge and Senate," June 1, 1555, in *Calendar of State Papers Relating To English Affairs in the Archives of Venice, Volume 6: 1555–1558,*

ed. Rawdon Brown (London: Her Majesty's Stationery Office, 1877), 93.

7. A biography can be found in Javier Virues Ortega, "Una aproximación a la vida de Juan Huarte de San Juan: los primeros años de práctica professional (1560–1578)," *Psicothema* 18 (2006): 232–237. Also see Rocío G. Sumillera's introduction to Juan Huarte de San Juan, *The Examination of Men's Wits*, trans. Richard Carew, ed. Rocío G. Sumillera (Cambridge, UK: Modern Humanities Research Association, 2014).

8. Geoffrey Parker, *Imprudent King: A New Life of Philip II* (New Haven, CT: Yale University Press, 2014).

9. I use the English translation here: Juan Huarte de San Juan, *Examen de ingenios: The Examination of Mens Wits*, trans. Richard Carew (London, 1596), ESTC S2748.

10. Huarte, *Examen*, 263.

11. Huarte, *Examen*, 20.

12. Huarte, *Examen*, 253.

13. Huarte, *Examen*, 264.

14. Huarte, *Examen*, 274.

15. Huarte, *Examen*, 268–284.

16. Huarte, *Examen*, 286.

17. Huarte, *Examen*, 284.

18. Huarte, *Examen*, 299.

19. Huarte, *Examen*, 268.

20. Huarte, *Examen*, 263.

21. Huarte, *Examen*, 240–241.

22. Huarte, *Examen*, 271.

23. S. Mendyk, "Carew, Richard (1555–1620), Antiquary and Poet," *Oxford Dictionary of National Biography*. September 23, 2004, https://www.oxforddnb.com/view/10.1093/ref:odnb/9780198614128.001.0001/odnb-9780198614128-e-4635.

24. Colin Martin and Geoffrey Parker, *The Spanish Armada* (Harmondsworth, UK: Hamish Hamilton, 1988), 23.

25. Richard Carew, *A Herrings Tayle* (London, 1598), ESTC S104891. The EEBO copy is the British Library copy and is missing two pages; the undigitized Bodleian copy is complete.

26. Richard Carew, *The Survey of Cornwall* (London, 1602), 156–158, ESTC S107479.

27. Carew, *A Herrings Tayle*, A2r.

28. Carew, *A Herrings Tayle*, C1v.

29. Carew, *A Herrings Tayle*, B2r.

30. Carew, *A Herrings Tayle*, B1v.

31. Carew, *A Herrings Tayle*, B4r.

32. Carew, *A Herrings Tayle*, Cr.

33. Huarte, *Examen*, 316–317.

34. On wind and humoral health, see Gail Kern Paster, *Humoring the Body: Emotions and the Shakespearean Stage* (Chicago: University of Chicago Press, 2004), 8–9.

35. Huarte, *Examen*, 303.

36. See, e.g., Hildegard of Bingen, *Hildegard of Bingen: On Natural Philosophy and Medicine. Selections from Cause et Cure*, ed. and trans. Margaret Berger (Cambridge, UK: D. S. Brewer, 1999), 45; Katherine M. Kueny, *Conceiving Identities: Maternity in Medieval Muslim Discourse and Practice* (Albany: SUNY Press, 2013), 204–206; Maaike Van der Lugt, *Le ver, le démon, et la vierge: les théories médievales de la génération extraordinaire* (Paris: Les Belles Lettres, 2004), 107–112.

37. Jonathan Gil Harris, "All Swell That End Swell: Dropsy, Phantom Pregnancy, and the Sound of Deconception in *All's Well That Ends Well*," *Renaissance Drama* 35 (2006): 169–189.

38. Martin and Parker, *The Spanish Armada*, 258.

39. Edward Tenance, "A Strategy of Reaction: The Armadas of 1596 and 1597 and the Spanish Struggle for European Hegemony," *English Historical Review* 118 (2003): 866–867, 876.

40. Carew, *The Survey of Cornwall*, 158.

41. Carew, *A Herrings Tayle*, D3r.

42. For complementary but different discussions of the Armada portraits, see Andrew Belsey and Catherine Belsey, "Icons of Divinity: Portraits of Elizabeth I," in *Renaissance Bodies: The Human Figure in English Culture 1540–1660*, eds. Lucy Gent and Nigel Llewellyn (London: Reaktion, 1997), 11–35; Roy Strong, *Gloriana: The*

Portraits of Queen Elizabeth I (London: Thames and Hudson, 1987), 131–133.

43. See, for example, "Medal Commemorating the Defeat of the Spanish Armada," 1588, Royal Maritime Museum, Greenwich, UK, ID: MEC0012, https://www.rmg.co.uk /collections/objects/rmgc-object-37452.

44. Belsey and Belsey, "Icons of Divinity," 12.

45. P. D. A. Harvey, *Medieval Maps* (London: British Library, 1991), 39-43. These complex overlapping circular shapes have been noted before but thought of differently. Belsey and Belsey, "Icons of Divinity," 17–18.

46. Harvey, *Medieval Maps*, 45.

47. Henry Peacham, *The Gentlemens Exercise* (1612), 131, ESTC S114350.

48. Carew, *A Herrings Tayle*, D4v.

49. Giles Milton, *Big Chief Elizabeth: The Adventures and Fate of the First English Colonists in America* (New York: Farrar, Straus & Giroux, 2000), 11, 71, 233.

50. Kris Lane, *Potosí: The Silver City That Changed the World* (Oakland: University of California Press, 2019), 49.

51. See, e.g., *Le roman de la rose*, ca. 1365, manuscript, Special Collection Research Center, University of Chicago Library, MS. 1380, fol. 102v. A digital surrogate is available at *Roman de la Rose* Digital Library, Sheridan Libraries, Johns Hopkins University, https://dlmm.library.jhu.edu/viewer/ #rose/UC1380/102v/image.

52. I have found the following works to be useful for understanding the allegories of nature: Rebecca Ann Davis, *Piers Plowman and the Books of Nature* (Oxford: Oxford University Press, 2016); George D. Economou, *The Goddess Natura in Medieval Literature* (Cambridge, MA: Harvard University Press, 1972); Kellie Robertson, *Nature Speaks: Medieval Literature and Aristotelian Philosophy* (Philadelphia: University of Pennsylvania Press, 2017); Hugh White, *Nature and Salvation in Piers Plowman* (Woodbridge, UK: Boydell & Brewer, 1988).

53. Rebecca Fett, *It Starts with the Egg: How the Science of Egg Quality Can Help You Get Pregnant Naturally, Prevent Miscarriage, and Improve Your Odds in IVF*, 2nd ed. (Surfside, FL: Franklin Fox, 2019, first published 2014), 11, 60.

54. Yusuf Onundi et al., "A Multidisciplinary Investigation of the Technical and Environmental Performances of TAML/Peroxide Elimination of Bisphenol A Compounds from Water," *Green Chemistry* 19 (2017): 4234.

55. Fett, *It Starts with the Egg*, 44–45.

56. Fett, *It Starts with the Egg*, 61.

57. M. M. Gomez-Ramos, A. I. García-Valcárcel, J. L. Tadeo, A. R. Fernández-Alba, and M. D. Hernando, "Screening of Environmental Contaminants in Honey Bee Wax Comb Using Gas Chromatography–High-Resolution Time-of-Flight Mass Spectrometry," *Environmental Science and Pollution Research* 23 (2016): 4609–4620.

58. Radhinka Govindrajan, "Flatulence," in *Anthropocene Unseen: A Lexicon*, eds. Cymene How and Anand Pandian (Santa Barbara, CA: Punctum Books, 2020), 197.

59. Bruno Latour, "Agency at the Time of the Anthropocene," *New Literary History* 45 (2014): 1.

60. Dipesh Chakrabarty, "The Climate of History: Four Theses," *Critical Inquiry* 35 (2009): 208.

Chapter 5

1. Sheila Heti, *Motherhood: A Novel* (London: Penguin, 2018), 150.

2. SBinRI, "Cloudy Pee as a Sign?," Baby and Bump by Momtastic (Internet forum), accessed June 20, 2018, https://babyandbump.momtastic.com /threads/cloudy-pee-as-a-sign.1094713 (the hyperlinks to private medical services that accompanied in this thread when first accessed have now been removed).

3. "Period Trackers to Be Reviewed over Data Concerns," BBC, September 8, 2023, https://www.bbc.co.uk/news/technology-66740184. In the United States since the 2022 overturning of *Roe v. Wade* and in other countries where abortion is being criminalised, there are also legal concerns about how this data is being misapplied.

4. The fullest historical account of uroscopy in the Middle Ages is Laurence Moulinier-Brogi, *L'uroscopie au Moyen Âge: "lire dans un verre la nature de l'homme"* (Paris: Champion, 2012).

5. The early modern to nineteenth-century part of the story is told by Michael Stohlberg, *Uroscopy in Early Modern Europe*, trans. Logan Kennedy and Leonhard Unglaub (Farnham, UK: Ashgate, 2015).

6. Stohlberg, *Uroscopy*, 3.

7. Henri Daniel, *Liber Uricisiarum*, in *A Critical Edition of the Middle English* Liber Uricisiarum *in Wellcome MS 225*, ed. Joanne Jasin (PhD diss., Tulane University, 1983).

8. *Wellcome Apocalyse*, ca. 1420, manuscript, Wellcome Collection, London, MS. 49, fol. 42r. A digital surrogate is available at https://wellcomelibrary.org/item/b19684915, accessed September 28, 2023.

9. M. Teresa Tavormina, ed., "Three Middle English Verse Uroscopies," *English Studies* 91 (2010): 597.

10. Moulinier-Brogi, *L'uroscopie*, 138.

11. Moulinier-Brogi, *L'uroscopie*, 139, 156.

12. Girolamo Mercurio, cited in Rudolph M. Bell, *How to Do it: Guides to Good Living for Renaissance Italians* (Chicago: University of Chicago Press, 1999), 71–72.

13. Stohlberg, *Uroscopy*, 82–90.

14. Stohlberg, *Uroscopy*, 85, 164–165.

15. Thomas Brian, *The Pisse-Prophet, or Certain Pisse-Pot Lectures* (London, 1655), A2r. ESTC R23808.

16. Brian, *The Pisse-Prophet*, A3v–A4r, E2v–E3r.

17. Brian, *The Pisse-Prophet*, 82–96

18. These stories are collected in Roberto Zapperi, *The Pregnant Man* (London: Harwood Academic, 1991).

19. Ekkehard V, *Casus Sancti Galli* (ca. 1214), cited in Plinio Prioreschi, *A History of Medicine: Medieval Medicine* (Omaha, NE: Horatius Press, 2003), 583.

20. The story of Theranos is told in John Carreyrou, *Bad Blood: Secrets and Lies in a Silicon Valley Startup* (New York: Knopf, 2018).

21. Carreyou, *Bad Blood*, 12.

22. Stohlberg, *Uroscopy*, 82.

23. "De urinis," in *Middle English Medical Miscellany, Including Receipts and Charms*, Vol. 6 (Leech-Books, ca. 1400), Wellcome Collection, London, MS. 409, f. 63r, https://wellcomecollection.org/works/y7xcant4.

24. See, e.g., Mary Fissell, "Hairy Women and Naked Truths: Gender and the Politics of Knowledge in *Aristotle's Masterpiece*," *William and Mary Quarterly* 60 (2003): 43–74; *The Secrets of Generation: Reproduction in the Long Eighteenth Century*, eds. Raymond Stephanson and Darren N. Wagner (Toronto: University of Toronto Press, 2015), esp. 5–8.

25. *Aristotle's Masterpiece* (London: B. Harris, 1697), part 2, chap. 12, pp. 151–152, ESTC R230121.

26. "Kiestéine," *Journal de chimie médicale, de parmacie et de toxicologie* 5, no. 2 (1839): 64–65. Kyestein is also discussed by Ann Oakley, *The Captured Womb: A History of the Medical Care of Pregnant Women* (Oxford: Basil Blackwell, 1990, first published 1984), 19. For spelling I use *Oxford English Dictionary*, s.v. "kyestein (n.)," July 2023, https://doi.org/10.1093/OED/7853401169.

27. W. F. Montgomery, *An Exposition of the Signs and Symptoms of Pregnancy* (Philadelphia, PA: Blanchard and Lea, 1857), 252–253.

28. Elisha Kent Kane, "Experiments on Kiesteine," *American Journal of the Medical Sciences* 4 (1842): 13–38.

29. A biography is available in Mark Sawin, *Raising Kane: Elisha Kent Kane and the Culture of Fame in Antebellum America* (Philadelphia, PA: American Philosophical Society Press, 2009).

30. Kane, "Experiments on Kiesteine," 6.

31. Meguelonne Toussaint-Samat, *A History of Food* (London: Wiley-Blackwell, 2009, first published 1992), 463.

32. Kane, "Experiments on Kiesteine," 22–24.

33. Mark Marshall, "The Kyesteine Pellicle: An Early Biological Test for Pregnancy," *Bulletin of the History of Medicine* 22 (1948): 192–193.

34. Reverse engineering on digital pregnancy tests is discussed at Kristina Panos, "Digital Pregnancy Tests Use LEDs to Read between the Lines," *Hackaday* (blog), September 9, 2020, https://hackaday.com/2020/09/09/digital -pregnancy-tests-use-leds-to-read -between-the-lines.

35. On the embryoscope, see the "Remaking the Human Body: Biomedical Imaging Technologies, Professional and Lay Visions" project at Queen Mary's College, University of London. E.g., Josie Hamper and Manuela Perrotta, "Watching Embryos: Exploring the Geographies of Assisted Reproduction through Encounters with Embryo Imaging Technologies," *Social & Cultural Geography*, 24, no. 1 (May 2022): 1557–1575, https://doi.org/10 .1080/14649365.2022.2073467.

36. Also discussed by Donna J. Drucker, *Fertility Technology* (Cambridge, MA: MIT Press, 2023), 172–174.

37. This shift occurred whilst this book was in press. Human Fertilisation and Embryology Authority, "Time-Lapse Imaging and Incubation," accessed April 28, 2024, https://www.hfea.gov .uk/treatments/treatment-add-ons/time -lapse-imaging-and-incubation.

38. Human Fertilisation and Embryology Authority, "Time-Lapse Imaging," accessed November 19, 2022, inactive by April 28, 2024, https://web.archive .org/web/20201031163022/https://www

.hfea.gov.uk/treatments/treatment-add -ons/time-lapse-imaging.

39. On the ethics and the financial and emotional burdens of add-ons, see M. Perrotta and J. Hamper, "Patient Informed Choice in the Age of Evidence-Based Medicine: IVF Patients' Approaches to Biomedical Evidence and Fertility Treatment Add-Ons," *Sociology of Health & Illness* 45, no. 2 (2023): 225–241, https://doi.org /10.1111/1467-9566.13581.

40. Viviana A. Rotman Zelizer, *Pricing the Priceless Child* (New York: Basic Books, 1985), 11.

41. Miranda Ward, *Adrift: Fieldnotes from Almost-Motherhood* (London: Weidenfeld & Nicolson, 2021), 260.

42. Jessica Hepburn, *The Pursuit of Motherhood* (London: Troubador, 2014), 105–109.

43. eemmlette, "Free Psychic/Tarot Readings" (trying-to-conceive forum), December 20, 2010, Baby Center, accessed November 19, 2022, https:// community.babycenter.com/post /a25501647/free_psychictarot_readings ?page=3.

44. Theodor W. Adorno, *The Stars Down to Earth and Other Essays in Irrational Culture*, ed. Stephen Crook (London: Routledge, 1994), 50.

45. David S. Areford, *The Viewer and the Printed Image in Late Medieval Europe* (Farnham, UK: Ashgate, 2010), 11.

46. I borrow this phrase from Perrotta and Hamper, "Patient Informed Choice," 226.

47. Mike Sosteric, "A Sociology of Tarot," *Canadian Journal of Sociology / Cahiers Canadiens de Sociologie* 39, no. 3 (2014): 361.

Chapter 6

1. Mary Wollstonecraft Shelley, *Frankenstein; or, the Modern Prometheus* (London: Colburn and Bentley, 1831), 33.

2. There is a huge literature on fiction and eugenics. See, e.g., Angus McLaren,

Reproduction by Design: Sex, Robots, Trees, and Test-Tube Babies in Interwar Britain (Chicago: University of Chicago, 2012).

3. Philip Ball, *Unnatural: The Heretical Idea of Making People* (London: Vintage, 2012).

4. Ball, *Unnatural*, 123.

5. Donna J. Drucker, *Fertility Technology* (Cambridge, MA: MIT Press, 2023), 7.

6. Ball, *Unnatural*, 1–2.

7. Ariel Levy, *The Rules Do Not Apply* (London: Fleet, 2017), 86.

8. Further reading, see S. Brown, L. R. Fraga, G. Cameron, L. Erskine, and N. Vargesson, "The Primodos Components Norethisterone Acetate and Ethinyl Estradiol Induce Developmental Abnormalities in Zebra Fish Embryos," *Scientific Reports* 8 (2018): 2917; Jesse Olszynko-Gryn, "Drug Scandals and the Media: The Unresolved Case of Primodos," *The Guardian*, March 22, 2018; Jesse Olszynko-Gryn, "Primodos was a Revolutionary Oral Pregnancy Test. But Was It Safe?," *The Guardian*, October 13, 2016; Jesse Olszynko-Gryn, *A Woman's Right to Know: Pregnancy Testing in Twentieth-Century Britain* (Cambridge, MA: MIT Press, 2023), chap. 7; Jesse Olszynko-Gryn, Eira Bjørvik, Merle Weßel, Solveig Jülich, and Cyrille Jeane, "A Historical Argument for Regulatory Failure in the Case of Primodos and Other Hormone Pregnancy Tests," *Reproductive Biomedicine and Society Online* 6 (2018): 34–44.

9. Isabel Gal, Brian Kirman, and Jan Stern, "Hormonal Pregnancy Tests and Congenital Malformation," *Nature* 216 (October 7, 1967): 83; Michael Laurence, Mary Miller, Mary Vowles, Kathleen Evans, and Cedric Carter, "Hormonal Pregnancy Tests and Neural Tube Malformations," *Nature* 233 (October 15, 1971): 495–496.

10. Personal communication with Jesse Olszynko-Gryn.

11. Robert Lyall, *The Medical Evidence Relative to the Duration of Human Pregnancy* (London: Burgess and Hill, 1826), xvii, n.

12. Gardner Peerage Claim, in Main Papers, Session 1825: Minutes of Evidence, May 19, 1825–July 4, 1825, Parliamentary Archives, London, HL/PO/JO/10/8/711. See also, Gardner Peerage Claim, in Main Papers, Session 1826: Minutes of Evidence, March 2, 1826-April 6, 1826, Parliamentary Archives, London, HL/PO/JO/10/8/744.

13. "Law Intelligence," *The Morning Post*, January 25,1827.

14. Lyall, *The Medical Evidence*, iii.

15. "Review," *The Lancet* 10, no. 144 (June 3, 1826): 291.

16. Jeremy Bentham, *The Panopticon Writings*, ed. Miran Božovič (London: Verso, 1995), 33.

17. Bentham, *Panopticon*, 91.

18. M. NourbeSe Philip, *She Tries Her Tongue: Her Silence Softly Breaks* (Middletown, CT: Wesleyan University Press, 2015, first published 1989), 90.

19. Gardner Peerage Claim, June 2, 1825, 68.

20. Lyall, *The Medical Evidence*, xxiii.

21. W. F. Montgomery, *An Exposition of the Signs and Symptoms of Pregnancy* (Philadelphia, PA: Blanchard and Lea, 1857), 329.

22. Centre for the Study of the Legacies of British Slavery, Database, University College, London, accessed July 3, 2020, https://www.ucl.ac.uk/lbs/.

23. Maria Nugent, *A Journal of a Voyage to, and Residence in, the Island of Jamaica, from 1801 to 1805* (London: 1839), 182–183.

24. Centre for the Study of the Legacies of Britishi Slavery, Database.

25. Matthew Gregory Lewis, *Journal of a West India Proprietor* (London: John Murray, 1834), 62.

26. Kenneth Morgan, "Slave Women and Reproduction in Jamaica, c. 1776–1834," *History* 91 (2006): 231–253.

27. Shauna J. Sweeney, "Market Marronage: Fugitive Women and the Internal Marketing System in Jamaica, 1781–1834," *William and Mary Quarterly* 76 (2019): 197–222.

28. Lewis, *Journal*, 61.
29. Lewis, *Journal*, 217.
30. Lewis, *Journal*, 143.
31. Lewis, *Journal*, 111.
32. Lewis, *Journal*, 207.
33. Lucius Apuleius, *The Golden Ass*, trans. W. Adlington (London: Heinemann, 1919), book 4: 32–33, book 5: 1–10, 192–215.
34. Matthew Lewis, *The Monk*, ed. Howard Anderson, rev. Nick Groom (Oxford: Oxford University Press, 2016), 232.
35. Mary Prince, *The History of Mary Prince, a West Indian Slave* (London: Westley and Davis, 1831), 23.
36. Prince, *The History of Mary Prince*, 22.
37. Sasha Turner, *Contested Bodies: Pregnancy, Child Rearing and Slavery in Jamaica* (Philadelphia: University of Pennsylvania Press, 2017).
38. Sweeney, "Market Marronage," 206.
39. Angela Davis, "Reflections on the Black Woman's Role in the Community of Slaves," *Massachusetts Review* 13, no. 1/2 (1972): 97.
40. See Morgan, "Slave Women and Reproduction."
41. Diana Paton, "Maternal Struggles and the Politics of Childlessness under Pronatalist Caribbean Slavery," *Slavery and Abolition* 38 (2017): 251–268.
42. Lewis, *Journal*, 82.
43. Rachel O'Donnell, "The Politics of Natural Knowing: Contraceptive Plant Properties in the Caribbean," *Journal of International Women's Studies* 17, no. 3 (2016): 62.
44. Suzanne O. Bell and Mary Fissell, "A Little Bit Pregnant? Productive Ambiguity and Fertility Research," *Population and Development Review* 47, no. 2 (2021): 521–522.
45. Shiona McCallum, "Period Tracking Apps Warning over *Roe v. Wade* Case in US," BBC, May 7, 2022, https://www.bbc.co.uk/news/technology-61347934.
46. I base my fictional table on Montgomery, *An Exposition of the Signs and Symptoms of Pregnancy*, 455.
47. Kay Elder and Martin H. Johnson, "The Oldham Notebooks: An Analysis of the Development of IVF 1969–1978.

II. Treatment Cycles and Their Outcomes," *Reproductive Biomedicine and Society Online* 1 (2015): 9–18.
48. Kay Elder and Martin H. Johnson, "The Oldham Notebooks: An Analysis of the Development of IVF 1969–1978. IV. Ethical Aspects," *Repoductive BioMedicine and Society Online* 1 (2015): 34–35. All the information in this paragraph is based on this article.
49. Drucker, *Fertility Technology*, 141–146.
50. Human Fertilisation and Embryology Authority, "Ethnic Diversity in Fertility Treatment 2018: UK Ethnicity Statistics for IVF and DI Fertility Treatment," March 2021, https://www.hfea.gov.uk/about-us/publications/research-and-data/ethnic-diversity-in-fertility-treatment-2018.
51. Sarah S. Richardson, *The Maternal Imprint: The Contested Science of Maternal-Fetal Effects* (Chicago: University of Chicago Press, 2021), 1.
52. Saidiya Hartman, *Lose Your Mother: A Journey along the Atlantic Slave Route* (New York: Farrar, Straus & Giroux, 2007), 133.

Chapter 7

1. John Wyndham, *Consider Her Ways* (London: Penguin Books, 2014, first published 1961), 46–47.
2. Heidi Murkoff, Arlene Eisenberg, and Sandee Hathaway, *What to Expect When You're Expecting*, 3rd ed. (London: Pocket Books, 2002, first published 1984), 4.
3. Zita West, *Plan to Get Pregnant: Ten Steps to Maximum Pregnancy* (London: Dorling Kindersley, 2008), 118–125.
4. Angela Carter, Letters dated January 26, 1971, and February 8/9, 1971, Unpublished correspondence, British Library, London, Additional MS. 89102/2.
5. See, for example, Ouj Umeora, "Pseudocyesis in a Rural Southeast Nigerian Community," *Journal of Obstetrics and Gynaecology Research* 35, no. 4 (2009): 660.

6. Marisa Costa, "My Imaginary Pregnancy," The Wayback Machine, 2015, accessed November 19, 2022, https://web.archive.org/web /20160520042430/http://www.babble .com/pregnancy/my-imaginary -pregnancy-my-body-has-all-the -symptoms-but-the-babys-just-in-my -head/.

7. Maggie O'Farrell, *I Am, I Am, I Am: Seventeen Brushes with Death* (London: Headline, 2017), 260–261.

8. West, *Plan to Get Pregnant*, 38.

9. For an example of a study funded by Swiss Precision Diagnostics, the manufacturer of Clear Blue products, including digital fertility monitors, see, e.g., William Ledger et al., "Impact of Digital Home Ovulation Test Usage on Stress, Psychological Wellbeing and Quality of Life during Evaluation of Subfertility: A Randomised Controlled Trial," Swiss Precision Diagnostics, accessed November 19, 2022, https:// uk.clearblue.com/sites/default/files /wysiwyg/hcpro/publications/HCP _Publications/PUB-0090_v2.pdf.

10. Olivia Negris et al., "Emotional Stress and Reproduction: What Do Fertility Patients Believe?," *Journal of Assisted Reproduction and Genetics* 38 (2021): 877–887.

11. D. M. Wegner and S. Zanakos, "Chronic Thought Suppression," *Journal of Personality* 62 (1994): 637, 615.

12. West, *Plan to Get Pregnant*, 118.

13. Miranda Ward, *Adrift: Fieldnotes from Almost-Motherhood* (London: Weidenfeld & Nicolson, 2021), 99.

14. West, *Plan to Get Pregnant*, 153.

15. A full discussion of historical hysteria is available at Helen King, "Once upon a Text: Hysteria from Hippocrates," in *Hysteria beyond Freud*, ed. Sander L. Gilman, 3–90 (Berkeley: University of California Press, 1993).

16. Barbara Taylor, *The Last Asylum: A Memoir of Madness in Our Times* (London: Penguin, 2014), 171.

17. Taylor, *The Last Asylum*, 170.

18. See, e.g., King, "Once upon a Text"; Elaine Showalter, *The Female Malady: Women, Madness, and English Culture, 1830–1980* (London: Virago, 1987).

19. Siri Hustvedt, *The Shaking Woman or a History of My Nerves* (London: Hodder & Stoughton, 2010), 10.

20. American Psychiatric Association, *Diagnostic and Styatistical Manual of Mental Disorders: DSM-V*, 5th ed. (Washington, DC: American Psychiatric Publishing, 2013), code 300.89, F.45.8, 327. The word *hysteria* hasn't appeared in the *DSM* since 1968.

21. Ina May Gaskin, "Has Pseudocyesis Become an Outmoded Diagnosis?," *Birth: Issues in Perinatal Care* 39, no. 1 (2012): 77.

22. Thomas Hawkes Tanner, *Signs and Diseases of Pregnancy* (London: Henry Renshaw, 1860), 32.

23. Angela Carter, Letter dated January 26, 1971, Unpublished correspondence, British Library, London, Additional MS. 89102/2.

24. Fabrizio Benedetti, *Placebo Effects: Understanding the Mechanisms of Health and Disease* (Oxford: Oxford University Press, 2009), 38–42.

25. Elizabeth A. Wilson, *Psychosomatic: Feminism and the Neurological Body* (Durham, NC: Duke University Press, 2004), 5.

26. Wilson, *Psychosomatic*, 13.

27. In this chapter, I sometimes refer to Harvey's original Latin text: William Harvey, *Exercitationes de generatione animalium* (London, 1651), H1091 (Wing). I also cite a near-contemporary translation of Harvey's Latin text that is closer and more characterful than later translations: William Harvey, *Anatomical Exercitations Concerning the Generation of Living Creatures* (London, 1653), ESTC R13027, quotations here 25.

28. Harvey, *Anatomical Exercitations Concerning the Generation of Living Creatures*, 24–25.

29. Roger French, "Harvey, William (1578–1657), Physician and Discoverer of the Circulation of the Blood," *Oxford Dictionary of National Biography*, September 23, 2004.

30. William Harvey, *De motu locali animalium*, ed. and trans. Gwyneth Whitteridge (Cambridge, UK: Cambridge University Press, 1959), 50–51.

31. For a fuller discussion, see Helen King, *The Disease of Virgins: Green Sickness, Chlorosis and the Problems of Puberty* (London: Routledge, 2004).

32. Harvey, *Anatomical Exercitations Concerning the Generation of Living Creatures*, 28.

33. Harvey, *Anatomical Exercitations Concerning the Generation of Living Creatures*, 480.

34. Harvey, *Exercitationes de generatione*, 161.

35. Harvey, *Anatomical Exercitations Concerning the Generation of Living Creatures*, 24.

36. Harvey, *Anatomical Exercitations Concerning the Generation of Living Creatures*, 119.

37. Harvey, *Anatomical Exercitations Concerning the Generation of Living Creatures*, 546–547.

38. Harvey, *Anatomical Exercitations Concerning the Generation of Living Creatures*, 417.

39. Harvey, *Anatomical Exercitations Concerning the Generation of Living Creatures*, 415.

40. Harvey, *Anatomical Exercitations Concerning the Generation of Living Creatures*, 544.

41. Harvey, *Anatomical Exercitations Concerning the Generation of Living Creatures*, 540.

42. Charis Charalampous, *Rethinking the Mind-Body Relationship in Early Modern Literature, Philosophy and Medicine: The Renaissance of the Body* (London: Routledge, 2015), esp. 2; Gail Kern Paster, *Humoring the Body: Emotions and the Shakespearean Stage* (Chicago: University of Chicago Press, 2004), 12.

43. Miranda Anderson, *The Renaissance Extended Mind* (London: Palgrave Macmillan, 2015); Andy Clark and David Chalmers, "The Extended Mind," *Analysis* 58 (1998): 7–19.

44. Harvey, *Anatomical Exercitations Concerning the Generation of Living Creatures*, 540–541.

45. Harvey, *Anatomical Exercitations Concerning the Generation of Living Creatures*, 5.

46. Harvey, *Anatomical Exercitations Concerning the Generation of Living Creatures*, 541.

47. Thomas Laqueur, *Making Sex: Body and Gender from the Greeks to Freud* (Cambridge, MA: Harvard University Press, 1990), 144.

48. James G. Lennox, "The Comparative Study of Animal Development: William Harvey's Aristotelianism," in *The Problem of Animal Generation in Early Modern Philosophy*, ed. Justin E. H. Smith (Cambridge, UK: Cambridge University Press, 2006), 45.

49. G. S. Rousseau, "'A Strange Pathology': Hysteria in the Early Modern World, 1500–1800," in *Hysteria Beyond Freud*, ed. Sander L. Gilman (Berkeley: University of California Press, 1993), 131–132.

50. Harvey, *Anatomical Exercitations Concerning the Generation of Living Creatures*, 415.

51. William Harvey, *Works of William Harvey*, trans. Robert Willis (London: Sydenham Society, 1847), 83.

52. Harvey, *On Generation, Anatomical Exercitations Concerning the Generation of Living Creatures*, 71.

53. Eve Keller, "Making Up for Losses: The Workings of Gender in William Harvey's *de Generatione animalium*," in *Inventing Maternity: Politics, Science, and Literature, 1650–1865*, eds. Susan C. Greenfield and Carol Barash (Lexington: University Press of Kentucky, 1999), 51–3. Elizabeth Spiller, *Science, Reading, and Renaissance Literature: The Art of Making Knowledge, 1580–1670* (Cambridge, UK: Cambridge University Press, 2004), 90–95.

Conclusion: Seeing the Unbecoming

1. Angela Carter, Unpublished journal, 1965, British Library, London, Additional MS. 88899/1/90, fols. 73r–75r. Although Carter uses the term

foetus, her reference to the "first month" indicates that she is really thinking about the embryo.

2. William Harvey, *Anatomical Exercitations Concerning the Generation of Living Creatures* (London, 1653), ESTC R13027, 545.

3. Harvey, *Anatomical Exercitations Concerning the Generation of Living Creatures*, 546–547.

4. Hieronymus Fabricius, *The Embryological Treatises of Hieronymus Fabricius of Aquapendente*, ed. and trans. Howard B. Adelmann (Ithaca, NY: Cornell University Press, 1942), 96.

5. Harvey, *Anatomical Exercitations Concerning the Generation of Living Creatures*, 539.

6. Harvey, *Anatomical Exercitations Concerning the Generation of Living Creatures*, unpaginated preface.

7. Janina Wellmann, *The Form of Becoming: Embryology and the Epistemology of Rhythm, 1760–1830* (New York: Zone Books, 2017), 233.

8. Wellmann, *The Form of Becoming*, 157.

9. Rosemary Betterton, "Promising Monsters: Pregnant Bodies, Artistic Subjectivity, and Maternal Imagination," *Hypatia* 21 (2006): 85.

10. Jane Maienschein, *Embryos under the Microscope: The Diverging Meanings of Life* (Cambridge, MA: Harvard University Press, 2014), 14.

11. Maienschein, *Embryos under the Microscope*, 278.

12. Maienschein, *Embryos under the Microscope*, 279–280.

13. Maienschein, *Embryos under the Microscope*, 280.

14. J. Allan Mitchell, *Becoming Human: The Matter of the Medieval Child* (Minneapolis: University of Minnesota Press, 2014), 8.

15. Maienschein, *Embryos under the Microscope*, 278.

16. A., "Meet the Embryo," *Little Red Hen: A Tale of Trying for a Baby* (blog), Wordpress, July 17, 2016, https://littleredhensite.wordpress.com/2016/07/17/meet-the-embryo. See also the discussion of the spatial geography of embryo transfer in Josie Hamper and

Manuela Perrotta, "Watching Embryos: Exploring the Geographies of Assisted Reproduction through Encounters with Embryo Imaging Technologies," *Social & Cultural Geography*, 24, no. 1 (May 2022): 11, https://doi.org/10.1080/14649365.2022.2073467.

17. Clara Pinto-Correia, *The Ovary of Eve: Egg and Sperm and Preformation* (Chicago: University of Chicago Press, 1997), 283.

18. Nick Hopwood, *Embryos in Wax: Models from the Ziegler Studio* (Cambridge, UK: Whipple Museum, 2002), 33.

19. Hopwood, *Embryos in Wax*, 73.

20. Maienschein, *Embryos under the Microscope*, 280.

21. Maienschein, *Embryos under the Microscope*, 14; Fabricius, *The Embryological Treatises*, 238.

22. Fabricius, *The Embryological Treatises*, 237.

23. Fabricius, *The Embryological Treatises*, 464.

24. National Organisation for Rare Disorders, "Chromosome 15, Distal Trisomy 15q," April 10, 2009, https://rarediseases.org/rare-diseases/chromosome-15-distal-trisomy-15q.

25. Harry Angelman, "'Puppet' Children: A Report on Three Cases," *Developmental Medicine & Child Neurology* 7 (1965): 681–688.

26. For two examples on this enormous subject, see Rosi Braidotti, "Signs of Wonder and Traces of Doubt: On Teratology and Embodied Differences," in *Between Monsters, Goddesses and Cyborgs: Feminist Confrontations with Science, Medicine and Cyberspace*, eds. Nina Lykke and Rosi Bradiotti (London: Zed Books, 1996), 145–148; Marie-Hélène Huet, *Monstrous Imagination* (Cambridge, MA: Harvard University Press, 1993).

27. Harvey, *Anatomical Exercitations Concerning the Generation of Living Creatures*, 544.

28. Harvey, *Anatomical Exercitations Concerning the Generation of Living Creatures*, 546.

29. Harvey, *Anatomical Exercitations Concerning the Generation of Living Creatures*, unpaginated preface.

Bibliography

Manuscripts and Objects

Beacon Planning. "Heritage Statement." November 2015. Application number PP/15/07206. Royal Borough of Kensington and Chelsea, London. https://www.rbkc.gov.uk.

Carter, Angela. "The Baby." ca. 1961. Unpublished story. British Library, London. Additional MS. 88899/1/42.

Carter, Angela. Letters dated January 26, 1971, and February 8-9, 1971. Unpublished correspondence. British Library, London. Additional MS. 89102/2.

Carter, Angela. Unpublished journal. 1961–1962. British Library, London. Additional MS. 88899/1/87.

Carter, Angela. Unpublished journal. 1965. British Library, London. Additional MS. 88899/1/90.

"De urinis." In *Middle English Medical Miscellany, Including Receipts and Charms (Leech-Books, VI)*. ca. 1400. Wellcome Collection, London, MS. 409, ff. 55r–66r. https://wellcomecollection.org/works/y7xcant4.

Elkan, Edward. "Sketches from My Life." 1983. Unpublished memoir. Wellcome Collection, London. MS. 9151.

Family Planning Association. Pregnancy Diagnosis Laboratory. 1949–1965. Family Planning Association Archives. Wellcome Collection, London. SA/FPA/A3 11–13. https://wellcomecollection.org/works/cw7cud69.

Gardner Peerage Claim. In Main Papers, Session 1825: Minutes of Evidence, May 19, 1825–July 4, 1825. Parliamentary Archives, London. HL/PO/JO/10/8/711.

Gardner Peerage Claim. In Main Papers, Session 1826: Minutes of Evidence, March 2, 1826–April 6, 1826. Parliamentary Archives, London. HL/PO/JO/10/8/744.

"Medal Commemorating the Defeat of the Spanish Armada." 1588. Medal. Royal Maritime Museum, Greenwich, UK. ID: MEC0012. https://www.rmg.co.uk/collections/objects/rmgc-object-37452.

"Ring." 1300–1400. Bronze engraved with "O mater dei memanto" (O mother of God, remember me). Victoria and Albert Museum, London. V&A accession number 995-1871. https://collections.vam.ac.uk/item/O377756/ring.

Roman de la rose. ca. 1365. Manuscript. Special Collection Research Center, University of Chicago Library, Chicago. MS. 1380. *Roman de la Rose* Digital Library, Sheridan Libraries, Johns Hopkins University. https://dlmm.library.jhu.edu/viewer/#rose.

Roman de la rose. ca. 1525. Manuscript. Morgan Library and Museum, New York. MS. M.948. *Roman de la Rose* Digital Library, Sheridan Libraries, Johns Hopkins University. https://dlmm.library.jhu.edu/viewer/#rose.

Wellcome Apocalypse. ca. 1420. Wellcome Collection, London. MS. 49. https://wellcomecollection.org/works/du9ua6nd.

Nonmanuscript Sources

Adorno, Theodor W. *The Stars Down to Earth and Other Essays in Irrational Culture.* Edited by Stephen Crook. London: Routledge, 1994.

American Psychiatric Association. *Diagnostic and Styatistical Manual of Mental Disorders: DSM-V.* 5th ed. Washington, DC: American Psychiatric Publishing, 2013.

Amnesty International. *Struggle for Maternal Health: Barriers to Antenatal Care in South Africa.* London: Amnesty International, 2014. https://www.amnesty.org/en/documents/afr53/006/2014/en.

Anderson, Miranda. *The Renaissance Extended Mind.* London: Palgrave Macmillan, 2015.

Angelman, Harry. "'Puppet' Children: A Report on Three Cases." *Developmental Medicine & Child Neurology* 7 (1965): 681–688.

Apuleius, Lucius. *The Golden Ass.* Translated by W. Adlington. London: Heinemann, 1919.

Areford, David S. *The Viewer and the Printed Image in Late Medieval Europe.* Farnham, UK: Ashgate, 2010.

Aristotle's Masterpiece. London: B. Harris, 1697. ESTC R230121.

Ball, Philip. *Unnatural: The Heretical Idea of Making People.* London: Vintage, 2012.

BBC. "Period Trackers to Be Reviewed over Data Concerns." September 8, 2023. https://www.bbc.co.uk/news/technology-66740184.

BBC News. "Where Have All the Men Gone?" April 6, 2004. http://news.bbc.co.uk/1/hi/magazine/3601493.stm.

BBC World Service. "The MV Stirling Castle." In *On Your Behalf.* December 9, 1998. https://www.bbc.co.uk/sounds/play/p033jx6n.

Beinart, William, and Lotte Hughes. *Environment and Empire.* Oxford: Oxford University Press, 2007.

Bell, Rudolph M. *How to Do It: Guides to Good Living for Renaissance Italians.* Chicago, IL: University of Chicago Press, 1999.

Bell, Suzanne O., and Mary Fissell. "A Little Bit Pregnant? Productive Ambiguity and Fertility Research." *Population and Development Review* 47, no. 2 (2021): 505–526.

Belsey, Andrew, and Catherine Belsey. "Icons of Divinity: Portraits of Elizabeth I." In *Renaissance Bodies: The Human Figure in English Culture 1540–1660,* edited by Lucy Gent and Nigel Llewellyn, 11–35. London: Reaktion, 1997.

Benedetti, Fabrizio. *Placebo Effects: Understanding the Mechanisms of Health and Disease.* Oxford: Oxford University Press, 2009.

Benninghaus, Christina. "Silences: Coping with Infertility in Nineteenth-Century Germany." In *The Palgrave Handbook of Infertility in History,* edited by Gayle Davis and Tracey Loughran, 99–122. London: Palgrave, 2017.

Bentham, Jeremy. *The Panopticon Writings.* Edited by Miran Božovič. London: Verso, 1995.

Berridge, G. R. *The Politics of the South Africa Run: European Shipping and Pretoria.* Oxford: Oxford University Press, 1987.

Betterton, Rosemary. "Promising Monsters: Pregnant Bodies, Artistic Subjectivity, and Maternal Imagination." *Hypatia* 21 (2006): 80–100.

Bivin, George David, and M. Pauline Klinger. *Pseudocyesis.* Bloomington, IN: Principia, 1937.

Braidotti, Rosi. "Signs of Wonder and Traces of Doubt: On Teratology and Embodied Differences." In *Between Monsters, Goddesses and Cyborgs: Feminist Confrontations with Science, Medicine and Cyberspace,* edited by Nina Lykke and Rosi Braidotti, 135–152. London: Zed Books, 1996.

Brian, Thomas. *The Pisse-Prophet, or Certain Pisse-Pot Lectures.* London, 1655. ESTC R23808.

Brooke, Chris. "Why College Girls Are Missing Out on Motherhood." *Daily Mail,* October 1, 2004, 17.

Brown, Rawdon, ed. and trans. *Calendar of State Papers Relating to English Affairs in the Archives of Venice, Volume 6: 1555–1558.* 38 vols. (London: Her Majesty's Stationery Office, 1877).

Brown, S., L. R. Fraga, G. Cameron, L. Erskine, and N. Vargesson. "The Primodos Components Norethisterone Acetate and Ethinyl Estradiol Induce Developmental Abnormalities in Zebra Fish Embryos." *Scientific Reports* 8 (2018): 2917.

Calendar of Patent Rolls. Philip and Mary 1555–1557. Vol. 3. London: Her Majesty's Stationery Office, 1938.

Carew, Richard. *A Herrings Tayle.* London, 1598. ESTC S104891.

Carew, Richard. *The Survey of Cornwall.* London, 1602. ESTC S107479.

Carreyrou, John. *Bad Blood: Secrets and Lies in a Silicon Valley Startup.* New York: Knopf, 2018.

Cassady, Carolyn. *Off the Road: My Years with Cassady, Kerouac, and Ginsberg.* New York: Morrow, 1990.

Centre for the Study of the Legacies of British Slavery. Database. University College, London. Accessed July 3, 2020. https://www.ucl.ac.uk/lbs.

Chakrabarty, Dipesh. "The Climate of History: Four Theses." *Critical Inquiry* 35 (2009): 197–222.

Charalampous, Charis. *Rethinking the Mind-Body Relationship in Early Modern Literature, Philosophy and Medicine: The Renaissance of the Body.* London: Routledge, 2015.

Chrastil, Rachel. *How to Be Childless: A History and Philosophy of Life without Children.* Oxford: Oxford University Press, 2020.

Clark, Andy, and David Chalmers. "The Extended Mind." *Analysis* 58 (1998): 7–19.

Cobern, Joy. *Fish Hoek, Looking Back.* Fish Hoek, South Africa: Fish Hoek Printing and Publishing, 2003. https://gosouth.co.za/wp-content/uploads/2016/05/FISH-HOEK-Looking-Back-Pdf.pdf.

Cody, Lisa Freeman. *Birthing the Nation: Sex, Science, and the Conception of Eighteenth-Century Britons.* Oxford: Oxford University Press, 2005.

Cooper, Trevor G., Elizabeth Noonan, Sigrid von Eckardstein, Jacques Auger, H. W. Gordon Baker, Hermann M. Behre, Trine B. Haugen, Thinus Kruger, Christina Wang, Michael T. Mbizvo, and Kirsten M. Vogelsong. "World Health Organization Reference Values for Human Semen Characteristics." *Human Reproduction Update* 16, no. 3 (May/June 2010): 231–245. https://doi.org/10.1093/humupd/dmp048. Published November 24, 2009.

Costa, Marisa. "My Imaginary Pregnancy." 2015. Wayback Machine. https://web.archive.org/web/20160520042430/http://www.babble.com/pregnancy/my-imaginary-pregnancy-my-body-has-all-the-symptoms-but-the-babys-just-in-my-head.

Cowgill, Ursula A. "Marriage and Its Progeny in the City of York, 1538–1751." *Kroeber Anthropological Society Papers* 42 (1970): 47–87.

Daniel, Henri. *Liber Uricisiarum.* In *A Critical Edition of the Middle English Liber Uricisiarum in Wellcome MS 225,* edited by Joanne Jasin. PhD diss., Tulane University, 1983.

Davis, Angela. "Reflections on the Black Woman's Role in the Community of Slaves." *Massachusetts Review* 13, no. 1/2 (1972): 81–100.

Davis, Gayle, and Tracey Loughran, eds. *The Palgrave Handbook of Infertility in History.* London: Palgrave, 2017.

Davis, Rebecca Ann. *Piers Plowman and the Books of Nature.* Oxford: Oxford University Press, 2016.

de Voragine, Jacobus. *Golden Legend: Readings on the Saints.* Translated by William Granger Ryan. Princeton, NJ: Princeton University Press, 2012.

Douglas, Mary. *Purity and Danger: An Analysis of Concept of Pollution and Taboo.* London: Routledge, 2002, first published 1966.

Drucker, Donna J. *Fertility Technology.* Cambridge, MA: MIT Press, 2023.

Duden, Barbara. *Disembodying Women: Perspectives on Pregnancy and the Unborn.* Cambridge, MA: Harvard University Press, 1993.

Economou, George D. *The Goddess Natura in Medieval Literature.* Cambridge, MA: Harvard University Press, 1972.

Elder, Kay, and Martin H. Johnson. "The Oldham Notebooks: An Analysis of the

Development of IVF 1969–1978. II. Treatment Cycles and their Outcomes." *Reproductive Biomedicine and Society Online* 1 (2015): 9–18.

Elder, Kay, and Martin H. Johnson. "The Oldham Notebooks: An Analysis of the Development of IVF 1969–1978. IV. Ethical Aspects." *Reproductive Biomedicine and Society Online* 1 (2015): 34–45.

Elkan, Edward R. "The Xenopus Pregnancy Test." *British Medical Journal* 2 (1938): 1253–1274.

English, Isobel. *Every Eye.* London: Persephone, 2000, first published 1956.

Ephron, Nora. *Heartburn.* London: Virago, 1996, first published 1983.

Epstein, Randi Hutter. *Get Me Out: A History of Childbirth from the Garden of Eden to the Sperm Bank.* New York: Norton, 2010.

Evans, Jennifer. *Aphrodisiacs, Fertility and Medicine in Early Modern England.* Woodbridge, UK: Boydell, 2014.

Fabricius, Hieronymus. *The Embryological Treatises of Hieronymus Fabricius of Aquapendente.* Edited and translated by Howard B. Adelmann. Ithaca, NY: Cornell University Press, 1942.

"Fashion: A Guide to Chic for Maternity Clothes." *Vogue,* June 7, 1930, 82–83, 102, 106, 126.

Fett, Rebecca. *It Starts with the Egg: How the Science of Egg Quality Can Help You Get Pregnant Naturally, Prevent Miscarriage, and Improve Your Odds in IVF.* 2nd ed. Surfside, FL: Franklin Fox, 2019.

Fissell, Mary. "Hairy Women and Naked Truths: Gender and the Politics of Knowledge in *Aristotle's Masterpiece.*" *William and Mary Quarterly* 60 (2003): 43–74.

Foxe, John. *Acts and Monuments.* 1563 edition. John Foxe's The Acts and Monuments Online. Humanities Research Institute, University of Sheffield. https://www.dhi.ac.uk/foxe.

Freidenfelds, Lara. *The Myth of the Perfect Pregnancy: A History of Miscarriage in America.* Oxford: Oxford University Press, 2019.

French, Roger. "Harvey, William (1578–1657), Physician and Discoverer of the Circulation of the Blood." *Oxford Dictionary of National Biography.* September 23, 2004.

Friedan, Betty. *The Feminine Mystique.* London: Thread, 2021, first published 1963.

Froude, J. A. *History of England from the Fall of Wolsey to the Death of Elizabeth.* 12 vols. London: Longmans, 1858–1870.

Gal, Isabel, Brian Kirman, and Ian Stern. "Hormonal Pregnancy Tests and Congenital Malformation." *Nature* 216, no. 7 (October 1967): 83.

Gascoigne, Rodney. "Life at Sea with Union Castle." 2003. Wayback Machine. https://web.archive.org/web/20060212220823/http:/rgascoyne.canadianwebs.com/LifeAtSea.htm.

Gaskin, Ina May. "Has Pseudocyesis Become an Outmoded Diagnosis?" *Birth: Issues in Perinatal Care* 39, no. 1 (2012): 77–79.

Gelpi, Barbara Charlesworth. *Shelley's Goddess: Maternity, Language, Subjectivity.* Oxford: Oxford University Press, 1992.

Goldberg, P. J. P., ed. *Women in England c. 1275–1525.* Oxford: Oxford University Press, 1995.

Gomez-Ramos, M. M., A. I. García-Valcárcel, J. L. Tadeo, A. R. Fernández-Alba, and M. D. Hernando. "Screening of Environmental Contaminants in Honey Bee Wax Comb Using Gas Chromatography–High-Resolution Time-of-Flight Mass Spectrometry." *Environmental Science and Pollution Research* 23 (2016): 4609–4620.

Govindrajan, Radhika. "Flatulence." In *Anthropocene Unseen: A Lexicon,* edited by Cymene How and Anand Pandian, 197–200. Santa Barbara, CA: Punctum Books, 2020.

Gowing, Laura. *Common Bodies: Women, Touch and Power in Seventeenth-Century England.* New Haven, CT: Yale University Press, 2003.

Green, Monica H. *Making Women's Medicine Masculine.* Oxford: Oxford University Press, 2008.

Green, Monica H. "Secrets of Women." In *Women and Gender in Medieval Europe:*

An Encyclopaedia, edited by Margaret Schaus, 733–734. London: Routledge, 2006.

Grimm, Jacob, and Wilhelm Grimm. *The Complete Folk and Fairy Tales of the Brothers Grimm.* Translated by Margaret Hunt. Ballingslöv, Sweden: Wisehouse Classics, 2016.

Grimm, Jacob, and Wilhelm Grimm. *Kinder und Hausmärchen.* Göttingen, Germany: Dieterich, 1857.

Grosz, Elizabeth. *Volatile Bodies: Toward a Corporeal Feminism.* Bloomington: Indiana University Press, 1995.

Guida, M., G. A. Tommaselli, S. Palomba, M. Pellicano, G. Moccia, C. Di Carlo, and C. Nappi. "Efficacy of Methods for Determining Ovulation in a Natural Family Planning Program." *Fertility and Sterility* 72, no. 5 (1999): 900–904.

Gunn, Thom. *Selected Poems, 1950–1975.* London: Faber & Faber, 1979.

Gurdon, J. B., and N. Hopwood. "The Introduction of *Xenopus laevis* into Developmental Biology: Of Empire, Pregnancy Testing and Ribosomal Genes." *International Journal of Developmental Biology* 44 (2000): 43–50.

Hadley, Robin A. *How Is a Man Supposed to Be a Man: Male Childlessness—a Life Course Disrupted.* Oxford: Berghahn, 2021.

Halden, Grace, Mel Johnson, Shalaka Kamerkar, Nancy Milligan, Genevieve Roberts, and Rebecca Ward. "Independent Family Planning: Choosing Solo Parenthood through Gamete or Embryo Donation." Wellcome Trust, March 2023. https://www .drgracehalden.com/_files/ugd/8699d5 _e8afa75dcc4c42919081e495f5dd4aea.pdf.

Hamper, Josie, and Manuela Perrotta. "Watching Embryos: Exploring the Geographies of Assisted Reproduction through Encounters with Embryo Imaging Technologies." *Social & Cultural Geography* 24, no. 1 (May 22, 2022): 1557–1575. https://doi.org/10.1080 /14649365.2022.2073467.

Harper, Joyce. *Your Fertile Years: What You Need to Know to Make Informed Choices.* London: Sheldon Press, 2021.

Harris, Jonathan Gil. "All Swell That End Swell: Dropsy, Phantom Pregnancy, and the Sound of Deconception in All's Well That Ends Well." *Renaissance Drama* 35 (2006): 169–89.

Hartman, Saidiya. *Lose Your Mother: A Journey along the Atlantic Slave Route.* New York: Farrar, Straus & Giroux, 2007.

Harvey, Karen. *The Impostress Rabbit Breeder.* Oxford: Oxford University Press, 2020.

Harvey, P. D. A. *Medieval Maps.* London: British Library, 1991.

Harvey, William. *Anatomical Exercitations Concerning the Generation of Living Creatures.* London, 1653. ESTC R13027.

Harvey, William. *De motu locali animalium.* Edited and translated by Gwyneth Whitteridge. Cambridge, UK: Cambridge University Press, 1959.

Harvey, William. *Exercitationes de generatione animalium.* London, 1651. Wing H1091.

Harvey, William. *Works of William Harvey.* Translated by Robert Willis. London: Sydenham Society, 1847.

Hepburn, Jessica. *The Pursuit of Motherhood.* London: Troubador, 2014.

Heti, Sheila. *Motherhood: A Novel.* London: Penguin, 2018.

Hildegard of Bingen. *Hildegard of Bingen: On Natural Philosophy and Medicine. Selections from* Cause et Cure. Edited and translated by Margaret Berger. Cambridge, UK: D. S. Brewer, 1999.

Hill, John. *Lucina sine concubitu. A Letter Humbly Address'd to the Royal Society.* London: Cooper, 1750. ESTC T124780.

Homer. *The Iliad of Homer.* Translated by Alexander Pope. 2 vols. Edinburgh: A. Donaldson, 1769, first published 1715. ESTC T90525.

Hopwood, Nick. *Embryos in Wax: Models from the Ziegler Studio.* Cambridge, UK: Whipple Museum, 2002.

Huarte de San Juan, Juan. *Examen de ingenios: The Examination of Mens Wits.* Translated by Richard Carew. London, 1596. ESTC S2748.

Huarte de San Juan, Juan. *The Examination of Men's Wits.* Translated by Richard Carew. Edited by Rocío G. Sumillera.

Cambridge, UK: Modern Humanities Research Association, 2014.

Huet, Marie-Hélène. *Monstrous Imagination*. Cambridge, MA: Harvard University Press, 1993.

Human Fertilisation and Embryology Authority. "Ethnic Diversity in Fertility Treatment 2018: UK Ethnicity Statistics for IVF and DI Fertility Treatment." March 2021. https://www.hfea.gov.uk/about-us/publications/research-and-data/ethnic-diversity-in-fertility-treatment-2018.

Human Fertilisation and Embryology Authority. "Time-Lapse Imaging." Accessed November 19, 2022 [inactive by April 28, 2024]. https://web.archive.org/web/20201031163022/https://www.hfea.gov.uk/treatments/treatment-add-ons/time-lapse-imaging.

Human Fertilisation and Embryology Authority. "Time-Lapse Imaging and Incubation." Accessed April 28, 2024. https://www.hfea.gov.uk/treatments/treatment-add-ons/time-lapse-imaging-and-incubation.

Hustvedt, Siri. *The Shaking Woman or a History of My Nerves*. London: Hodder & Stoughton, 2010.

Inchbald, Elizabeth. *Every One Has His Fault*. Dublin, 1793. ETSC T20768.

Juster, Susan. "Mystical Pregnancy and Holy Bleeding: Visionary Experience in Early Modern Britain and America." *William and Mary Quarterly* 57, no. 2 (2000): 249–288.

Kane, Elisha Kent. "Experiments on Kiesteine." *American Journal of the Medical Sciences* 4 (1842): 13–38.

Karr, Mary. *Cherry: A Memoir*. London: Picador, 2017.

Kassell, Lauren, Michael Hawkins, Robert Ralley, John Young, Joanne Edge, Janet Yvonne Martin-Portugues, and Natalie Kaoukji, eds. *The Casebooks of Simon Forman and Richard Napier, 1596–1634: A Digital Edition*. The Casebooks Project, University of Cambridge. Accessed January 27, 2021. https://casebooks.lib.cam.ac.uk.

Keller, Eve. "Making Up for Losses: The Workings of Gender in William Harvey's *de Generatione animalium*." In *Inventing Maternity: Politics, Science, and Literature, 1650–1865*, edited by Susan C. Greenfield and Carol Barash, 34–56. Lexington: University Press of Kentucky, 1999.

Kerouac, Jack. *On the Road*. New York: Viking, 1955.

"Kiestéine." *Journal de chimie médicale, de parmacie et de toxicologie* 5, no. 2 (1839): 64–65.

King, Helen. *The Disease of Virgins: Green Sickness, Chlorosis and the Problems of Puberty*. London: Routledge, 2004.

King, Helen. "Once upon a Text: Hysteria from Hippocrates." In *Hysteria beyond Freud*, edited by Sander L. Gilman, 3–90. Berkeley: University of California Press, 1993.

Kueny, Katherine M. *Conceiving Identities: Maternity in Medieval Muslim Discourse and Practice*. Albany, NY: SUNY Press, 2013.

Lane, Kris. *Potosí: The Silver City That Changed the World*. Oakland: University of California Press, 2019.

Laqueur, Thomas. *Making Sex: Body and Gender from the Greeks to Freud*. Cambridge, MA: Harvard University Press, 1990.

Larsen, Ulla, and Sharon Yan. "The Age Pattern of Fecundability: An Analysis of French Canadian and Hutterite Birth Histories." *Social Biology* 47 (2000): 34–50.

Laskaya, Anne, and Eve Salisbury, eds. *The Middle English Breton Lays*. Kalamazoo, MI: Medieval Institute Publications, 1995.

Latour, Bruno. "Agency at the Time of the Anthropocene." *New Literary History* 45 (2014): 1–18.

Laurence, Michael, Mary Miller, Mary Vowles, Kathleen Evans, and Cedric Carter. "Hormonal Pregnancy Tests and Neural Tube Malformations." *Nature* 233 (October 15, 1971): 495–496.

"Law Intelligence." *The Morning Post*, January 25, 1827.

Ledger, William, Georgina Jones, Sarah Tiplady, Sheila Duffy, and Sarah Johnson. "Impact of Digital Home Ovulation Test Usage on Stress, Psychological Wellbeing and Quality of Life during Evaluation of

Subfertility: A Randomised Controlled Trial." Swiss Precision Diagnostics. Accessed November 19, 2022. https://uk.clearblue.com/sites/default/files/wysiwyg/hcpro/publications/HCP_Publications/PUB-0090_v2.pdf.

Lemon, Robert, ed. "Queen Mary—Volume 5: June 1555." In *Calendar of State Papers Domestic: Edward VI, Mary and Elizabeth, 1547–80*. London: Her Majesty's Stationery Office, 1856.

Lennox, James G. "The Comparative Study of Animal Development: William Harvey's Aristotelianism." In *The Problem of Animal Generation in Early Modern Philosophy*, edited by Justin E. H. Smith, 21–46. Cambridge, UK: Cambridge University Press, 2006.

Levy, Ariel. *The Rules Do Not Apply*. London: Fleet, 2017.

Lewis, Matthew Gregory. *Journal of a West India Proprietor*. London: John Murray, 1834.

Lewis, Matthew Gregory. *The Monk*. Edited by Howard Anderson. Revised by Nick Groom. Oxford: Oxford University Press, 2016.

Lyall, Robert. *The Medical Evidence Relative to the Duration of Human Pregnancy*. London: Burgess and Hill, 1826.

Machyn, Henry. *The Diary of Henry Machyn, Citizen and Merchant-Taylor of London, 1550–1563*. Edited by John Gough Nichols. London: Camden Society Publications, 1848.

Mahdawi, Arwa. "It Is Time to Reassess Our Obsession with Women's Fertility and the Number 35." *The Guardian*, April 10, 2021.

Maienschein, Jane. *Embryos under the Microscope: The Diverging Meanings of Life*. Cambridge, MA: Harvard University Press, 2014.

Mantel, Hilary. "Royal Bodies." *London Review of Books* 35, no. 4 (February 21, 2013).

Marshall, Mark. "The Kyesteine Pellicle: An Early Biological Test for Pregnancy." *Bulletin of the History of Medicine* 22 (1948): 178–195.

Martin, Colin, and Geoffrey Parker. *The Spanish Armada*. Harmondsworth, UK: Hamish Hamilton, 1988.

McLaren, Angus. *Reproduction by Design: Sex, Robots, Trees, and Test-Tube Babies in Interwar Britain*. Chicago, IL: University of Chicago, 2012.

McLaren, Angus. *Reproductive Rituals: The Perception of Fertility in England from the Sixteenth Century to the Nineteenth Century*. London: Methuen, 1984.

McCallum, Shiona. "Period Tracking Apps Warning over *Roe v. Wade* Case in US." BBC, May 7, 2022. https://www.bbc.co.uk/news/technology-61347934.

McClive, Cathy. "The Hidden Truths of the Belly: The Uncertainties of Pregnancy in Early Modern Europe." *Social History of Medicine* 15 (2002): 209–227.

McKay, Harriet. "'It's Fun in South Africa': Interior Design for the Union Castle Shipping Line, 1948–1977." In *The Politics of Design: Privilege and Prejudice in Aotearoa New Zealand, Australia and South Africa*, edited by Federico Freschi, Farieda Nazier, and Jane Venis, 231–253. Dunedin, New Zealand: Otago Polytechnic Press, 2022.

Mendyk, S. "Carew, Richard (1555–1620), Antiquary and Poet." *Oxford Dictionary of National Biography*. September 23, 2004. https://doi-org.ezproxy.lib.bbk.ac.uk/10.1093/ref:odnb/4635.

Meredith, Martin. *Diamonds, Gold, and War: The British, the Boers and the Making of South Africa*. New York: Simon and Schuster, 2007.

Milton, Giles. *Big Chief Elizabeth: The Adventures and Fate of the First English Colonists in America*. New York: Farrar, Straus & Giroux, 2000.

Minnis, Alastair. "Aspects of the Medieval French and English Traditions of the *De Consolatione Philosophiae*." In *Boethius: His Life, Thought and Influence*, edited by Margaret Gibson, 337–341. Oxford: Oxford University Press, 1981.

Mitchell, J. Allan. *Becoming Human: The Matter of the Medieval Child*. Minneapolis: University of Minnesota Press, 2014.

Mitchison, Naomi. *You May Well Ask: A Memoir 1920–1940*. London: Flamingo, 1986, first published 1979.

Montgomery, William Fetherstone. *An Exposition of the Signs and Symptoms of*

Pregnancy. London: Sherwood, Gilbert & Piper, 1837.

Montgomery, William Fetherstone. *An Exposition of the Signs and Symptoms of Pregnancy*. Philadelphia, PA: Blanchard and Lea, 1857.

Morgan, Kenneth. "Slave Women and Reproduction in Jamaica, c. 1776–1834." *History* 91 (2006): 231–253.

Morroni, Chelsea, and Jennifer Moodley. "The Role of Urine Pregnancy Testing in Facilitating Access to Antenatal Care and Abortion Services in South Africa: A Cross-Sectional Study." *BMC Pregnancy and Childbirth* 6 (2006): 1–3. https://doi .org/10.1186/1471-2393-6-26.

Moulinier-Brogi, Laurence. *L'uroscopie au Moyen Âge: "lire dans un verre la nature de l'homme."* Paris: Champion, 2012.

Murkoff, Heidi, Arlene Eisenberg, and Sandee Hathaway. *What to Expect When You're Expecting*. 3rd ed. London: Pocket Books, 2002, first published 1984.

National Organisation for Rare Disorders. "Chromosome 15, Distal Trisomy 15q." Accessed November 19, 2022. https://rarediseases.org/rare-diseases /chromosome-15-distal-trisomy-15q.

Navarro, Mireya. "Here Comes the Mother-to-Be." *New York Times*, March 13, 2005.

Negris, Olivia, Angela Lawson, Dannielle Brown, Christopher Warren, Isabel Galic, Alexandria Bozen, Amelia Swanson, and Tarun Jain. "Emotional Stress and Reproduction: What Do Fertility Patients Believe?" *Journal of Assisted Reproduction and Genetics* 38 (2021): 877–887.

Nelson, Maggie. *The Argonauts*. London: Melville House, 2015.

Nolsoe, Eir. "What Is the Ideal Age to Have Children?" YouGov, June 21, 2021. https:// yougov.co.uk/topics/lifestyle/articles-reports /2021/06/21/what-ideal-age-have-children.

Nugent, Maria. *A Journal of a Voyage to, and Residence in, the Island of Jamaica, from 1801 to 1805*. London, 1839.

Oakley, Ann. *The Captured Womb: A History of the Medical Care of Pregnant Women*. Oxford: Basil Blackwell, 1990, first published 1984.

O'Donnell, Rachel. "The Politics of Natural Knowing: Contraceptive Plant Properties in the Caribbean." *Journal of International Women's Studies* 17, no. 3 (2016): 59–79.

O'Farrell, Maggie. *I Am, I Am, I Am: Seventeen Brushes with Death*. London: Headline, 2017.

Office for National Statistics. "Standardised Mean Age of Mother by Birth Order, 1938–2020 England and Wales." Information on Births by Parents' Characteristic Statistics. UK Statistics Authority, January 13, 2022. https://www.ons.gov.uk/file?uri =/peoplepopulationandcommunity /birthsdeathsandmarriages /livebirths/datasets /birthsbyparentscharacteristics/2020 /finalparentscharacteristics2020workbook .xlsx.

Olszynko-Gryn, Jesse. "Drug Scandals and the Media—The Unresolved Case of Primodos." *The Guardian*, March 22, 2018.

Olszynko-Gryn, Jesse. "The Feminist Appropriation of Pregnancy Testing in 1970s Britain." *Women's History Review* 28 (2019): 869–894.

Olszynko-Gryn, Jesse. "Primodos Was a Revolutionary Oral Pregnancy Test. But Was It Safe?" *The Guardian*, October 13, 2016.

Olszynko-Gryn, Jesse. *A Woman's Right to Know: Pregnancy Testing in Twentieth-Century Britain*. Cambridge, MA: MIT Press, 2023.

Olszynko-Gryn, Jesse, Eira Bjørvik, Merle Weßel, Solveig Jülich, and Cyrille Jeane. "A Historical Argument for Regulatory Failure in the Case of Primodos and Other Hormone Pregnancy Tests." *Reproductive Biomedicine and Society Online* 6 (2018): 34–44.

Onundi, Yusuf, Bethany A. Drake, Ryan T. Malecky, Matthew A. DeNardo, Matthew R. Mills, Soumen Kundu, Alexander D. Ryabov, Evan S. Beach, Colin P. Horwitz, Michael T. Simonich, Lisa Truong, Robert L. Tanguay, L. James Wright, Naresh Singhal, and Terrence J. Collins. "A Multidisciplinary Investigation of the Technical and Environmental Performances of TAML/ Peroxide Elimination of Bisphenol

A Compounds from Water." *Green Chemistry* 19 (2017): 4234–4262.

The Pad, a New Ballad, Sung by Mr Dighton. London: 42 Long Lane, ca. 1795.

Panos, Kristina. "Digital Pregnancy Tests Use LEDs to Read between the Lines." *Hackaday* (blog), September 9, 2020. https://hackaday.com/2020/09/09/digital-pregnancy-tests-use-leds-to-read-between-the-lines.

Park, Katherine. *The Secrets of Women: Gender, Generation, and the Origins of Human Dissection*. Chicago: Zone Books, 2006.

Parker, Geoffrey. *Imprudent King: A New Life of Philip II*. New Haven, CT: Yale University Press, 2014.

Paster, Gail Kern. *Humoring the Body: Emotions and the Shakespearean Stage*. Chicago, IL: University of Chicago Press, 2004.

Paton, Diana. "Maternal Struggles and the Politics of Childlessness under Pronatalist Caribbean Slavery." *Slavery and Abolition* 38 (2017): 251–268.

Peacham, Henry. *The Gentlemens Exercise*. 1612. ESTC S114350.

Pérez, Alfredo. "General Overview of Natural Family Planning." *Genus* 54 (1998): 75–93.

Perrotta, Manuela, and Josie Hamper. "Patient Informed Choice in the Age of Evidence-Based Medicine: IVF Patients' Approaches to Biomedical Evidence and Fertility Treatment Add-Ons." *Sociology of Health & Illness* 45 (2023): 225–241. https://doi.org/10.1111/1467-9566.13581.

Philip, M. NourbeSe. *She Tries Her Tongue: Her Silence Softly Breaks*. Middletown, CT: Wesleyan University Press, 2015, first published 1989.

Pine, Emilie. *Notes to Self*. Dublin: Tramp Press, 2018.

Pinto-Correia, Clara. *The Ovary of Eve: Egg and Sperm and Preformation*. Chicago, IL: University of Chicago Press, 1997.

Pollard, A. F. *The History of England from the Accession of Edward VI to the Death of Elizabeth*. London: Longmans, 1910.

Porter, Linda. *Mary Tudor: The First Queen*. London: Little, Brown, 2007.

Price, Max. "Health Care as an Instrument of Apartheid Policy in South Africa." *Health Policy and Planning* 3 (1982): 158–170.

Prince, Mary. *The History of Mary Prince, A West Indian Slave*. London: Westley and Davis, 1831.

Prioreschi, Plinio. *A History of Medicine: Medieval Medicine*. Omaha, NE: Horatius Press, 2003.

Radcliffe, Ann Ward. *The Mysteries of Udolpho*. Edited by Bonamy Dobrée. Oxford: Oxford University Press, 1980, first published 1794.

Raine-Fenning, Nicholas. "Hard Evidence: Does Fertility Really Drop Off a Cliff at 35?" *The Conversation*, July 15, 2014.

Rapp, Rayna. "Real-Time Fetus: The Role of the Sonogram in the Age of Monitored Reproduction." In *Cyborgs and Citadels: Anthropological Interventions into Techno-Humanism*, edited by G. Downey, J. Dumit, and S. Traweek, 31–48. Seattle: University of Washington Press, 1997.

Reid-Peršin, Tina. "The People of Lamberhurst Are Horrified." *Tina Reid-Peršin* (blog). September 24, 2012. https://tinamreid.wordpress.com/category/photos-ill-never-take-2/page/4.

Remmington, Janet. "Solomon Plaatje's Decade of Creative Mobility, 1912–1922: The Politics of Travel and Writing in and beyond South Africa." *Journal of Southern African Studies* 39 (2013): 425–446.

"Review of *The Pad*: A Farce, in One Act, by Robert Woodbridge," in *The Monthly Review: or Literary Journal Enlarged* 2, no. 11 (1793): 348–349. https://hdl.handle.net/2027/hvd.hxjg9t.

Rich, Adrienne. *Of Woman Born: Motherhood as Experience and Institution*. New York: Norton, 1995, first published 1976.

Richards, Judith M. *Mary Tudor*. London: Routledge, 2008.

Richards, Judith M. "Reassessing Mary Tudor: Some Concluding Points." In *Mary Tudor: Old and New Perspectives*, edited by Susan Doran and Thomas Freeman, 206–224. London: Macmillan, 2011.

Richardson, Sarah S. *The Maternal Imprint: The Contested Science of Maternal-Fetal Effects*. Chicago: University of Chicago Press, 2021.

Robertson, Kellie. *Nature Speaks: Medieval Literature and Aristotelian Philosophy.* Philadelphia: University of Pennsylvania Press, 2017.

Rosen, Cari. *The Secret Diary of a New Mum Aged 43¼.* London: Vermillion, 2011.

Rotman Zelizer, Viviana A. *Pricing the Priceless Child.* New York: Basic Books, 1985.

Rousseau, G. S. "'A Strange Pathology': Hysteria in the Early Modern World, 1500–1800." In *Hysteria beyond Freud,* edited by Sander L. Gilman, 91–221. Berkeley: University of California Press, 1993.

Sage, Lorna. *Bad Blood.* London: Fourth Estate, 2000.

Sawin, Mark. *Raising Kane: Elisha Kent Kane and the Culture of Fame in Antebellum America.* Philadelphia, PA: American Philosophical Society Press, 2009.

Seedat, Aziza. *Crippling a Nation: Health in Apartheid South Africa.* London: International Defence and Aid Fund for South Africa, 1984.

Sellar, Walter Carruthers, and Robert Julian Yeatman. *1066 and All That: A Memorable History of England.* London: Methuen, 1930.

Seymour, M. C., ed. *On the Properties of Things: John Trevisa's Translation of Bartholomaeus Anglicus,* De Proprietatibus Rerum: *A Critical Text.* 3 vols. Oxford: Clarendon Press, 1975–1988.

Sharp, Jane. *The Midwives Book or the Whole Art of Midwifery Discovered.* London, 1671. ESTC R203554.

Shelley, Mary Wollstonecraft. *Frankenstein; or, the Modern Prometheus.* London: Colburn and Bentley, 1831.

Shigley, S. B. "Great Expectations: Infertility, Disability, and Possibility." In *The Palgrave Handbook of Infertility in History,* edited by Gayle Davis and Tracey Loughran, 37–55. London: Palgrave, 2017.

Showalter, Elaine. *The Female Malady: Women, Madness, and English Culture, 1830–1980.* London: Virago, 1987.

Skedd, Susan. "Women Teachers and the Expansion of Girls' Schooling in England,

c. 1760–1820." In *Gender in Eighteenth-Century England: Roles, Representations and Responsibilities,* edited by Hannah Barker and Elaine Chalus, 101–125. London: Routledge, 1997.

Skovsholm, Klavs. "The Right to Vote in South-Africa—A Hundred Years of Experience." *Law and Politics in Africa, Asia and Latin America* 32 (1999): 236–252.

Sosteric, Mike. "A Sociology of Tarot." *Canadian Journal of Sociology / Cahiers Canadiens de Sociologie* 39, no. 3 (2014): 357–392.

Spicer, Kate. "Leaving It Too Late." *The Sunday Times,* October 2, 2011.

Spiller, Elizabeth. *Science, Reading, and Renaissance Literature: The Art of Making Knowledge, 1580–1670.* Cambridge, UK: Cambridge University Press, 2004.

Stephanson, Raymond, and Darren N. Wagner, eds. *The Secrets of Generation: Reproduction in the Long Eighteenth Century.* Toronto: University of Toronto Press, 2015.

Stohlberg, Michael. *Uroscopy in Early Modern Europe.* Translated by Logan Kennedy and Leonhard Unglaub. Farnham, UK: Ashgate, 2015.

Stoppard, Miriam. *Conception, Pregnancy and Birth: The Childbirth Bible for Today's Parents.* Revised ed. London: Dorling Kindersley, 2008.

Strong, Roy. *Gloriana: The Portraits of Queen Elizabeth I.* London: Thames and Hudson, 1987.

Sweeney, Shauna J. "Market Marronage: Fugitive Women and the Internal Marketing System in Jamaica, 1781–1834." *William and Mary Quarterly* 76 (2019): 197–222.

Tanner, Thomas Hawkes. *On the Signs and Diseases of Pregnancy.* London: Henry Renshaw, 1860.

Tavormina, M. Teresa, ed. "Three Middle English Verse Uroscopies." *English Studies* 91 (2010): 591–622.

Taylor, Barbara. *The Last Asylum: A Memoir of Madness in Our Times.* London: Penguin, 2014.

Tenance, Edward. "A Strategy of Reaction: The Armadas of 1596 and 1597 and the Spanish Struggle for European Hegemony." *English Historical Review* 118 (2003): 855–882.

Thomas, Keith. "The Meaning of Literacy in Early Modern England." In *The Written Word: Literacy in Transition*, edited by Gerd Baumann, 97–131. Oxford: Clarendon Press, 1986.

Topsell, Edward. *The Historie of Serpents*. London: William Jaggard, 1608. ESTC S122051.

Toussaint-Samat, Meguelonne. *A History of Food*. London: Wiley-Blackwell, 2009, first published 1992.

Turner, Sasha. *Contested Bodies: Pregnancy, Child Rearing and Slavery in Jamaica*. Philadelphia: University of Pennsylvania Press, 2017.

Tuttle, Leslie. *Conceiving the Old Regime: Pronatalism and the Politics of Reproduction in Early Modern France*. Oxford: Oxford University Press, 2010.

Umeora, Ouj. "Pseudocyesis in a Rural Southeast Nigerian Community." *Journal of Obstetrics and Gynaecology Research* 35 (2009): 660–665.

"Union Castle Line (Race Segregation)." House of Commons Debate, December 6, 1948. Hansard, vol. 459, cols. 30–31. https://api.parliament.uk/historic-hansard /commons/1948/dec/06/union-castle-line -race-segregation.

Union-Castle Mail Steamship Company. "South Africa, East and West Africa." 1930. Brochure. Cayzer Family Archive. https://cayzer.com/business/shipping /union-castle-s-s-company/union-castle -line-motorships-brochure.

Urwin, Rosamund. "Having a Baby Takes a Bit of Forward Planning." *London Evening Standard*, January 31, 2011, 17.

Van der Lugt, Maaike. *Le ver, le démon, et la vierge: les théories médievales de la génération extraordinaire*. Paris: Les Belles Lettres, 2004.

van Sittert, Lance, and G. John Measey. "Historical Perspectives on Global Exports and Research of African Clawed Frogs (*Xenopus laevis*)." *Transactions of the Royal Society of South Africa* 71 (2016): 157–166.

Virues Ortega, Javier. "Una aproximación a la vida de Juan Huarte de San Juan: los primeros años de práctica professional (1560–1578)." *Psicothema* 18 (2006): 232–237.

Wabiri, Njeri, Matthew Chersich, Olive Shisana, Duane Blaauw, Helen Rees, and Ntabozuko Dwane. "Growing Inequities in Maternal Health in South Africa: A Comparison of Serial National Household Surveys." *BMC Pregnancy and Childbirth* 16 (2016). https://doi.org/10.1186/s12884-016-1048-z.

Ward, Miranda. *Adrift: Fieldnotes from Almost-Motherhood*. London: Weidenfeld & Nicolson, 2021.

Wegner, D. M., and S. Zanakos. "Chronic Thought Suppression." *Journal of Personality* 62 (1994): 615–640.

Weldon, Ché, Atherton L. De Villiers, and Louis H. Du Preez. "Quantification of the Trade in *Xenopus laevis* from South Africa, with Implications for Biodiversity Conservation." *African Journal of Herpetology* 56 (2007): 77–83.

Wellmann, Janina. *The Form of Becoming: Embryology and the Epistemology of Rhythm, 1760–1830*. New York: Zone Books, 2017.

Wells, A. W. *South Africa: A Planned Tour of the Country To-Day*. London: J. M. Dent, 1949, first published 1939.

Weschler, Toni. *Taking Charge of Your Fertility: The Definitive Guide to Natural Birth Control, Pregnancy Achievement, and Reproductive Health*. London: Harper Collins, 2006, first published 1995.

West, Zita. *Plan to Get Pregnant: Ten Steps to Maximum Pregnancy*. London: Dorling Kindersley, 2008).

White, Hugh. *Nature and Salvation in Piers Plowman*. Woodbridge, UK: Boydell & Brewer, 1988.

Whitelock, Anna. *Mary Tudor: Princess, Bastard, Queen*. London: Bloomsbury, 2009.

Williams, Kate. *Becoming Queen: The Tragic Death of Princess Charlotte and the Unexpected Rise of Britain's Greatest Monarch*. New York: Ballantine, 2008.

Wilson, Elizabeth A. *Psychosomatic: Feminism and the Neurological Body*. Durham, NC: Duke University Press, 2004.

Withycombe, Shannon. *Lost: Miscarriage in Nineteenth-Century America*. New Brunswick, NJ: Rutgers University Press, 2018.

Wollstonecraft, Mary. *A Vindication of the Rights of Man; A Vindication of the Rights of Woman; An Historical and Moral View of the French Revolution*. Edited by Janet Todd. Oxford: Oxford University Press, 1993.

Woodbridge, Robert. *The Pad, a Farce, in One Act*. London: J. Parsons, 1793. ESTC T043545.

Wright, Thomas, and James Orchard Halliwell, eds. *Reliquiæ antiquæ: Scraps from Ancient Manuscripts*. 2 vols. London: John Russell Smith, 1845.

Wrigley, E. A. *Population and History*. New York: McGraw-Hill, 1969.

Wrigley, E. A., and Roger Schofield. *The Population History of England, 1541–1871: A Reconstruction*. London: Edward Arnold, 1981.

Wyndham, John. *Consider Her Ways*. London: Penguin Books, 2014, first published 1961.

Zapperi, Roberto. *The Pregnant Man*. London: Harwood Academic, 1991.

Zephaniah, Benjamin, "I'm 64 and my Infertility still Brings me to Tears", inews.co.uk, August 5, 2022. https://web.archive.org/web/20220812031319/https://inews.co.uk/opinion/benjamin-zephaniah-64-infertility-tears-1772217.

Zwarenstein, H. "The Frog Pregnancy Test: The First of Its Kind in the World." *Bulletin of the Adler Museum of the History of Medicine* 11 (1985): 9–10.

Index